T0213515

Multidimensional Approaches to Impacts of Changing Environment on Human Health

Multidimensional Approaches to Impacts of Changing Environment on Human Health

Edited by
Joystu Dutta, Srijan Goswami and Abhijit Mitra

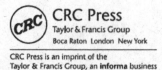

CRC Press
Taylor & Francis Group
Boca Raton London New York

CRC Press is an imprint of the
Taylor & Francis Group, an **informa** business

First edition published 2022
by CRC Press
6000 Broken Sound Parkway NW, Suite 300, Boca Raton, FL 33487-2742

and by CRC Press
2 Park Square, Milton Park, Abingdon, Oxon OX14 4RN

Library of Congress Cataloging-in-Publication Data
Names: Dutta, Joystu, editor. | Goswami, Srijan, editor. | Mitra, Abhijit, editor.
Title: Multidimensional approaches to impacts of changing environment on human health /
edited by Joystu Dutta, Srijan Goswami, Abhijit Mitra.
Description: First edition. | Boca Raton: CRC Press, 2022. |
Includes bibliographical references and index.
Identifiers: LCCN 2021009269 (print) | LCCN 2021009270 (ebook) |
ISBN 9780367558499 (hbk) | ISBN 9780367558512 (pbk) | ISBN 9781003095422 (ebk)
Subjects: LCSH: Environmental health. | Public health–Environmental aspects.
Classification: LCC RA565 .M85 2022 (print) | LCC RA565 (ebook) | DDC 613/.1–dc23
LC record available at https://lccn.loc.gov/2021009269
LC ebook record available at https://lccn.loc.gov/2021009270

ISBN: 978-0-367-55849-9 (hbk)
ISBN: 978-0-367-55851-2 (pbk)
ISBN : 978-1-003-09542-2 (ebk)

DOI: 10.1201/9781003095422

Typeset in Times
by Newgen Publishing UK

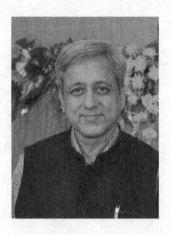

Dr. Sujit Kumar Dutta
April 24, 1953–December 25, 2020
****

This book is dedicated to the loving memory of Professor Dr. Sujit Kumar Dutta, a loving soul who left untimely for his heavenly abode after suffering from COVID-19.

He will be remembered forever as a great human being.

Contents

UNIT I Impacts of Changing Environment on Human Health

UNIT II Impact of Increasing Environmental Pollution on Human Health

UNIT III   Climate Change and Human Health: A Perspective

UNIT IV   Industrial Safety and Occupational Health Issues

UNIT V   Food Safety and Impacts on Health and Environment

UNIT VI Successful Models of Waste Management

UNIT VII Pandemics: Challenges and Way Forward

UNIT VIII Perspectives on Environmental and Human Health Management

Preface

Natural catastrophes and war bring mankind to the edge of existential crisis only to fight back again on the trajectory of progress and development in every sphere of modern life. History has enough such proofs of human struggles for existence. Is it an inherent adaptation strategy of man? We cannot draw such conclusions without scientific evidence. Our collective hope says that no dark phase lasts forever. Death gives way to life as night unleashes a new day. COVID-19 has been an unstoppable and cruel killer in 2020. It has been a year now and millions of active cases are still reported every day across the globe with thousands of deaths. This is a watershed moment in our struggle for existence in the modern world where technology and medical science have undergone unimaginable developments. We have stopped relying on nature-based solutions. We have only the slightest idea where these unwarranted consumption patterns and unsustainable lifestyles are leading us. Humongous modern luxuries are meaningless if our health system is compromised and our immunity is weak. The COVID-19 pandemic has exposed this truth in the hardest manner as we have witnessed the dance of death and health emergencies globally. Industrial developments and economic growth would stand silent and still if health infrastructure breaks down, as is evident from the stringent lockdowns imposed worldwide to contain the viral strains of COVID-19. Anthropogenic interferences on the natural world have taken a toll on Mother Earth, with species becoming extinct every minute. This is the time we must put our ears to the ground and listen to the voices from the field and embrace nature in harmony. Sustainable development is the need of the hour. This book is a timely and honest attempt in such a direction. We as authors would be delighted if this highly necessary book is read by hundreds of young minds globally whose actions would bring a positive change to our world and usher in a better tomorrow. Seven billion dreams matter and seven million hopes and voices cannot die! Let's make our Mother Earth a great place to live again!

Dr. Joystu Dutta, Dr. Srijan Goswami and Dr. Abhijit Mitra

About the Editors

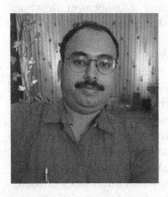

Joystu Dutta

Dr. Joystu Dutta is currently posted as an Assistant Professor and Head, Department of Environmental Science, Sant Gahira Guru University, Sarguja, a state university with the Government of Chhattisgarh. His main activities are teaching, research and extension besides supervising administrative activities in various capacities. He is a member of the International Union for Conservation of Nature (IUCN) Commission of Ecosystem Management. He is a Department of Science and Technology (DST) Inspire Fellow and also holds UNESCO scholarships as well as a University Grants Commission (UGC) National Educational Testing (NET) Lectureship in Environmental Sciences. He has written over 20 research papers in national and international journals. He has participated in collaborative research projects with organizations such as Forest Research Institute Dehradun, Gujarat Institute of Desert Ecology, Chhattisgarh Forest Department and Ramsar Culture Network, to name a few, as well as short-term consultancy-based projects with organizations such as Sahapedia and forest departments. Previously he was attached to the Reliance Foundation, Corporate Social Responsibility (CSR) Wing of Reliance Industries Limited, Mumbai as Assistant Programme Manager. He has more than two years of work experience in the field of rural development, advocacy and corporate communications. He has also done an internship as Young Development Professional with the Reliance Foundation. He has received Gold Medals during his graduation as well as post-graduation studies. He has also received several accolades for excellent professional achievements, such as Vice Chancellor's Best Employee Award and Young Scientist Award from the Indian Environmental Science Academy, among many others. He voraciously writes in journals and newsletters and is on the reviewer and editorial board of various national and international journals. Dr. Dutta loves to work with communities at grass root level. During leisure, Joystu is busy reading story books, writing poems and plays, travelling to new places and swimming. He is also an established stage actor and writes as well as direct plays for his students. His university team has received a National Award from Digital India Programme, Ministry of Information and Broadcasting Government of India for Best Play at university level. Currently, Dr. Dutta is pursuing his doctoral research in environmental toxicology as well as engaging with Voice of Environment, a Guwahati-based non-government organization which works in the sector of environmental awareness and sustainable conservation approaches.

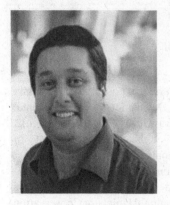

Srijan Goswami

Dr. Srijan Goswami is the Head and Senior Faculty, Department of Paramedical Sciences, Delhi Paramedical and Management Institute (DPMI), Behala, Kolkata, India and Founder of the Indian School of Complementary Therapy and Allied Sciences, Kolkata, India (non-government and non-profit organization). Presently he is associated as the Guest Faculty of Immunology and Physiology at the Department of Zoology (post-graduate courses), Serampore College, India. He was formerly associated as an Assistant Professor at the Department of Biotechnology and Molecular Biology, Institute of Genetic Engineering, Badu, India till July 2018 and as a Lecturer at the Department of Computer Science, Webel Informatics Limited, Basirhat College Unit India till June 2016. Dr. Goswami is a Physician of Biochemic System of Medicine and also holds specialization in Medical Biotechnology and Clinical Nutrition. He received his professional training on Community Nutrition and Child Care, Medical Microbiology and Medical Biochemistry from reputed medical colleges in Kolkata, India and holds a Post Graduate Diploma in Software Engineering (PGDSE) from West Bengal Electronics Industry Development Corporation Limited (WEBEL), India. Dr. Goswami has around seven years of experience in the field of teaching and research and has had about 20 research papers published in national and international journals. He has independently and successfully guided about ten under-graduate and post-graduate students to complete their research work and publications in the past three years. He acted as an Examination Superintendent for National Digital Literacy Mission at Pravda Infotech Pvt. Ltd, India in 2016. He has a qualified Ph.D. Entrance Examination conducted by the Department of Biotechnology, Maulana Abul Kalam Azad University of Technology (MAKAUT), in 2018. Dr. Goswami has received three Letters of Commendation for Global Community Services and a Certificate of Honor for his contribution to the field of Science and Knowledge from *International Journal of Agricultural Research, Sustainability and Food Sufficiency* (IJARSFS), *International Journal of Advances in Medical Sciences and Biotechnology* (IJAMSB) and *International Journal of Health, Safety and Environment* (IJHSE) in 2019 and 2020. The *Current Research in Nutrition and Food Science* (Enviro Research Group) and *Academia Scholarly Journals* awarded him the Certificate of Excellence as Reviewer in 2020. He is actively associated as Editorial Review Board Member of 15 international journals and holds the post of Honorary Vice-Principal and Head of the Department of Physiology at Shree Krishna Biochemic College, Kolkata, India. Currently, Dr. Goswami is pursuing his second professional M.Sc. in Clinical Dietetics. His domain of expertise includes molecular biology, medical-informatics, clinical nutrition, immunonutrition, mechanism of drug action, nutraceuticals and functional foods, holistic science and One Health.

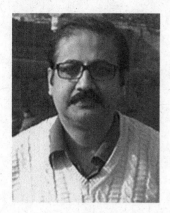

Abhijit Mitra

Dr. Abhijit Mitra, Associate Professor and Former Head, Department of Marine Science, University of Calcutta (India), has been active in the sphere of Oceanography since 1985. He obtained his Ph.D. as National Educational Testing (NET)-qualified scholar in 1994 after securing a Gold Medal in M.Sc. (Marine Science) from the University of Calcutta. Subsequently he joined Calcutta Port Trust and World Wildlife Fund (WWF), in various capacities to carry out research programs on environmental science, biodiversity conservation and climate change and carbon sequestration. Presently Dr. Mitra is serving Techno India University as Director of Research. He has to his credit about 553 scientific publications in various national and international journals, and 42 books at post-graduate standard. Dr. Mitra is presently the member of several committees, such as Pacific Congress on Marine Science and Technology (PACON) International, the International Union for Conservation of Nature (IUCN) and Svalbard Integrated Artic Earth Observing System (SIOS), and has successfully completed about 19 projects on biodiversity loss in fishery sector, coastal pollution, alternative livelihood, climate change and carbon sequestration. Dr. Mitra also visited as faculty member and invited speakers at several foreign Universities of Singapore, Kenya, Oman and the USA. In 2008, Dr. Mitra was invited as visiting fellow at the University of Massachusetts at Dartmouth, USA, to deliver a series of lectures on climate change. Dr. Mitra also successfully guided 38 Ph.D. students. Presently his domain of expertise includes environmental science, mangrove ecology, sustainable aquaculture, alternative livelihood and climate change and carbon sequestration.

List of Contributors

Abha Arya
Symbiosis Institute of Health Sciences,
Symbiosis International (Deemed)
University, Pune, India

Ratul Arya Baishya
Mega Mission Society; Samagra
Gramya Unnayan Yojana, Guwahati,
Assam, India

Dhanya B.
Associate Professor, Indian Institute of
Forest Management, Bhopal, India

Rameshwari A. Banjara
Department of Chemistry,
Rajiv Gandhi Government Post
Graduate College, Ambikapur,
Chhattisgarh, India

Anjali Barwal
National Institute of Disaster
Management, Ministry of Home
Affairs, GoI, New Delhi, India

Asani Bhaduri
Cluster Innovation Centre, University
of Delhi, India

Arghya Chakravorty
School of Bio-Sciences & Technology,
Vellore Institute of Technology,
Vellore, India

Anurag Chanda
Fingers Crossed Foundation, Asansol,
West Bengal, India

Moharana Choudhury
Voice of Environment (VoE),
Guwahati, Assam, India

Antara Das
School of Environmental Studies,
Jadavpur University, Kolkata, India

Debojyoti Das
Science Policy Research Unit,
University of Sussex, UK

C. R. Desai
HPS Wellness, Shiatsu Research and
Training Institute (SRTI), Satayushi
Institute of Enhanced Living,
Pune, India

Joystu Dutta
Sant Gahira Guru University, Sarguja,
Ambikapur- Chhattisgarh, India

Sujit K. Dutta
Department of Management and
Social Sciences. Assam Down Town
University, Guwahati, Assam, India

Alka Ekka
Department of Biotechnology,
Guru Ghasidas University Bilaspur,
Chhattisgarh, India

Upasona Ghosh
Indian Institute of Public Health,
Bhubaneshwar, India

Srijan Goswami
Indian School of Complementary
Therapy and Allied Sciences, Ichapur,
Kolkata, India

Ushmita Gupta Bakshi
Community Nutrition and Child Care,
Indian School of Complementary Therapy
and Allied Sciences, Kolkota, India

Madhurima Joardar
School of Environmental Studies,
Jadavpur University, Kolkata, India

Mohamed Kamal
EcoConServ Environmental Solutions
(ECS), Zamalek, Cairo, Egypt

Ashish Kumar
Department of Biotechnology, Sant
Gahira Guru Vishwavidyalaya, Sarguja
Ambikapur, Chhattisgarh, India

Maneet Kumar Chakrawarti
Antimicrobial Research Laboratory,
School of Environmental Sciences,
Jawaharlal Nehru University, New
Delhi, India

Anil Kumar Gupta
National Institute of Disaster
Management, Ministry of Home Affairs,
Government of India, New Delhi, India

Chetan Kumar Joshi
Government College, Sikar,
Rajasthan, India

Santosh Kumar Sethi
Department of Biotechnology
Gangadhar Meher University,
Sambalpur, Odisha, India

Nawin Kumar Tiwary
Department of Environmental Studies,
Indraprastha College for Women,
University of Delhi, India

Himani Kumari
Antimicrobial Research Laboratory,
School of Environmental Sciences,
Jawaharlal Nehru University, New
Delhi, India

Abhinav Mehta
TGIS, Vastrapur, Ahmedabad,
Gujarat, India

Jyoti Mehta
Department of Environmental
Sciences, Central University of
Jharkhand, Ranchi, Jharkhand, India

Rojita Mishra
Department of Botany, Polasara
Science College, Polasara, Ganjam,
Odisha, India

Abhijit Mitra
Department of Marine Science,
University of Calcutta, Kolkata, India

Madhur Mohan Ranga
Department of Environmental
Science, UTD, Sant Gahira Guru
Vishwavidalaya, Surguja, India

Rinku Moni Devi
Indian Institute of Forest Management,
Bhopal, India

Pritam Mukherjee
Department of Oceanography, Techno
India University, West Bengal,
Kolkata, India

Kasturi Mukhopadhyay
Antimicrobial Research Laboratory,
School of Environmental Sciences,
Jawaharlal Nehru University, New
Delhi, India

Amrita Kumari Panda
Department of Biotechnology, Sant
Gahira Guru University, Ambikapur,
Chhattisgarh, India

Sheetal Patil
School of Development, Azim Premji
University, Bangalore, India

Sonali Rajput
Antimicrobial Research Laboratory,
School of Environmental Sciences,
Jawaharlal Nehru University, New
Delhi, India

Shrey Rakholia
TGIS, Vastrapur, Ahmedabad,
Gujarat, India

Surbhi Ranga
Zydus Medical College and Hospital,
Dahod, Gujarat, India

Shreelata Rao Seshadri
School of Development, Azim Premji
University, Bangalore, India

Rehab A. Rayan
Department of Epidemiology, High
Institute of Public Health, Alexandria
University, Egypt

Nilanjana Roy Chowdhury
School of Environmental Studies,
Jadavpur University, Kolkata, India

Tarit Roychowdhury
School of Environmental Studies,
Jadavpur University, Kolkata, India

Bingshati Sarkar
Indian School of Complementary
Therapy and Allied Sciences,
Kolkota, India

Chandini Sayeed
Indian School of Complementary
Therapy and Allied Sciences,
Kolkota, India

Chandra Shekhar Sanwal
Herbal Research and Development
Institute, Mandal Gopeshwar Chamoli,
Uttarakhand, India

Rajat Shubhro Mukherjee
Deutsche Gesellschaft für
Internationale Zusammenarbeit,
Delhi, India

Govind Singh
Jindal School of Environment and
Sustainability, O.P. Jindal Global
University, Sonipat, Haryana, India

Madhuri Singh
Antimicrobial Research Laboratory,
School of Environmental Sciences,
Jawaharlal Nehru University, New
Delhi, India

Prem Prakash Singh
Mahali Bhagat Government College,
Kusmi, Balrampur, Chhattisgarh, India

Satpal Singh Bisht
Department of Zoology, Kumaun
University, Nainital, Uttarakhand,
India

Atisha Sood
National Institute of Disaster
Management, Ministry of Home
Affairs, GoI, New Delhi, India

Sushma
Department of Farm Forestry, UTD,
SantGahira Guru Viswavidyalaya,
Sarguja, Ambikapur, India

Raghvendra S. Vanjari
Research Center, Azim Premji
University, Bangalore, India

Sufia Zaman
Department of Oceanography, Techno
India University, West Bengal,
Kolkata, India

Unit I

Impacts of Changing Environment on Human Health

1 Air Pollutants and Acid Precipitation
Impact on Ecology and Human Health

Joystu Dutta* and Prem Prakash Singh

CONTENTS

1.1 INTRODUCTION

Acid deposition refers to the transport of acids and acidifying compounds from the atmosphere to the Earth's surface as wet deposition (snow, rain, fog, mist, sleet, hail, dew, etc.) and dry deposition (gas, dry particles, vapor, and aerosols containing high amounts of nitric and sulfuric acids), which is more common at high elevations or in coastal areas. "Acid rain" is a popular term that refers to wet acidic atmospheric depositions. Almost 50% of the acidic pollutants in the atmosphere fall back through dry deposition. Wet deposition ("acid rain" or "acid precipitation"), also called "the unseen plague," is also not uncommon. Our atmosphere naturally contains acid anhydrides as non-metal oxides at a low concentration; anthropogenic activities have greatly increased the concentration, leading to acid rain. Rapid and unplanned industrialization is the main cause of acid rain in India (Mohan and Kumar, 1998).

* Corresponding author: Joystu Dutta. joystu.dutta@gmail.com

DOI: 10.1201/9781003095422-1

Climate change concerns across the globe overshadow local concerns of acid precipitation, leading to lack of mitigation and adaptation strategies. In 1872, Robert Angus Smith published the book *Air and Rain: The Beginnings of a Chemical Climatology*. This book presents his studies on the chemistry of atmospheric precipitation. It further includes studies of acid rain in northern British cities during 1852, as a consequence of the burning of coal rich in sulfur. The popular term "acid rain" actually appeared in the 1960s when the first consequences of the phenomenon were reported on trees and fish. Robert Smith is regarded as the "Father of Acid Rain" (Thorpe, 1884; Oden, 1967; Gibson and Farrar, 1973; Gorham, 1982; Hamlin, 2004; United States Geological Survey, USGS, 2013). Little attention was paid to his work until the 1950s, when biologists noticed an alarming decline of fish populations in the lakes of southern Norway and traced the problem to acid rain. Similar findings were made in the 1960s in North America (the Adirondacks, Ontario, Quebec) (Almer et al., 1974; Nair and Prenzel, 1978; Nd, 1983; Sutcliffe and Carrick, 1973; Muniz, 1984, 1991). These findings spurred intense research towards understanding the origin of the acid rain phenomenon (Liu et al., 2019).

Over the last 25 years, much attention has been devoted to acid rain. Acid rain primarily results from emissions of sulfur- (S) and nitrogen- (N) containing oxides from anthropogenic emissions, industrial exhausts, vehicular emissions as well as large-scale deforestation activities across the globe (Zhao et al., 2009; US Environmental Protection Agency (US EPA), 2018). Acid deposition is today one of the most pressing issues of the century and has the focus of the scientific community because of its potential impact on ecosystems contributing to water acidification, soil mineral depletion, plant and animal disappearance, forest damage, cultural heritage erosion, and other problems (Menz and Seip, 2004; Liu et al., 2019).

Pollutants causing acidification play a crucial role in other environmental problems such as eutrophication, ground level ozone perturbation, and climate change (Manisalidis et al., 2020; Mohajan, 2018). In North America, Central Europe, and South-east Asia, acid rain has been a severe environmental issue for decades, and therefore has received much attention (Kuylenstierna et al., 2001; Zhao et al., 2009). Aquatic communities thriving in many siliceous mountain ranges of central Europe, such as the Black Forest, Harz, Erzgebirge, and Bohemian ranges, have faced consequences of acid rain and further signs of biological recovery have also been observed in these degraded ecosystems (Meybohm and Ulrich, 2007). Decreasing SO_2 emissions due to stringent environmental regulations in North America and Europe, as observed from 1990 to 2016, are responsible for such ecosystem recovery (U.S. Environmental Protection Agency (US EPA), 2018; European Monitoring and Evaluation Programme (EMEP), 2019). Many international agreements, such as Clean Air Act and Convention on Long-range Transboundary Air Pollution legislation, have played a pivotal role in reducing anthropogenic emissions of NO_x and SO_x (US EPA, 2018; EMEP, 2019).

Acid rain has impacted ecosystems globally, leading to far-reaching consequences during the last century in the post-industrial revolution era. Lake ecosystems have lost their food web complexity and stability due to reduced biodiversity. Zooplankton and phytoplankton communities have disappeared while acid precipitation over surface waters has created a major loss to the entire ecological makeup of areas under the effects of acid precipitation (Keitel, 1995). Acid rain leads to various ecological and economic consequences. It is therefore termed an "industrial plague" (Singh and Agrawal, 2008). Acid rain damages flora and the morphological structure of plants (Murray et al., 2004; Singh and Agrawal, 2004; Balasubramanian, 2007) and inhibits or reduces physiological activities (Ferenbaugh, 1976; Murray et al., 2004; Singh and Agrawal, 1996, 2004, 2008; Wyrwicka and Skłodowska, 2006) as well as plant productivity (Singh and Agrawal, 1996, 2004), eventually leading to canopy cover reduction, crown damage, and drying up of the plant body (Tomlinson, 1983). Acid deposition brings unalterable changes in the physico-chemical properties of the soil and kills soil microbial fauna by increasing ion exchange between H^+ in acids and nutrient cations such as K^+, Na^+, Mg^{2+}, and Al^{3+} as well as metal ions such as Al^{3+}, Pb^{2+}, Hg^{2+}, and Cd^{2+} (Irving, 1983; Zhang et al., 2007).

The term "polluted air" means a condition of the atmosphere where pollutants are present beyond recommended limits, leading to adverse effects on the biosphere and environment as a whole. Growing awareness about the negative effects of air pollution on the environment and human health gave rise to international and national legislation on emission reductions (Reis et al., 2012; Maas and Grennfelt, 2016; UNECE, 2016). According to the Convention on Long-Range Transboundary Air Pollution, often abbreviated as Air Convention or CLRTAP, air pollution means the direct or indirect introduction of unwanted substances into the atmosphere due to natural processes and anthropogenic activities, which damage human health, living sources, ecosystems, and material property and disturb the proper use of the natural and human environment. Ninety percent of all air pollutants come from natural sources, such as soil and rock erosion, volcanic activity, natural fires, sea water spray, and biological processes, while anthropogenic sources contribute about 10%. Their amounts are, however, continually increasing and this ratio is thus rising. Its change adversely affects the equilibrium formed between natural sources and the processes of removal of pollutants from the atmosphere. Besides this, as a consequence of human activity, much more highly aggressive substances frequently enter the atmosphere, which may threaten many biological processes on Earth.

Air pollutants comprise primary and secondary air pollutants (Figure 1.1). Primary air pollutants are emitted directly from sources. They include, but are not limited to, particulate matter (PM), sulfur dioxide (SO_2), nitric oxides (NO_x), hydrocarbon (HCs), volatile organic compounds (VOCs), carbon monoxide (CO), and ammonia (NH_3). Secondary air pollutants are produced by the chemical reactions of two or more primary pollutants or by reactions with normal atmospheric constituents. Examples of secondary air pollutants are ground level ozone, formaldehyde, smog, and acid mist. Air pollutants other than PM present primarily as gases. VOCs are chemicals that contain carbon and/or hydrogen and evaporate easily. VOCs are a family of organic compounds that are volatile in

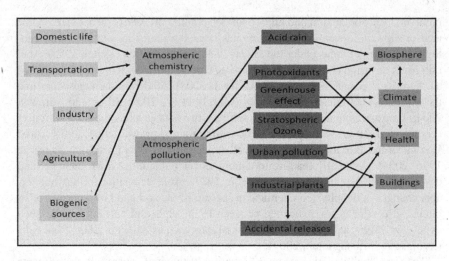

FIGURE 1.1   Categorization of air pollutants.

nature. They are mainly lower (C1–C4) paraffin, olefins, aldehydes (e.g., formaldehyde), ketones (e.g., acetone) and aromatics (e.g., benzene, toluene, benzaldehyde, phenol). Polycyclic aromatic hydrocarbons (PAH) (boiling point 218°C) are also a type of VOC. Methane (CH_4), CO, and halogenated organics such as 1,1,1-trichloroethane and chlorofluorocarbons (CFCs) are not considered as VOCs. VOCs are the main air emissions from the oil and gas industry, as well as indoor consumer products and construction materials, such as new fabrics, wood, and paints. VOCs are a major contributing factor to ground level ozone, a common air pollutant, and a proven public health hazard. Sulfur dioxide (SO_2) and nitric oxides (NO_x) are two major gaseous air pollutants generated through combustion processes. CO and HC are generated from incomplete combustion and are converted into CO_2 through a complete combustion process. Secondary air pollutants are those formed through complex physical and/or chemical reactions, e.g., coagulation and condensation or photochemical reactions. Acid formation in the atmosphere facilitated by NO_x and SO_x in the presence of water vapor leads to acid rain formation. Sixty-seven percent of total SO_2 emissions (20 million tons) and 22% of total NO_x emissions in the USA are from anthropogenic sources according to reports published by US electric power industry. The most acidic rain falls in northeastern USA, where the pH averages 4–4.2 (Mohajan, 2018). The principal oxide of carbon is carbon dioxide (CO_2) which is present in normal air with a relatively constant concentration of about 0.03%. Reaction of CO_2 with moisture then produces "normal rain," with a pH of about 5.6. Rain with a pH lower than 5.6 is considered to be acidic.

Elemental sulfur is relatively inert and harmless to human beings and in fact is needed in some quantity for life. It occurs naturally in the environment, mostly in the form of sulfates like $CaSO_4$. SO_2 tends to be preferred at higher temperatures while sulfur trioxide (SO_3) is preferred at lower temperatures (Bowman, 1991). Pollutants containing sulfur are as follows: SO_2, SO_3, sulfuric acid, hydrogen sulfide, carbon disulfide, and various organic compounds of sulfur.

An essential portion of sulfur in the atmosphere comes from hydrogen sulfide. It makes up 46.1%, whereas the proportions of sulfur corresponding to SO_2 and to sulfites together with sulfates are 33.2 and 20.7%, respectively. Sulfur-based pollutants in the air are formed as a result of a sequence of complex chemical reactions in the atmosphere, as detailed in Box 1.1 according to the published reports of Zevenhoven and Kilpinen (2002).

Fuel sulfur is first heated and devolatilized through R1. Both solids and gases (vapors) are produced through this reaction. The solid phase char sulfur can be oxidized through the following reactions, where H_2S, SO_2, and CO_2 are

---

BOX 1.1 SEQUENCE OF STEP REACTIONS OF NITROGEN AND SULFUR-BASED POLLUTANTS IN THE ATMOSPHERE

$$Fuel - S_S \rightarrow H_2S + COS + ... + Char - S_S \qquad \text{R1}$$

$$Char - S \rightarrow O_2 \rightarrow SO_2 \qquad \text{R2}$$

$$Char - S \rightarrow CO_2 \rightarrow COS \qquad \text{R3}$$

$$Char - S \rightarrow H_2O \rightarrow H_2S \qquad \text{R4}$$

$$H_2S - 1\frac{1}{2}O_2 \rightarrow SO_2 \rightarrow H_2O \qquad \text{R5}$$

$$H_2S - CO_2 \rightarrow COS \rightarrow H_2O \qquad \text{R6}$$

$$H_2S - CO \rightarrow H_2 \rightarrow COS \qquad \text{R7}$$

$$H_2S - COS \rightarrow CS_2 \rightarrow H_2O \qquad \text{R8}$$

$$CS_2 - C \rightarrow \frac{2}{X}S_X \qquad \text{R9}$$

$$SO_2 + \frac{1}{2}O_2 \leftrightharpoons SO_3 \qquad \text{R10}$$

$$N_2 + O_2 \rightarrow NO, NO_z \qquad \text{R11}$$

$$O + N_2 \leftrightharpoons NO + N \qquad \text{R12}$$

$$N + O_2 \leftrightharpoons NO + O \qquad \text{R13}$$

$$N + OH \leftrightharpoons NO + H \qquad \text{R14}$$

$$CH_4 + O_2 + N_2 \rightarrow NO, NO_z, CO_2, H_2O \; Species \qquad \text{R15}$$

$$R_X N + O_2 \rightarrow NO, NO_z, CO_2, H_2O \, trace \; Species \qquad \text{R16}$$

produced: R2, R3, R4. The gas phases produced during the above three reactions can further react through R5–R9. In these products, the concentrations of SO_2 and SO_3 at equilibrium can still be determined by the overall reaction in Equation R10.

Since most combustion processes are at high temperatures, SO_2 is the predominant form of SO_x emitted from systems containing sulfur. Nearly all fossil fuels contain sulfur atoms. Some of the sulfur in fuels is eventually oxidized to SO_2 and SO_3. Sulfur in coal is present in both organic and inorganic forms, the latter being pyretic sulfur (FeS_2), and sulfates (Na_2SO_4, $CaSO_4$, $FeSO_4$). Sulfides, mercaptanes, bisulfides, thiophenes, and thiopyrones are some of the forms of organic sulfur which are present in unrefined oils and heavy fuel oils (Zevenhoven and Kilpinen, 2002). The more sulfur in the fuel, the higher level of SO_2 emission. SO_2 is mainly formed when the sulfur elements are oxidized by O_2 and SO_2 can be oxidized to SO_3.

On a worldwide basis, natural production of SO_2 far exceeds man-made sources. However, in industrialized nations, sulfur oxides generated by humans often far exceed the natural production of SO_2 (Mohajan, 2018). Global SO_2 emission trends over the last decade have affected global as well as regional atmospheric composition, leading to changes in air quality, atmospheric deposition and the radiative forcing of sulfate aerosols (Aas et al., 2019). Electric power generation is by far the largest single source of SO_2 emissions. Approximately 60–70% of total SO_2 emitted in the atmosphere is responsible for global acid deposition. More than 90% of SO_2 in the atmosphere is created from human activities, such as industrial combustion (69.4%), transportation (3.7%), coal burning (2–3%), and smelting of metal sulfide ores (mostly copper, lead, and zinc) to obtain pure metals (about 14%). The remaining 10% of SO_2 is emitted from volcanic eruptions, forest fires, sea spray, rotting vegetation, plankton, organic decay, and so forth. When coal and wood were major fuels, much of the acidity produced by combustion was neutralized by smoke and fly ash. A portion of the sulfur compounds in air are oxidized to sulfate (SO_4^-) and react with other materials to form fine particulate aerosols. The most common form appears to be ammonium sulfate, with the ammonia presumably derived from volatilization from biological materials.

Most fuels contain nitrogen. The amount of nitrogen in fuel varies with the fuel type. As summarized in the reaction sequences, typical coal and oil contain chemically bound organic nitrogen, which is different from that found in natural gas. Most of the world's nitrogen occurs naturally in the atmosphere as an inert gas contained in air, which consists of approximately 78% N_2 by volume. Of the various emissions of nitrogen compounds which enter into the atmosphere NO, NO_2, N_2O and NH_3, NH:, are the most important species. Natural sources considerably exceed sources from anthropogenic activity (Robinson and Robbins, 1972). The oxides of nitrogen in air are complex and usually referred to as NO_x. Nitrogen oxides (NO_x) represent the following seven oxides of nitrogen as per US EPA (1983):

1. Nitric oxide (NO)
2. Nitrogen dioxide (NO_2)
3. Nitrous oxide (N_2O)
4. Dinitrogen dioxide (N_2O_2)
5. Dinitrogen trioxide (N_2O_3)
6. Dinitrogen tetroxide (N_2O_4)
7. Dinitrogen pentoxide (N_2O_5).

The US Environmental Protection Agency defines nitrogen oxides as "all oxides of nitrogen except nitrous oxide".[1] However, NO_x often refer only to NO and NO_2 in most of the environmental legislation imposed worldwide. These two forms of nitrogen oxides are the major contributors to air pollution worldwide, as has been observed in scientific investigations in recent times (Zevenhoven and Kilpinen, 2002). NO_x emissions are among the primary air pollutants because of their contribution to smog formation, acid rain, and ozone depletion in the upper atmosphere.

Nitrous oxide (N_2O) contributes to ozone destruction in the stratosphere and is a relatively strong greenhouse gas (GHG) (Portmann et al., 2012). Although it is not an important factor in most of the high-temperature industrial combustion sources considered here, it is important at lower temperatures (705–950°C), especially when solid fuels are used.

There are three generally accepted mechanisms for NO_x production: thermal, prompt, and fuel. Thermal NO_x is formed by the high-temperature reaction (hence the name thermal NO_x) of nitrogen with oxygen, by the well-known Zeldovich mechanism (Zeldovich, 1946). It is sometimes referred to as Zeldovich NO_x (Dean and Bozzelli, 2000). It is given by the simplified reaction (R11 in Box 1.1). The two predominant reactions are R12 and R13). The extended Zeldovich mechanism includes a third equation (R14).

Thermal NO_x increases exponentially with temperature. Above about 2000°F (1100°C), it is generally the predominant mechanism in combustion processes, making it important in most high-temperature heating applications. Prompt NO_x is formed by the relatively fast reaction (hence the name prompt NO_x) between nitrogen, oxygen, and hydrocarbon radicals. It is sometimes referred to as Fenimore NOx after C.P. Fenimore from the General Electric Research and Development Center in Schenectady, NY, who first coined the term "prompt NOx" and showed experimentally the presence of this mechanism (Fenimore, 1971). It is given by the overall reaction R15 in Box 1.1. In reality, this very complicated process consists of hundreds of reactions. Hydrocarbon radicals are intermediate species formed during the combustion process. Prompt NO_x is generally an important mechanism in lower-temperature combustion processes, but it is generally much less important compared to thermal NO_x formation at the higher temperatures found in most industrial combustion processes. It is also generally important in very fuel-rich conditions, which are not normally encountered except under certain circumstances.

Fuel NO_x is formed by the direct oxidation of organonitrogen compounds contained in the fuel (hence the name fuel NO_x). It is given by the overall reaction R16 in Box 1.1. In reality, there are many intermediate reactions for this formation mechanism. Fuel NO_x is not a concern for high-quality gaseous fuels like natural gas or propane, which normally have no organically bound nitrogen. The conversion of fuel-bound nitrogen to NO_x ranges from 15 to 100%. The conversion efficiency is generally higher the lower the nitrogen content in the fuel. Controlling excess oxygen is an important strategy for minimizing fuel NO_x emissions.

The principal source of nitrogen oxides is high-temperature combustion where nitrogen and oxygen naturally present in the air combine to form NO_x. In clean air, nitric oxide is known to have a half-life of a few days, but in polluted air it may be converted rapidly into nitrogen dioxide, which is soluble in water. As with SO_2, natural emission of NO_x on a global basis far exceeds human contributions but automobiles and other combustion processes overwhelm these sources in industrial areas. About 95% of NO_x is emitted from anthropogenic activities; in the automobile sector (56%), in fertilizer industries (5%), and fuel combustion (34%), etc. The remaining 5% is emitted by natural processes such as forest fires, lightning, soil erosion, and so on (Almaraz et al., 2018; Mohajan, 2018). At present, sulfur oxides in the air generally exceed nitrogen oxides but increased emissions of NO_x are expected to increase the nitric acid component in rain. Additionally, NO_x combines with VOCs to form ground level ozone (smog). Thus, in reality acid rain is a mixture of acids dissolved in water, reactive gaseous oxides, and fine particulate sulfate and nitrate aerosols. In addition air contains other pollutants such as ozone, hydrocarbons, and heavy metals which may interact in a synergistic fashion with various components in acid rain; consequently, acid rain must be considered as only a part of the larger problem of air pollution.

1.2   EFFECTS OF ACID DEPOSITION

Increasing concentrations of hydrogen ions (H^+) in soil or water leads to acidification. It can cause metals and their compounds to ionize, producing ions (such as Al^{3+}) and leading to serious health effects (Figure 1.2). The toxic concentration causes damage to cells of plants, animals, and microorganisms. Acid rain incidents across the globe have little environmental effect on the biosphere because acid rain is rapidly neutralized after it falls. In particular, acid rain falling over the oceans is rapidly neutralized by the large supply of CO_3^{2-} ions. In areas where the biosphere is sensitive to acid rain, there has been ample evidence of the negative effects of acid rain on freshwater ecosystems, soil, forest, infrastructure (materials and structures), and human health.

The effects of acidic deposition include the following:

1. Acidification of surface waters (freshwater rivers, lakes, and oceans) and subsequent damage to aquatic ecosystems
2. Acidification of soil and damage to forests

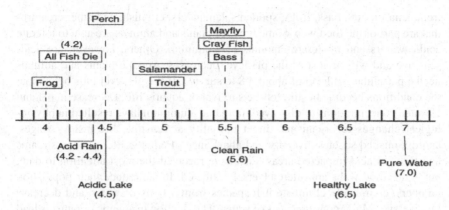

FIGURE 1.2 Aquatic animals and their critical pH levels.

3. Damage to materials and structures
4. Damage to human health

1.2.1 ACIDIFICATION OF SURFACE WATERS (FRESHWATER RIVERS, LAKES, AND OCEANS) AND SUBSEQUENT DAMAGE TO AQUATIC ECOSYSTEMS

The first and most obvious ecological effects of acid rain are most clearly seen in aquatic environments such as streams, lakes, ponds, marshes, and wetlands where it can be harmful to fish and other wildlife (Schindler, 1988; Driscoll et al., 2003). The first reports of the effects of acid precipitation on freshwater ecosystems worldwide were well documented by Giddings and Galloway (1976). Acid precipitation over a freshwater ecosystem directly impacts biodiversity. Freshwater resources represent the smallest proportion of the Earth's surface area available for acidic deposition. Yet, the best-known effect is acidification of freshwater aquatic systems. Tens of thousands of lakes and streams in North America and Europe are more acidic than they were a few decades ago as a result of acid deposition (Schindler, 1988). Acidification of freshwaters has resulted in losses of fish and other aquatic organisms (Schindler, 1988). Ocean acidification processes can mess with a fish's mind, leading to misbalance of its nervous system and reflex abilities (Fischetti, 2012). In the Adirondack Mountains, the Department of Environmental Conservation has found that fish populations are endangered in more than half of all the lakes and ponds in the region and more than 200 lakes have become totally fishless. Indeed, surface water acidification as a result of acid rain has had demonstrable effects on organisms at several trophic levels, including fish, zooplankton, and benthic organisms. As acid rain flows through the soil, acidic rain water can leach aluminum from soil clay particles and then flow into streams and lakes. The more acid that is introduced to the ecosystem, the more aluminum is released. Unfortunately, this increase in acidity and aluminum levels can be deadly to aquatic wildlife, including phytoplankton, mayflies, rainbow trout, small mouth bass, frogs, spotted salamanders, crayfish, and other creatures that are part of the food web. Some types of plants and animals are able to tolerate acidic waters and moderate amounts of aluminum. Others, however, are acid-sensitive and will be lost as the pH level decreases. Aquatic plants and animals need a particular pH level of about 4.8 to survive. If the pH level falls below that the conditions become hostile for the survival of aquatic life. Decrease in pH and elevated concentrations of dissolved inorganic aluminum have resulted in physiological changes to organisms, direct mortality at sensitive life history stages, and diminished species diversity and abundance of aquatic life in many streams and lakes in acid-impacted areas. Fish have received the most attention to date, but entire food webs are often adversely affected. It can reduce their population numbers, completely eliminate fish species from a body of water, and decrease biodiversity. Major consequences of water pH reduction in aquatic organisms lead to disruption of their chemosensory abilities, as the detection of chemical cues underpins a wide range of decision-making processes; for example, a reduction to low pH has been shown to interfere with predator avoidance and the detection of foraging cues. In India, acidification of freshwater ecosystems is well studied (Aggarwal et al., 2001; Duan et al., 2016).

Studies demonstrate effects of acidic deposition on fish at three ecosystem levels:

1. Effects on single organisms (condition factor – the relationship between the weight and the length of a fish). Fish condition factor is related to several chemical indicators of acid–base status, including minimum pH. This analysis suggests that fish in acidic streams use energy to maintain internal chemistry that would otherwise be used for growth.
2. Population-level effects (increased mortality). Bioassay experiments show greater mortality in chronically acidic streams than in high-acid-neutralizing capacity streams. Eggs and fry are sensitive life history stages for fish.
3. Community-level effects (reduced species richness). The species richness of fish and other aquatic organisms decreases with decreasing acid-neutralizing capacity and pH.

1.2.1.1 Ocean Acidification and Consequences

Carbon dioxide concentration in the Earth's atmosphere now exceeds 380 ppm, which is more than 80 ppm above the maximum values of the past 740,000 years (Petit et al., 1999; ÉPICA, 2004), if not 20 million years (Raven et al., 2005). Mean oceanic CO_2 values are expected to reach 1000 μatm CO_2 by the year 2100 and 1900 μatm CO_2 by the year 2300 as a result of global anthropogenic emissions and increasing rates of GHG concentration in the atmosphere (Caldeira and Wickett, 2003; Meehl et al., 2007). Of all CO_2 emitted globally due to land use changes, fossil fuel burning, and cement production in the past 200 years, only about half has remained in the atmosphere. Oceans have been the largest sinks of CO_2 and sequester the lion's share of GHG in the atmosphere. A concern of many scientists is that rising levels of atmospheric CO_2 are causing an increasing acidification of oceans resulting in constant decline in pH values (IPCC, 2007, 2014; Kroeker et al., 2013). Average ocean surface pH records a decline of 0.32 and 0.77 units respectively (Caldeira and Wickett, 2005). Shifting of ocean chemistry is expected to show a profound impact on marine biodiversity worldwide (Secretariat of the Convention on Biological Diversity, 2014), resulting in a direct impact on fish physiology as observed during a scientific investigation (Heuer and Grosell, 2014, 2016). Gattuso et al., (2015) demonstrated that coral reefs are the most sensitive marine ecosystems globally. In a landmark review of the potential impacts of different Intergovernmental Panel on Climate Change (IPCC) scenarios on oceans and associated ecosystem services, irrespective of the IPCC scenario (RCP2.6/RCP8.5), acidification leads to bleaching of corals globally (Hoegh-Guldberg et al., 2007; Hooidonk et al., 2013).

1.2.2 ACIDIFICATION OF SOIL AND DAMAGE TO FORESTS

Soil acidification is a phenomenon determined by natural and anthropogenic factors. The decomposition of organic matter, the imbalance of the nitrogen, sulfur, and carbon cycles, the excess in cation uptake on anions, and N fixation by legumes influence the concentration of protons [H^+] in soil solution. Anthropogenic factors such as the use of fertilizers (nitrogen, phosphorus, and potassium: NPK), the use of acidifiers and aerosols (H_2S, H_2SO_4, HF, and Cl_2), and the emission of gases (CO_2, NO_2, and SO_2) into the atmosphere by use of fossil energy give rise to environmental pollution. Such molecules find their way into soil and water bodies in the form of acid rain, causing acidification of soils and the release of Al ions in a form easily absorbed by the plant root system, which is extremely toxic. Also, nutrient deficiency (P, Mg, and K) and toxicity by other metals (Mn and Fe) may occur.

Acid rain has become of increasing concern today in Europe and North America because of the *die-back* of forest trees, a harmful process also known as *forest decline*. Acid rain can be extremely harmful to forests; acid rain that seeps into the ground can dissolve nutrients, such as magnesium and calcium, essential minerals for vegetation growth. Acid rain also causes aluminum to be released into the soil, which makes it difficult for trees to take up water. It makes trees vulnerable to disease, extreme weather, and insects by destroying their leaves, damaging the bark, and arresting their growth. Trees that are located in mountainous regions at higher elevations, such as spruce or fir trees, are at greater risk because they are exposed to acidic clouds and fog, which contain greater amounts of acid than rain or snow. Acidic deposition has contributed to the decline of red spruce and sugar maple trees in the eastern USA and shifts in the distribution of tree species. Symptoms of tree decline include poor condition of the canopy, reduced growth, and unusually high levels of mortality. Acidic deposition impacts red spruce through loss of membrane calcium due to direct leaching from foliage or reduced uptake of calcium from soil. The loss of membrane calcium makes red spruce more susceptible to winter injury. Acidic deposition results in loss of soil-available calcium and magnesium and less uptake by sugar maple. This condition may make sugar maple more susceptible to insect or drought stress. Declines of red spruce and sugar maple in the northeastern USA have occurred during the past five decades (Gavin et al., 2008).

1.2.3 DAMAGE TO MATERIALS AND STRUCTURES

Acid rain of pH value 3–5 is known as "stone cancer." It has been observed that numerous buildings and historical monuments have been damaged worldwide because of acid rain. The Taj Mahal of Agra, India, which is widely regarded as one of the seven wonders of the world was also a victim of acid rain due to extreme air pollution in and around the area. Acid rain itself has little effect on material damage. Most damage is caused by dry deposition or sorption of gases, particularly SO_2 and NO_x, which then react with dew or other moisture. Other environmental factors contributing to damage are sunlight, temperature freezing and thawing, microorganisms such as fungal attack, and salt deposition. The marble and limestone of archeological monuments and historical structures and statues are being slowly eaten up by atmospheric acid precipitation. Buildings and outdoor monuments are being gradually eroded away as a result of acid rain. Calcium carbonate and sulfuric acid (the primary acid components of the rain) result in the dissolution of $CaCO_3$ to give aqueous ions, which in turn are washed away in the water flow.

$$CaCO_3 + H_2SO_4 \rightarrow Ca^{2+} (aq) + SO_4^{2-} + H_2O + CO_2$$

1.2.4 DAMAGE TO HUMAN HEALTH

Approximately 7 million people across the world die every year from exposure to polluted air while ambient air pollution was responsible for more than 4.2 million deaths in 2016. Household air pollution caused as a result of cooking with adulterated oils and fuels caused an estimated 3.8 million deaths in the same period. The situation is worse in low-income countries, where 98% of cities fail to meet World Health Organization air quality standards. Acid rain can harm humans both directly and indirectly (Goyer et al., 1985; Kumar, 2017). Acid dissolution in surface drinking water sources as well as ground-water resources causes neural damage, pulmonary diseases (asthma and bronchitis), brain damage, kidney problems, cancer, and Alzheimer's disease. There is little clinical evidence or investigations of any direct effect of acid rain such as increased acidity of rainfall on human health. The notion that acid rain will burn skin or dissolve clothing has no basis in fact. However, varied impacts of acid precipitation on human health and ecological resources are beyond any doubt.

1.3 MITIGATION, CONCLUSIONS, AND WAY FORWARD

During the last 25 years there has been an increase in the awareness of environmental atmospheric pollution and acid precipitation worldwide, as is evident from various scientific investigations across multi-temporal and multi-spatial environmental matrices. Strategies to combat air pollution and acid precipitation must include investment in sustainable and green technologies that reduce our dependence on fossil fuels, strengthening of public health infrastructure and surveillance systems, and mass education on the health risks of air pollution, acid precipitation, and climate change. The post-COVID-19 era seems to be more challenging and exciting, with our responsibility to fight global climate change becoming more pertinent and urgent. Given below are a few solutions, which can greatly reduce the threat of acid rain, if strictly followed by all stakeholders – governments, corporate, non-governmental organizations and, most importantly, the general public.

1.3.1 USE OF CLEAN FUEL TECHNOLOGIES

Embracing clean fuel technologies is urgently needed in every country across the globe irrespective of its financial position or socio-economic scenario. The Kyoto Protocol speaks of "similar but differentiated responsibilities" to be performed by all countries. Consumption of clean fuel technology stands on the most urgent priority platform currently. According to the World Resources Institute Report (WRI, 2017) findings, India is responsible for approximately 6.65% of total global carbon emissions, ranked fourth after China (26.83%), the USA (14.36%), and the EU (9.66%), and further approved by the findings of CESI (2017) and Pappas (2017). Combustion strategies are also being developed by Indian Institutes of Technology and Indian Institutes of Science, Education and Research across India that would greatly reduce the formation and subsequent release of NO_x and SO_x; the two major culprits of degrading air pollution indices in large cities across the world, from New York to New Delhi and Seoul to Beijing. There are several options for reducing SO_2 emissions, including using coal containing less sulfur and washing the coal. Specific disincentives need to be imposed on industries that use high-end energy, and add on to the emissions and carbon footprints. Machineries with anti-pollution techniques that would have zero emission effects need to be installed. One of the most fundamental solutions is to utilize clean fuel technologies that burn fuels more cleanly, or to burn coal more efficiently. This will greatly reduce the quantity of acids released in the atmosphere. Clean coal technologies (CCT) include a number of innovative new technologies designed to use coal in a more efficient and cost-effective manner while enhancing environmental protection. Technologies include fluidized-bed combustion, integrated gasification combined cycle (IGCC), limestone injection, multistage burner, enhanced flue gas desulfurization (EFGD) (or *scrubbing*), coal liquefaction, and coal gasification. Coal cleaning by washing has been standard practice in developed countries such as the USA, Australia, Russia, Germany, France, Italy, and the UK for some time. It reduces emissions of ash and sulfur dioxide when the coal is burned. Furthermore, electrostatic precipitators and fabric filters can remove 99% of fly ash from flue gases and such technologies are in widespread use. In addition, EFGD reduces the output of SO_2 to the atmosphere and low-NO_x burners allow coal-fired plants to reduce nitrogen oxide emissions. Both technologies are widely used in developed economies and have also been embraced in developing economies during the last decade. Other technologies such as IGCC and pressurized fluidized bed combustion (PFBC) enable higher thermal efficiencies for the future. Pulverized coal consumption forms the new mandate for marine vessels. Ultra clean coal (UCC) from new processing technologies reduce ash below 0.25% and sulfur to very low levels, which means that pulverized coal might be used as fuel for large marine vessels and tankers, in place of heavy fuel oil. Scrubbers used in industrial power plants efficiently reduce air pollution while locking down the air pollutants and toxic gases. These scrubbers reduce the amount of sulfur released through smoke by 90–95%. Tall chimneys are mandated for heavy industries to avoid air pollution at lower atmosphere by the Government of India. Power plants can also switch to fuels; for example, burning natural gas creates much less SO_2 than burning coal. Similar to scrubbers on power plants, catalytic converters reduce NO_x emissions from cars. Vehicular exhausts form another humongous source of air pollution beside industrial exhausts. Green buildings can significantly reduce domestic power and electricity consumption in large towns and cities. The Green Rating for Integrated Habitat Assessment (GRIHA) initiative by The Energy and Resources Institute (TERI) New Delhi is a welcome step in such a direction. The Ministry Of Environment, Forest and Climate Change (MOEFCC) headquarters in New Delhi is also a significant and excellent example of green building in India.

1.3.2 USE OF ALTERNATIVE RENEWABLE ENERGY SOURCES

The primary objective for deploying renewable energy in India is to advance economic development, improve energy security, improve access to energy, and mitigate climate change (Kumar and Majid, 2020). Nuclear power, hydropower, wind energy, geothermal energy, solar energy, wave energy, and biofuels are alternative energy sources suggested worldwide in the era of low-carbon lifestyle and global commitments toward the reduction of GHG concentrations in the atmosphere as well as lowering the temperature by 1.5°C, as per the Paris Climate Agreement. Nuclear, solar, and hydropower have been proved to be most promising for India in coming times, taking the huge energy demand and consumption pattern into consideration (Mishra et al., 2015; Dawn et al., 2016).

India is experiencing a stupendous energy demand to fulfill the mammoth economic development plans that have been implemented since the last decade. Arranging extra quantum of energy is a vital pre-requisite for economic or industrial growth of any kind in modern times (Kumar et al., 2019). Almost all of the electricity that powers modern life comes from burning fossil fuels such as coal, natural gas, and oil. However, exhaust emissions from these fuels are the main causes of acid deposition released into the atmosphere. From an environmental point of view this would be unsustainable unless advanced CCT with carbon sequestration is deployed. CCT is based on an IGCC that converts coal to gas that is then used in a turbine to provide electricity with CO_2 and pollutant removal before the fuel is burned. Alternative energies are also available to power automobiles, including electric vehicles, biofuel-powered engines in automobiles, natural gas-powered vehicles, battery-powered cars, fuel cells, and combinations of alternative and gasoline-powered vehicles. All sources of energy have environmental costs as well as benefits.

1.3.3 Use of Lime

Liming is one of the urgent practical steps needed to counteract the effect of acidification and to ensure the restoration of species assemblages as well as the preservation of functional processes until spontaneous recovery of streams occurs (Tixier and Guérold 2005). Powdered limestone added to water and soil to neutralize acid is commonly used in Norway and Sweden. However, it is more expensive and a short-term remedy. Acid deposition penetrates deeply into the fabric of an ecosystem, changing the chemistry of the soil as well as the chemistry of streams.

1.4 CASE STUDY: ACID PRECIPITATION AND ALUMINUM TOXICITY

Aluminum is the third most abundant element found in the Earth's crust (Gupta et al., 2013). Aluminum occurs naturally in the air, water, and soil. Mining and processing of aluminum elevates its level in the environment (Agency for Toxic Substances and Disease Registry (ATSDR), 2008). In recent years, humans have probably experienced a burgeoning exposure to biologically reactive aluminum, with possible relevant consequences for human health and disease (Andia, 1996; Merce et al., 2009; Crisponi and Nurchi, 2011; Crisponi et al., 2012, 2013). This potentially dangerous exposure is related to a great extent to atmospheric acidification due to acid rain, which is causing progressive acidification of the soil, followed by a massive export of aluminum from the crust of the Earth to surface waters, putting vegetables, animals and humans in contact with absorbable cationic aluminum species, probably for the first time in their history (Kopacek et al., 2009). Owing to acid rain, numerous metal ions, including aluminum, are escaping from mineral deposits where they had been stored for billions of years as hydroxy-aluminosilicates (HAS) (Exley et al., 1997, 2002), increasing the biological availability of aluminum to living organisms. According to this hypothesis, acid rain is acting as a key to the lock for aluminum release, causing its appearance in polluted waters. The mobilization of toxic aluminum ions, resulting from changes in the pH of soil and water caused by acid rain and increasing acidification of the surrounding atmosphere, has an adverse effect on the environment. This is manifested by the drying of forests, plant poisoning, crop decline or failure, death of aquatic animals, and also by various imbalances in the function of human and animal systems (Barabasz et al., 2002).

Recent investigations on environmental toxicology revealed that aluminum may present a major threat for humans, animals, and plants in causing many diseases (Campbell and Bondy, 2000; Barabasz et al., 2002). Many factors, including pH of water and organic matter content, greatly influence the toxicity of aluminum. Recent research reveals a similar mode of Al action in all living organisms (plant, animals, and humans), namely interference with the secondary messenger system (phosphoinositide and cytosolic Ca^{2+} signaling pathways) and enhanced production of reactive oxygen species resulting in oxidative stress (Rengel, 2004; Kochian et al., 2005; Krewski et al., 2007;). Aluminum uptake by plants is relatively quick (across the intact plasma membrane in <30 min and across the tonoplast in <1 h, despite a huge proportion of Al being bound in the cell wall. Aluminum absorption in the animal/human digestive system is low (only about 0.1% of daily Al intake stays in the body), except when aluminum is complexed with organic ligands (e.g., citrate, tartrate, glutamate). Aluminum accumulates in bones and brain, with Al citrate and Al transferrin crossing the complex blood–brain barrier and accumulating in brain cells (Rengel, 2004). The interaction of Al^{3+} with apoplastic, plasma membrane, and symplastic targets leads to toxicity and distracts the physical and cellular processes in plants. Common manifestations are root growth inhibition, cellular modification in leaves, small and dark green leaves, yellowing and death of leaves, chlorosis, purpling, and foliar necrosis (Gupta et al., 2013). A pH < 5 can lead to soil acidity which is a major concern around the world that affects crop production. Due to aluminum toxicity, crop production was constrained to 67% of total acid soil area in the world. Due to acid soils (pH < 5), silicon is leached, leaving behind aluminum in solid form, known as aluminum oxyhydroxides, such as gibbsite and boehmite. These unstable forms of aluminum discharge phytotoxic Al^{3+}, which is well known as $Al(OH)^{3+}$ in soil (Abate et al., 2013).

Aluminum in high concentrations is very toxic for aquatic animals, especially for gill-breathing organisms such as fish, causing osmoregulatory failure by destroying plasma and hemolymph ions. The activity of gill enzyme, essential for the uptake of ions, is inhibited by the monomeric form of aluminum in fish (Rosseland et al., 1990). Living organisms in water, such as seaweeds and crawfish, are also affected by Al toxicity (Bezak-Mazur et al., 2001). Aluminum has no biological role and is a toxic non-essential metal to microorganisms (Olaniran et al., 2013). Enzymes such as hexokinase, phosphodiesterase, alkalic phosphatase, and phosphoxidase are inhibited by aluminum since it has a greater affinity to DNA and RNA. Metabolic pathways in the living organism involving calcium, phosphorus, fluorine, and iron metabolism are affected by aluminum. Symptoms that indicate the presence of higher amounts of aluminum in the human body are nausea, mouth ulcers, skin ulcers, skin rashes, vomiting, diarrhea, and arthritic pain (Figure 1.3). These symptoms have however been reported to be mild and short-lived (Clayton, 1989). The main routes of aluminum consumption by humans are through inhalation, ingestion, and dermal contact and sources of exposure are drinking water, food, beverages, and aluminum-containing drugs. Aluminum is naturally present in

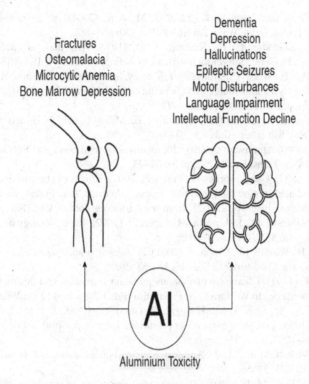

Fractures
Osteomalacia
Microcytic Anemia
Bone Marrow Depression

Dementia
Depression
Hallucinations
Epileptic Seizures
Motor Disturbances
Language Impairment
Intellectual Function Decline

Al

Aluminium Toxicity

FIGURE 1.3 Aluminum toxicity leading to series of health consequences.

food. A causal role for aluminum in human pathology has been clearly established in at least three diseases: dialysis dementia (Alfrey et al., 1976), osteomalacia (Bushinsky et al., 1995), and microcytic anemia without iron deficiency (Touam et al., 1983; Campbell and Bondy, 2000).

NOTE

1   www3.epa.gov/ttncatc1/dir1/fnoxdoc.pdf.

REFERENCES

Aas, W., Mortier, A., Bowersox, V., et al. (2019). Global and regional trends of atmospheric sulfur. Sci Rep 9: 953. https://doi.org/10.1038/s41598-018-37304-0.

Abate, E., Hussien, S., Laing, M., Mengistu, F. (2013). Aluminium toxicity tolerance in cereals: Mechanisms, genetic control and breeding methods. Afr J Agric Res 8(9): 711–722.

Agency for Toxic Substances and Disease Registry (ATSDR). (2008). Public Health Statement Aluminium. ATSDR Publication CAS#7429-90-5. Atlanta, GA. www.atsdr.cdc.gov/ToxProfiles/tp22-c1-b.pdf.

Aggarwal, S. G., Chandrawanshi, K., Patel, R. M., et al. (2001). Acidification of surface water in central India. Water Air Soil Pollut 130: 855–862.

Alfrey, A. C., LeGendre, G. R., Kaehny, W. D. (1976). The dialysis encephalopathy syndrome. Possible aluminium intoxication. N Engl J Med 294: 184–188.

Almaraz, M., Bai, E., Wang, C., Trousdell, J., Conley, S., Faloona, I., Houlton, B. Z. (2018). Agriculture is a major source of NOx pollution in California. Sci Adv 4(1): eaao3477. https://doi.org/10.1126/sciadv.aao3477.

Almer, B., Dickson, W., Ekström, C., Hörnström, E., Miller, U. (1974). Effects of acidification on Swedish lakes. Ambio 3: 30–36.

Andia, J. B. (1996). Aluminum toxicity: Its relationship with bone and iron metabolism. Nephrol Dial Transplant 11 (Suppl 3): 69–73.

Balasubramanian, G., Udayasoorian, C., Prabu, P. (2007). Effects of short-term exposure of simulated acid rain on the growth of Acacia Nilotica. J Trop Forest Sci 19(4): 198–206. Retrieved January 31, 2021, from www.jstor.org/stable/43595388.

Barabasz, W., Albinska, D., Jaskowska, M., Lipiec, J. (2002). Ecotoxicology of aluminium. Pol J Environ Stud 11(3): 199–203.

Bezak-Mazur, E., Widiak, M., Ciupa, T. (2001). A speciation analysis of aluminium in the River Silnica. Pol J Environ Stud 10(4): 263–268.

Bowman, C. T. (1991). Chemistry of gaseous pollutant formation and destruction. Fossil fuel combustion. In W. Bartok, A. F. Sarofim (Eds.), New York: John Wiley.

Bushinsky, D. A., Sprague, S. M., Hallegot, P., Girod, C., Chabala, J. M., Levi-Setti, R. (1995). Effects of aluminium on bone surface ion composition. J Bone Miner Res 10: 1988–1997.

Caldeira, K., Wickett, M. E. (2003). Anthropogenic carbon and ocean pH. Nature 425, 365. doi: 10.1038/425365a.

Caldeira, K., Wickett, M. E. (2005). Ocean model predictions of chemistry changes from carbon dioxide emissions to the atmosphere and ocean. J Geophys Res 110: 2156–2202. doi: 10.1038/nature13798.

Campbell, A., Bondy, S. C. (2000). Aluminium induced oxidative events and its relation to inflammation: A role for the metal in Alzheimer's disease. Cell Mol Biol (Noisy-le-grand) 46: 721–730.

CESI, Canadian Environmental Sustainability Indicators (2017). Global greenhouse gas emissions. Available at www.ec.gc.ca/indicateurs-indicators/54C061B5-44F7-4A93-A3EC-5F8B253A7235/GlobalGHGEmissions_EN.pdf.

Clayton, D. B. (1989). Water pollution at Lowermoore North Cornwall: Report of the Lowermoore incident health advisory committee: Truro, Cornwall District Health Authority.

Crisponi, G., Nurchi, V. M. (2011). Thermodynamic remarks on chelating ligands for aluminium related diseases. J Inorg Biochem 105: 1518–1522.

Crisponi, G., Nurchi, V. M., Bertolasi, V., Remelli, M., Faa, G. (2012). Chelating agents for human diseases related to aluminium overload. Coord Chem Rev 256: 89–104.

Crisponi, G., Fanni, D., Gerosa, C., Nemolato, S., Nurchi, V. M., Crespo-Alonso, M., Lachowicz, J. I., Faa, G. (2013). The meaning of aluminium exposure on human health and aluminium-related diseases. BioMol Concepts 4(1): 77–87.

Dawn, S., Tiwari, P. K., Goswami, A. K., Mishra, M. K. (2016). Recent developments of solar energy in India: Perspectives, strategies and future goals. Renew Sustain Energy Rev 62: 215–235.

Dean, A. M., Bozzelli, J. W. (2000). Combustion chemistry of nitrogen. In W. C. Gardiner (Ed.), Gas-phase combustion chemistry. New York: Springer, Chapter 2.

Driscoll, C., Driscoll, K., Mitchell, M., Raynal, D. (2003). Effects of acidic deposition on forest and aquatic ecosystems in New York State. Environment Pollut 123: 327–336.

Duan, L., Yu, Q., Zhang, Q., Wang, Z., Pan, Y., Larssen, T., Tang, J., Mulder, J. (2016). Acid deposition in Asia: emissions, deposition, and ecosystem effects. Atmosph Environ 146: 55–69.

ÉPICA. (2004) Community members. Nature 429: 623.

European Monitoring and Evaluation Programme (EMEP). (2019). Officially Reported Emission Trends. Available online at: www.emep.int/ (accessed 21 January 2019).

Exley, C., Pinnegar, J. K., Taylor, H. (1997). Hydroxyaluminosilicates and acute aluminium toxicity in fish. J Theor Biol 189: 133–139.

Exley, C., Schneider, C., Doucet, F. (2002). The reaction of aluminium with silicic acid in acidic solution: An important mechanism in controlling the biological availability of aluminium. Coord Chem Rev 228: 127–135.

Fenimore, C. P. (1971). Formation of nitric oxide in premixed hydrocarbon flames. Thirteenth Symposium (International) on Combustion. Pittsburgh, PA: The Combustion Institute, pp. 373–380.

Ferenbaugh, R. W. (1976). Effects of simulated acid rain on Phaseolus vulgaris L. (Fabaceae). Am J Bot 63: 283–288.

Fischetti, M. (2012). Ocean acidification can mess with a fish's mind. Available online at: www.scientificamerican.com/article/ocean-acidification-can-m/

Gattuso, J.-P., Magnan, A., Billé, R., Cheung, W. W. L., Howes, E. L., Joos, F., Allemand, D., Bopp, L., Cooley, S. R., Eakin, C. M., Hoegh-Guldberg, O., Kelly, R. P., Pörtner, H.-O., Rogers, A. D., Baxter, J., Laffoley, D., Osborn, D., Rankovic, A., Rochette, J., Sumaila, U. R., Treyer, S., Turley, C. (2015). Oceanography. Contrasting futures for ocean and society from different anthropogenic CO_2 emissions scenarios. Science 349 (6243):aac4722. doi: 10.1126/science.aac4722. PMID: 26138982.

Gavin, D., Beckage, B., Osborne, B. (2008). Forest dynamics and the growth decline of red spruce and sugar maple on Bolton Mountain, Vermont: A comparison of modeling methods. Can J Forest Res 38: 2635–2649. doi:10.1139/X08-106.

Gibson, A., Farrar, W. V. (1973). Robert Angus Smith, FRS, and sanitary science. Notes Records R Soc 28(2): 241–262. doi:10.1098/rsnr.1974.0017.

Giddings, J., Galloway, J. H. (1976). Effects of acid precipitation on aquatic and terrestrial ecosystems. In: Literature Reviews on Acid Precipitation. Ithaca, NY: Center for Environmental Quality Management and the Water Resources and Marine Science Center, Cornell University, pp. 1–40.

Gorham, E. (1982). Robert Angus Smith, F.R.S., and 'chemical climatology.' Notes Records R Soc Lond 36(2): 267–272. doi:10.1098/rsnr.1982.0016. PMID 11615878.

Goyer, R., Bachmann, J., Clarkson, T., Ferris, B., Graham, J., Mushak, P., Perl, D., Rall, D., Schlesinger, R., Sharpe, W. (1985). Potential human health effects of acid rain: Report of a workshop. Environ Health Perspect 60: 355–368. doi:10.1289/ehp.8560355.

Gupta, N., Gaurav, S. S., Kumar, A. (2013). Molecular basis of aluminium toxicity in plants: A review. Am J Plant Sci 4: 21–37.

Hamlin, C. (2004). Smith, (Robert) Angus (1817–1884). In: Oxford Dictionary of National Biography. Oxford: Oxford University Press. Retrieved 10 August 2007. doi:10.1093/ref:odnb/25893.

Heuer, R. M., Grosell, M. (2014). Physiological impacts of elevated carbon dioxide and ocean acidification on fish. Am J Physiol Regul Integr Comp Physiol 307: R1061–R1084. doi: 10.1152/ajpregu.00064.2014.

Heuer, R. M., Grosell, M. (2016). Elevated CO_2 increases energetic cost and ion movement in the marine fish intestine. Sci Rep 6: 34480. doi: 10.1038/srep34480.

Hoegh-Guldberg, O. et al. (2007). Coral reefs under rapid climate change and ocean acidification. Science 318: 1737. doi: 10.1126/science.1152509.

Hooidonk, R. V., Maynard, J. A., Menzello, D., Planes, S. (2013). Opposite latitudinal gradients in projected ocean acidification and bleaching impacts on coral reefs. Global Change Biol doi: 10.1111/gcb.12394.

IPCC. (2007). Climate change 2007: synthesis report. In Core Writing Team, R. K. Pachauri, A. Reisinger (Eds.), Contribution of Working Groups I, II and III to the Fourth Assessment Report of the Intergovernmental Panel on Climate Change. Geneva: IPCC, p. 104.

IPCC. (2014). "Climate change 2014: Synthesis report. In Core Writing Team, R. K. Pachauri, A. Reisinger (Eds.), Contribution of Working Groups I, II and III to the Fifth Assessment Report of the Intergovernmental Panel on Climate Change. Geneva: IPCC, p. 151.

Irving, P. M. (1983). Acidic precipitation effects on crops: A review and analysis of research. J Environ Qual 12: 442–453.

Keitel, M. (1995). Langzeitbetrachtung der Gewässerversauerung – Fallstudie im Erzgebirge. Wasser Boden 47: 27–33.

Kochian, L. V., Pineros, M. A., Hoekenga, O. A. (2005). The physiology, genetics and molecular biology of plant aluminum resistance and toxicity. Plant Soil 274: 175–195.

Kopacek, J., Hejzlar, J., Kana, J., Norton, S. A., Porcal, P., Turek, J. (2009). Trends in aluminium export from a mountainous area to surface waters, from deglaciation to the recent: Effects of vegetation and soil development, atmospheric acidification, and nitrogen-saturation. J Inorg Biochem 103: 1439–1448.

Krewski, D., Yokel, R. A., Nieboer, E., Borchelt, D., Cohen, J., Harry, J., Rondeau, V. (2007). Human health risk assessment for aluminium, aluminium oxide, and aluminium hydroxide. J Toxicol Environ Health B Crit Rev 10(S1): 1–269.

Kroeker, K. J., Kordas, R. L., Crim, R., Hendriks, I. E., Ramajo, L., Singh, G. S., et al. (2013). Impacts of ocean acidification on marine organisms: Quantifying sensitivities and interaction with warming. Glob Chang Biol 19: 1884–1896. doi: 10.1111/gcb.12179.

Kumar, C. R. J., Majid, M. A. (2020). Renewable energy for sustainable development in India: current status, future prospects, challenges, employment, and investment opportunities. Energ Sustain Soc 10: 2. https://doi.org/10.1186/s13705-019-0232-1.

Kumar, C. R. J., Kumar, V. D., Majid, M. A. (2019). Wind energy programme in India: Emerging energy alternatives for sustainable growth. Energy Environ 30(7): 1135–1189.

Kumar, S. (2017). Acid rain – the major cause of pollution: Its causes, effects. Int J Appl Chem 13(1): 53–58.

Kuylenstierna, J. C. I., Rodhe, H., Cinderby, S., Hicks, K. (2001). Acidification in developing countries: Ecosystem sensitivity and the critical load approach on a global scale. Ambio 30: 20–28.

Liu, Z., Yang, J., Zhang, J., Xiang, H., Wei, H. (2019). A bibliometric analysis of research on acid rain. Sustainability 11: 3077. https://doi.org/10.3390/su11113077.

Maas, R., Grennfelt, P. E. (2016). (Eds.), Towards Cleaner Air. Scientific Assessment Report EMEP Steering Body and Working Group on Effects of the Convention on Long-Range Transboundary Air Pollution, www.unece.org/fileadmin/DAM/env/lrtap/ExecutiveBody/35th_session/CLRTAP_Scientific_Assessment_Report_-_Final_20-5-2016.pdf.

Manisalidis, I., Stavropoulou, E., Stavropoulos, A., Bezirtzoglou, E. (2020). Environmental and health impacts of air pollution: A review. Front Public Health 8: 14. https://doi.org/10.3389/fpubh.2020.00014.

Meehl, G. A., Stocker, T. F., Collins, W. D., Friedlingstein, P., Gaye, A. T., Gregory, J. M., et al. (2007). Global climate projections. In Climate Change 2007: The Physical Science Basis. Contribution of Working Group I to the Fourth Assessment Report of the Intergovernmental Panel on Climate Change 2007. Cambridge: Cambridge University.

Menz, F. C., Seip, H. M. (2004). Acid rain in Europe and the United States: An update. Environ Sci Policy 7(4): 253–265. https://doi.org/10.1016/j.envsci.2004.05.005.

Merce, A. L. R., Felcman, J., Recio, M. A. L. (2009). Molecular and supramolecular bioinorganic chemistry: Applications in medical sciences. New York: Nova Biomedical Books.

Meybohm, A., Ulrich, K. U. (2007). Response of drinking-water reservoir ecosystems to decreased acidic atmospheric deposition in SE Germany: Signs of biological recovery. Water Air Soil Pollut: Focus 7: 275–284. https://doi.org/10.1007/s11267-006-9069-7.

Mishra, M. K., Khare, N., Agrawal, A. B. (2015). Small hydro power in India: Current status and future perspectives. Renew Sustain Energy Rev 51: 101–115.

Mohajan, H. (2018). Acid rain is a local environment pollution but global concern. MPRA Paper 91622. Munich: University Library of Munich, Germany.

Mohan, M., Kumar, S. (1998). Review of acid rain potential in India: Future threats and remedial measures. Curr Sci 75(6): 579–593. www.jstor.org/stable/24100562.

Muniz, I. P. (1984). The effects of acidification on Scandinavian freshwater fish fauna. Phil Trans R Soc Lond B 305: 517–528.

Muniz, I. P. (1991). Freshwater acidification: Its effects on species and communities of freshwater microbes, plants and animals. Proc R Soc Edinburgh 97b: 227–235.

Murray, A. M., Percival, D. C., Stratton, G. W. (2004). Impact of simulated acid rain on photochemistry, morphology, and yield of the wild blueberry (Vaccinium angustifolium Ait.). Can J Plant Sci 84: 877–880.

Nair, V. D., Prenzel, J. (1978). Calculations of equilibrium concentration of mono- and polynuclear hydroxyaluminium species at different pH and total aluminium concentrations. Z Pflanzenernähr Bodenk 141: 741–751.

Oden, S. (1967). The acidification of air and precipitation and its consequences in the natural environment. Ecology Committee. Bulletin no. 1. Stockholm: Swedish National Science Research Council.

Olaniran, A. O., Balgobind, A., Pillay, B. (2013). Bioavailability of heavy metals in soil: Impact on microbial biodegradation of organic compounds and possible improvement strategies. Int J Mol Sci 14(5): 10197–10228.

Pappas, D. (2017). Energy and industrial growth in India: The next emissions superpower? Energy Procedia 105: 3656–3662.

Petit, J. R. et al. (1999). Climate and atmospheric history of the past 420,000 years from the Vostok ice core, Antarctica. Nature 399: 429.

Portmann, R. W., Daniel, J. S., Ravishankara, A. R. (2012). Stratospheric ozone depletion due to nitrous oxide: influences of other gases. Philos Trans R Soc Lond Ser B, Biol Sci 367(1593): 1256–1264. https://doi.org/10.1098/rstb.2011.0377.

Ramadan, A. E. K. (2004). Acid Deposition Phenomena. Prospects of Oil, Gas and Petrochemical Industries in the Arab Region: Opportunities and Challenges, Vols. 1 and 2 (p. 1534). Egypt.

Raven, J. et al. (2005). Acidification due to increasing carbon dioxide. Pohcy Document 12/05. London: Royal Society.

Reis, S. et al. (2012). From acid rain to climate change. Science 338: 1153–1154. https://doi.org/10.1126/science.1226514.

Rengel, Z. (2004). Aluminium cycling in the soil–plant–animal–human continuum. Biometals 17: 669–689.

Robinson, E., Robbins, R. C. (1972). In: Air pollution control, part 11. W. Strauss (ed.). New York: Wiley.

Rosseland, B. O., Eldhuset, T. D., Staurnes, M. (1990). Environmental effects of aluminium. Environ Geochem Health 12(1–2): 17–27.

Schindler, D. W. (1988). Effects of acid rain on freshwater ecosystems. Science 239(4836): 149–157.

Secretariat of the Convention on Biological Diversity. (2014). History of the Convention on Biological Diversity. www.cbd.int/history/default.shtml,

Singh, A., Agrawal, M. (1996). Response of two cultivars of *Triticum aestivum L.* to simulated acid rain. Environ Pollut 91: 161–167.

Singh, B., Agrawal, M. (2004). Impact of simulated acid rain on growth and yield of two cultivars of wheat. Water Air Soil Pollut 152: 71–80.

Singh, A., Agrawal, M. (2008). Acid rain and its ecological consequences. J Environ Biol 29: 15–24.

Sutcliffe, D. W., Carrick, T. R. (1973). Studies on mountain streams in the English Lake District. 111. Aspects of water chemistry in Brownrigg Well, Whelpside Ghyll. Freshwat Biol 3: 561–568.

Thorpe, T. E. (1884). Robert Angus Smith. Nature 30(761): 104–105.

Tixier, G., Guérold, F. (2005). Plecoptera response to acidification in several headwater streams in the Vosges Mountains (northeastern France). Biodivers Conserv 14: 1525–1539. 10.1007/s10531-004-9790-3.

Tomlinson, G. H., (1983). 2nd. Air pollutants and forest decline. Environ Sci Technol. Jun 1; 17(6):246A–56A. doi: 10.1021/es00112a716. PMID: 22656466.

Touam, M., Martinez, F., Lacour, B., Bourdon, R. et al. (1983). Aluminium-induced, reversible microcytic anemia in chronic renal failure: Clinical and experimental studies. Clin Nephrol 19: 295–298.

UNECE. (2016). Towards cleaner air. Scientific Assessment Report 2016: North America. Available online at: www.unece.org/fileadmin/DAM/env/documents/2016/AIR/Publications/LRTAP_Assessment_Report_-_North_America.pdf.

United States Geological Survey, USGS (2013). Acid rain: Do you need to start wearing a rainhat? http://ga.water.usgs.gov/edu/acidrain.html.

U.S. Environmental Protection Agency (US EPA). (2018). Our nation's air: Air quality improves as America grows. Available online at: https://gispub.epa.gov/air/trendsreport/2018 (accessed 21 January 2019).

US EPA. (1983). Control techniques for nitrogen oxides emissions from stationary sources, 2nd edn. Washington, D.C.: U.S. EPA.

WRI. (2017). Forging Ahead. WRI 2017-2018 Annual Report. Washington, DC: World Resources Institute. https://wriorg.s3.amazonaws.com/s3fs-public/uploads/wri-2017-annual-report.pdf.

Wyrwicka, A., Skłodowska, M. (2006). Influence of repeated acid rain treatment on antioxidative enzyme activities and on lipid peroxidation in cucumber leaves. Environ Exp Bot, 56: 198–204.

Zeldovich, Y. B. (1946). Acta Physicochem (USSR) 21: 557.

Zevenhoven, R., Kilpinen, P. (2002). Flue gas and fuel gas, 2nd edn. Report TKK ENY-4, The Nordic energy research programme. Norway: Solid Fuel Committees, pp. 3–4.

Zhang, J., Ouyang, Y., Ling, D. (2007). Impacts of simulated acid rain on cation leaching from the Latosol in south China. Chemosphere 67: 2131–2137.

Zhao, Y., Duan, L., Xing, J., Larssen, T., Nielsen, C. P., Hao, J. (2009). Soil acidification in China: Is controlling SO_2 emissions enough? Environ Sci Technol 43: 8021–8026.

2 Human Health in a Changing Environment

Exploring the Biological and Socioeconomic Impacts

*Rajat Shubhro Mukherjee**

CONTENTS

2.1 INTRODUCTION

The severity and nature of the effects and impacts of environmental and climatic changes define the risk such environmental hazards pose. However, the same severity and nature of such impacts also reveal that the risk is not only limited to the nature of the hazard but also to exposure of people and property to such hazards and the vulnerability or susceptibility to harm of such people and property (IPCC, 2014, p. 54). This is the intricate and fragile causal as well as co-relational nature of the impact of environmental and climatic changes on human health. For the purpose of this chapter, the terms climate change and environmental change refer to the larger shift in our climate towards a more disconcerting direction, focusing especially on anthropogenic reasons for the shift in environmental and climatic conditions.

It has long been known that large-scale environmental factors pose a significant threat to human health, but it is only recently that a greater focus has been afforded to factors larger in scale than toxicological and microbiological (McMichael et al., 2003, p. 3). This ecological perspective of human health focuses on a slender balance of life-supporting properties present within the biosphere that requires

* Corresponding author: Rajat Shubhro Mukherjee. rajat.shubhro.mukherjee@gmail.com

DOI: 10.1201/9781003095422-2

to be preserved to have a healthier ecosystem. According to the World Health Organization (McMichael, Nyong, & Corvalan, 2008, p. 191), these health hazards manifest in three distinct steps chronologically corresponding to the change in socioeconomic conditions. This correlation refers to how a changing environment, whether through particulate matter pollution, contamination of air, water, or soil, or climate change due to greenhouse gas (GHG) emissions, has varying and changing effects on the human body and society at large. As per the World Health Organization, as a society becomes more educated and wealthier the profile of environmental and climatic hazards also changes.

As per Figure 2.1 individuals and households move from heavy air pollution and water and air-borne pollutions at lower levels of individual and household income (Category A) to fine particulate pollutants, chlorofluorocarbons (CFCs), and heavy metals at middle-income levels (Category B), and finally to GHGs, soil quality depletion, desertification, and depletion in fresh water supply, and biodiversity loss (Category C) (McMichael et al., 2003, p. 4). The shift depicted in Figure 2.1 also shows that as socioeconomic conditions change the hazards also change from being local to being global. Heavy particulate matter air pollution, water pollution, and household waste have a more localised effect, where people share the same water source and the same air which may be polluted by factories and indiscriminate and mismanaged disposal and at times burning of garbage.

As society moves up in per capita gross national product reaching middle-income levels, the causes for environmental degradation also shift to CFC-based pollution, fine particulate matter air pollution, and heavy-metal contamination in water sources, soil, and even air. These effects manifest at larger scales like

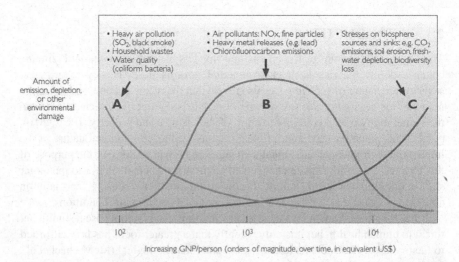

FIGURE 2.1 Change in environmental profile with changing per capita gross national product (GNP) (McMichael et al., 2003).

nations and continental and sub-continental regions. At higher levels of income, the other causes of environmental change give way to GHG-based stresses on our biosphere which result in an increase in global temperature, depletion in habitat and resources, and unpredictability of extreme weather events. These effects are at the largest scales affecting the entire biosphere of the planet, both terrestrial and aquatic. McMichael mentions that these effects moved chronologically, with the local effects manifesting during industrialisation, regional effects taking hold during the period of economic boom when society experiences economic development, and global effects taking hold when society has achieved higher living standards with higher GHG emissions (McMichael et al., 2003). These effects can be seen to exist currently amongst various countries. A country like India may see all these three categories coexisting. Category A is visible in slums, industrial peri-urban regions, and poorer settlements. Category B can be seen in regions with higher levels of construction, driven mostly by increasing incomes and levels of consumption. Category C has a greater effect and has grown together with living conditions. Excessive use of fossil fuels and using materials with a high GHG emission footprint have contributed to the growth of category C. A big reason behind the growth of Category C, according to McMichael, is the shift away from conditions that caused environmental degradation under Categories A and B. This transition can be seen in countries which are currently in their developing stages. In countries with steady-state growth and developed socioeconomic indicators, which have moved away from Categories A and B, the impact of Category C is becoming more visible. This coexistence of multiple categories of climatic and environmental change has heterogeneous impacts across the globe, with stark differences between the effects of environmental change on low-income nations versus high-income nations (25% versus 17% of deaths related to environmental change respectively) (McMichael, Nyong, & Corvalan, 2008, p. 191).

These categories of change in climatic and environmental profiles are indicative of the health impacts that may be caused and the kinds of exposure and vulnerability those experiencing these changes will suffer. The essay at hand shall describe and discuss the manifestation of health impacts under two categories, namely, health impacts that have a short-term impact with severe outcomes, or acute health impacts; and long-term impacts where the health conditions degrade over longer periods of time. This may have moderate or severe outcomes, or chronic health impacts. Finally, this essay shall look at how climate and environmental change, the resulting health impacts, and the socioeconomic wellbeing of people interact and become an interconnected and complex situation.

2.2 SPECTRUM OF HEALTH IMPACTS OF A CHANGING ENVIRONMENT

When having a discussion on health impacts of a changing environment, it is important to understand why health is impacted because of the change in the first place. In Figure 2.1 the categories of environmental change represent the addition of such compounds to the overall biosphere; the excess or presence of such factors may have effects on human bodily functions or such environmental aspects that impact human health. Categories A, B, and C or any other form of environmental pollution, contamination, or change impact human health through the air breathed in, the water consumed, the soil in which food is grown and later consumed, or by changing the local or global environment making the habitat incapable of supporting life. These impacts can be as direct as breathing heavy or fine particulate matter or toxic gases, ingesting heavy metals, or being physically exposed to chemical compounds which directly impact bodily function, viz. radioactivity. These impacts can be indirect, for example rising temperature causing food shortage, facilitating breeding of diseases or disease-carrying vectors, or impacting habitat by desertification, floods, and other similar environmental adversities that may result in indirect health impacts due to change in living conditions.

Figure 2.2 shows an intricate interrelationship amongst various environmental and climatic hazards and how they come together to impact human health. It is this intricacy that requires concerted efforts to reduce health burdens, as every pathway depicted here and the variables from which they emerge affect and in return are affected by every other variable and pathways, hence making interventions ever so complex.

This section shall discuss the different health impacts that may occur because of a changing environment. To facilitate the discussion, this section shall be divided into two subtopics that discuss human health impacts by looking at the nature of

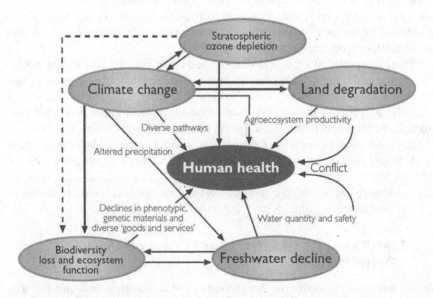

FIGURE 2.2 Interrelationships between major environmental and climate change with human health (McMichael et al., 2003).

exposure of the impact arising out of the change. As mentioned in Section 2.1, the health impacts shall be divided into acute and chronic as addressing the two requires different strategies towards research and development and policy making.

2.2.1 ACUTE HEALTH IMPACTS

Crombet and Lage define acute diseases as those where the initiation of the disease is sudden, the causes are limited, the symptoms are external and perceivable, and the disease lasts for a brief period as its clinical course is short, especially if the disease is responsive to medical interventions and therapies (Crombet & Lage, 2016, p. 105). Acute conditions are usually caused by microbial infections, but can also occur due to injury, change in ecosystem conditions, or misuse of drugs. The main characteristics of an acute health condition is a rapid onset, with distinct symptoms and a need for urgent care.

The acute health impacts of the changing environment can be further categorised. First are those caused by particulate, orgnanic, and inorganic contamination of the ecosystem (air, water, soil), for example the contamination of river and other local water sources with *Escherichia coli* due to dumping of untreated human and solid waste into such water bodies (Pandey et al., 2014), or contamination of air with heavy and fine particulate matter, or toxic gases like oxides of sulphur, nitrogen, and other such noxious gases which can cause severe respiratory ailments including bronchitis, other respiratory infections, and even congenital ailments when such pollutants enter the bloodstream of pregnant women (Kim, Chen, Zhou, & Huang, 2018, p. 89).

Second are those changing conditions that facilitate the spread of infection, for example, vector-borne diseases and other infectious diseases whose breeding and spread can be correlated to the change in climate and the environment. These diseases emerge as both a direct and an indirect effect of some aspect of the changing environment. These diseases are then transmitted through direct or indirect (mediated by a vector or vehicle) zoonoses (transmission from animals to humans) or direct or indirect anthroponoses (transmission from humans to humans which may follow zoonoses) (Patz et al., 2003, p. 106). Indirect anthroponoses like vector-borne diseases, especially those caused by mosquitoes, happen in regions which did not usually have mosquito infestation. Warmer regions in Europe, like Italy, have always seen the effects of mosquito-borne diseases, but rising global temperatures and subsequently increasing rainfall have created conditions suitable for mosquitoes to breed even in latitudes which are usually too cold for them (Semenza & Suk, 2018, p. 3). Diseases like dengue fever, Zika, and Chikungunya spread by mosquitoes of the genus *Aedes* have not grown in colder European countries; the warming of the climate has contributed to their spread. Even rarer forms of zoonotic disease threats are emerging due to environmental change, namely the occurrence of ancient anthrax which had lain dormant in dead animals burried under the permafrost in regions such as Siberia, Northern Canada, Alaska, and Greenland (Walsh, deSmalen, & Mor, 2018). The thawing of the permafrost, which as its name suggests should be permanently frozen, is revealing ancient dead animals which were preserved in the ice, but as these animal corpses have emerged, the threat of anthrax – a highly infectious disease – has increased. A recent outbreak in 2016 in the Yamal Peninsula of Siberia is attributed to climate change-led thawing of the permafrost (Timofeev et al., 2019).

There are also insights from a climate and environmental change perspective into the spread of SARS COV2 and COVID-19. SARS COV2 belongs to the Coronaviridae family of encased, positive-sense, single-strand viruses whose genome is made of ribonucleic acid (RNA). These viruses are identifiable under an electron microscope due to their peplomers or protein spikes that bind to specific receptors on the body cells of amphibians, birds, and mammals. Viruses from this family are known to cause the common cold, severe acute respiratory syndrome (SARS), Middle East respiratory syndrome (MERS), and now COVID-19, and there is a prevalent belief that COVID-19's spread may be aided by climate change (Harmooshi, Shirbandi, & Rahim, 2020). The mechanism of spread of SARS COV2 is understood but an understanding of environmental conditions is still not very clear. For example, one study has shown that when humidity changes from 30% to 50% the half-life of thhe virus increases from 27 hours to 67 hours, but at 80% humidity the half-life drops to merely 3 hours (Harmooshi, Shirbandi, & Rahim, 2020, p. 7). At different levels of humidity a change in temperature, for example a drop of 6°C at 80% humidity, may add 3 hours to the virus' half-life (Harmooshi, Shirbandi, & Rahim, 2020). An overall rise in temperature at the global level affecting periodic relative humidity levels may affect how the virus, and other similar viruses, may affect future generations. It has been observed that the pathogenicity of viruses like avian influenza virus or the H5N1 virus increases with warming of temperature as it affects the humidity and the risk of migratory birds catching the disease and zoonotic patterns change based on these factors (Morin et al., 2018, p. 245). In agricultural regions the transmission of H5N1 is rooted in changing enviromental and climatic patterns, as it affects how migratory birds which are carriers of this virus interact with other farm birds. With the ever-expanding need for food for an ever-expanding population, human–animal conflict is also increasing, and with increase in global temperatures the cultivation period of certain crops like paddy has also expanded, allowing migratory birds and free-range birds to interact more often, creating far more chances of zoonosis and ultimately anthroponosis (Morin et al., 2018).

Climate change is affecting the way pathogens are surviving in the atmosphere, how vectors are spreading to places where they had not been due to lack of temperature conducive for breeding, and by changing the exposure period to such pathogens. This is indicative of a change in hazard. On the other hand, particulate matter pollution of the air and the presence of toxic chemicals are affecting our bodies in ways that reduce immunity to withstand diseases by increasing the body's vulnerability to infection, such as impact of pollution on how the lungs are infected with respiratory diseases, especially in children who have a larger lung surface area (Kim, Chen, Zhou, & Huang, 2018, p. 76). These acute health impacts have a severe short-term effect on health conditions, increasing the periodic morbidity of the local population. Climate and environmental change provides more opportunities for conditions, such as acute infections and other diseases, to give a health shock to a large number of people, and with deterioration over time, these instances may only increase in frequency.

2.2.2 CHRONIC HEALTH IMPACTS

Chronic ailments and diseases are defined as those whose initiation is "insidious" (Crombet & Lage, 2016, p. 105). The causes of such diseases are at times internal and multiple with external factors enabling internal factors to flair up as a disease. Chronic conditions have a slower clinical course than acute diseases and the treatment process is more complex with no guarantee of restoration to the previous healthy state, with symptoms and effects lasting the lifetime of the patient (Crombet & Lage, 2016). The burgeoning health burden of chronic diseases is a recent phenomenon and it has a lot to do with changes in multiple interconnected factors. The health burden of acute diseases formed the greater share of disease-related mortality. Pathogens causing severe acute syndromes, like septicaemia, cholera, due to lack of antibiotics, or influenza, rabies, and other diseases due to lack of vaccines, were the more immediate cause of mortality (Crombet & Lage, 2016). As medical science grew and drugs like penicillin derived from fungus or the pox vaccine derived from cow pox became popular in combating public health problems, suddenly such diseases which were seen as ailments of the ageing or weak body came forth as real public health problems, like cancer, chronic obstructive pulmonary disease (COPD), cardiac diseases, pancreatic, renal, and hepatic diseases, neurological and psychological disorders, and others (Crombet & Lage, 2016, p. 106). With improvements in diagnosis, pathology, and the overall science of epidemiology it was further understood that these ailments, which developed in and stayed with the body for a long time, had a strong relationship with the environment and human behaviour.

Chronic diseases which are strongly connected with the changing environment may or may not have a causal relationship with the change in the environment and may have multiple pathways to affect human health. On one hand there are diseases which are directly caused by the influence of the environment, like particulate matter pollution causing COPD, or cancer due to exposure to ionising radiation, chemicals that cause build-up of free radicals in the body causing damage to deoxyribonucleic acid (DNA). On the other hand, there are diseases that come about due to how the changing environment puts stress on our body, whether through the availability of nutrition by impacting agriculture, through bodily stresses caused by migration when land is lost due to rising ocean levels, flash floods and landslides, or desertification, or psychological stress occurring due to the impending socioeconomic and physical danger of climate and environmental change (Mash, 2010). These physical dangers may extend anywhere from heat stroke and heat-related accidents due to climate change-led heat waves to the same heat wave causing droughts and famines and causing mass morbidity due to lack of nutrition (Kjellstrom, Butler, Lucas, & Bonita, 2010, p. 98).

Chronic diseases and climate change interact through three distinct pathways, namely through non-communicable diseases and ailments like heat stroke, cancer, and cardiovascular diseases; communicable diseases like tuberculosis (TB); and injuries like death due to drowning in flash floods, accidents during extreme weather events like cyclones, and other such factors. The impact of these interactions can be further divided into direct and indirect, with physical effects being direct and psychosocial effects being indirect, for example increase in farmer suicides due to substantive crop losses after adverse weather events (Kjellstrom, Butler, Lucas, & Bonita, 2010).

Climate and environmental change have very distinct and well-studied effects on the human body via the non-communicable pathway. Diseases like COPD, autoimmune disorders like asthma and type 1 diabetes, and cancer have been directly linked to how climatic and environmental factors affect our health in the long term. The presence of particulate matter has long been linked with respiratory diseases; for example, due to increases in annual average temperatures the presence of pollen in the air is prolonged, triggering an autoimmune response where the body's own immune system attacks the body itself (Verbanas, 2020). Particulate matter pollution also makes the lungs vulnerable to multiple diseases like chronic bronchitis due to damage to the lung tissue (Kim, Chen, Zhou, & Huang, 2018). Type 1 diabetes has also been linked to reduced temperatures and a low-sunlight environment (low levels of vitamin D), especially in an oceanic climate (Chen et al., 2017). Type 1 diabetes is most prevalent amongst adolescent children. Besides these, the changing environment has caused a significant rise in incidence of cancer, through heavy metal and radioactive contamination of soil, air, and water sources (McMichael et al., 2003). Another source of carcinogenic effects of environmental change is ultraviolet radiation-led cancer of the skin, eye, and other body parts, due to the depletion of stratospheric ozone caused by chlorofluorocarbon emissions (McMichael, Lucas, Ponsonby, & Edwards, 2003, p. 173).

Under the communicable pathway chronic diseases like TB have been observed to have a strong interrelation with climate change. Studies have revealed that temperature, humidity, and rainfall are factors that affect TB the most, with low temperature and low relative humidity and low levels of average rainfall contributing to the highest levels of TB, indicating highest incidences during late spring and early summer (Kuddus, McBryde, & Adegboye, 2019). With climate change affecting seasonal patterns, extending the spring season across the globe, the burden of TB has also been affected, with examples from Bangladesh and China (Kuddus, McBryde, & Adegboye, 2019, p. 6). This debilitating disease is also highly contagious and communicable, being one of the longest-running pandemics in the world, affecting poorer population centres disproportionately.

Lastly, for climate and environmental changes that cause injuries, the most siginificant reasons in recent times have been flash floods and subsequent landslides, droughts, and wild fires (Wehner, Arnold, Knutson, Kunkel, & LeGrande, 2017).

Extreme precipitation due to changes in seasonal patterns causing flash floods, extreme storms due to more extreme temperature gradients between land and water, and rapid glacial thawing due to rising global temperatures causing rivers to overflow are responsible for severe loss of life and may cause severe injuries. These changes are a direct result of changes in climate and how that affects the delicate water cycle. In addition, human-led environmental change, like deforestation, destroying flood plains, and other such activities may cause landslides during flash floods (Wehner, Arnold, Knutson, Kunkel, & LeGrande, 2017, p. 240). Besides floods, climate change may also contribute to droughts and desertification. Droughts can be caused by lack of water in three different ways, namely: (1) meteorologial drought, or lack of precipitation; (2) agricultural drought, or lack of soil water; and (3) hydrological drought, or lack of runoff water source. These may be directly cause loss of rain and drying of water supply due to extreme temperatures, changes in wind patterns, and ocean currents, which ultimately change precipitation patterns creating dry spells which may even cause wild fires, as seen in California, in the United States, and in Australia, causing severe loss of animal and human life (Wehner, Arnold, Knutson, Kunkel, & LeGrande, 2017).

The discussion on chronic diseases enabled by climate and environmental change demonstrates the pervasive nature of environmental and climatic degradation and the interconnectivity of various factors causing long-term, severe, and at times irreparable damage. Furthermore, the insidious nature of chronic human health and wellbeing-related problems makes it difficult to pinpoint the exact pathway of the effect of environmental change, further complicating mitigating strategies. The toll of climate change-related chronic health impact on human wellbeing is very high, difficult to predict, and much more difficult to prevent as compared to acute diseases which may have equally severe and at times larger scope of effect.

2.3 SOCIOECONOMIC EFFECTS OF CLIMATE AND ENVIRONMENTAL CHANGE-INDUCED HEALTH IMPACTS

The health and physical impacts of climate and environmental change may force populations, especially impoverished ones, to undertake migration to escape the health and physical impacts. This migration itself may have a distinct biological effect on the human body due to extreme stress. This impact is yet to be understood but in psychosocial stress the body releases stress-related hormones and other proteins which may damage or shorten telomeres present at the ends of chromosomes. The length of the telomeres represents the biological age of the body at the cellular level (Savolainen, 2016). Shortening of telomeres during such migrations may affect the average age of the individual, as has been observed with the stress migration of the Saharia tribe in Central India (Zahran et al., 2015). These stress-causing situations demonstrate drastic shortening of the telomeres, making the body seem to age at a cellular level and creating the threat of multiple complications like chronic illnesses amongst children, Alzheimer disease amongst the older population, and possible threat of cancer and cardiovascular diseases later in life (Shammas, 2011, p. 30).

These kinds of "bio-psychosocial" stresses can be witnessed across the world, especially in the context of changing environment, like mass exoduses after droughts, floods, wild fires, and as witnessed recently, exodus of migrant labourers during a pandemic. The phenotype (physical properties of organisms) effects and peculiarities due to these bio-psychosocial stress on the genotype (genetic makeup of organisms) can be seen across the poorer regions of the world, especially in a country like India, stemming from multiple reasons (Majumdar & Basu, 2015). These bio-psychosocial stresses lead to health shocks, loss of habitat and livelihoods, and destruction of essential infrastructure and social networks, which ultimately affect the socioeconomic status of already vulnerable populations across regions most susceptible to such climatic and environmental changes. A well-documented socioeconomic impact of the changing environment is poverty, social oppression, and gender atrocities. Within the social makeup of developing societies in socially vulnerable regions (especially those with lower levels of literacy and higher levels of poverty, like in India) women are made responsible for collecting firewood, herbs, or flowers of economic value, and most importantly water (Government of India, 2014). With environmental degradation these resources become scarce, affecting the livelihoods of households that depend on such resources, forcing women to travel farther out to find these resources, affecting their health and their opportunity to earn a better living or get educated (Lal, 2016).

The exposure caused by climate and environmental change affecting macro-economic and socioeconomic aspects is mediated through human systems and the impact could be severe with greater pollution of air, water, and soil, rising temperatures, and irregular precipitation affecting food production and cost across equatorial and tropical regions in the world where highly populous habitats exist (Watts et al., 2015). This affects food inflation in the region, forces migration which affects economic growth and restorative efforts towards environmental adversity, and ultimately renders the human capital incapable of coping with the changes due to lack of nutrition and ability to work, further slipping into poverty and intergenerational disparity (Watts et al., 2015, p. 8). This forms a vicious cycle where the public policy formulation to tackle the immediate problems of environmental change, of low productivity, low income and consumption levels, and overall stagnation of local economies has to undertake the same actions to pick up economic growth that caused the problems in the first place, like improving income and consumption, like industrial activities, clearing of land for expansion of agriculture, cheaper solutions to waste management, and engaging in high-carbon-emission activities to improve economic output (Watts et al., 2015, p. 13).

The understanding here is that environmental and climatic degradation affects those specific aspects of the biosphere that interact with our bodies in a way that impacts our quality of life, ability to maintain a healthy and functioning body, and to have a functioning society that is not beset with such debilitating health problems. These societal level problems ultimately affect how the economic and social systems function, and how any disruption to these systems will resonate across generations. This becomes a problem when larger and larger numbers of people are affected by the changing environment and climate, under the pretext that the activities that are changing the environment would bring socioeconomic prosperity, which is not true.

2.4 CONCLUSION

This essay provides an overview of the array of health impacts that are caused by a change in the environment away from a range that is conducive for optimal functioning of life, the balance of the ecosystem, and interconnected aspects of human society. What the essay attempts to achieve is to provide a simplified understanding of how the changing environment impacts human health and the adverse effects of changing health on the broader aspects of social and economic dynamics.

This essay began by describing the profile of various forms of environmental change, the causes and societal chronology of environmental degradations, and how different human groups interact with these changes and degradation of the environment and the climate. The essay further explains how health is impacted in both an acute and chronic manner where the effects of various forms of communicable and non-communicable diseases are enhanced and enabled because of these changes and injuries become more common and devastating because of the degrading ecosystem. The essay goes further to briefly explain how human socioeconomic systems are also intricately connected with how human health is impacted by the environment and how a change for the worst further entrenches the problems that socioeconomic systems and institutions face. The requirement for robust policy making is apparent within this section as only preventive, restorative, and adaptive policy making can ensure that society, from the global to the household level, can prevent health-based injury and socioeconomic misery. Only robust institutions, public and private expenditure, and widespread awareness could shield human health and society from the adverse impacts of a changing environment.

REFERENCES

Chen, Yin-ling, Yong-cheng Huang, Yong-chao Qiao, Wei Ling, Yan-hong Pan, Li-jun Geng, Jian-long Xiao, Xiao-Xi Zhang, and Hai-lu Zhao. 2017. "Climates on incidence of childhood type 1 diabetes mellitus in 72 countries." *Nature* 7: 1–17.
Crombet, Tania, and Agustin Lage. 2016. "Immunotherapy for transforming advanced cancer into a chronic disease: How far are we?" In *Immune Rebalancing: The Future of Immunosuppression*, edited by Diana Boraschi and Giselle Penton-Rol, 105–120. Havana: Academic Press.
Government of India. 2014. *Drinking Water, Sanitation, Hygiene and Housing Condition in India 2012*. New Delhi: Ministry of Statistics and Programme Implementation, Government of India.

Harmooshi, Narges Nazari, Kiarash Shirbandi, and Fakher Rahim. 2020. *Environmental Concern Regarding the Effect of Humidity and Temperature on SARS-COV-2 (COVID-19) Survival: Fact or Fiction.* Ahvaz: Ahvaz Jundishapur University of Medical Sciences.

IPCC. 2014. *Climate Change 2014: Synthesis Report.* Geneva: IPCC.

Kim, Dasom, Zi Chen, Lin-Fu Zhou, and Shou-Xiong Huang. 2018. "Air pollutants and early origins of respiratory diseases." *Chronic Diseases and Translational Medicine* 4: 75–94.

Kjellstrom, Tord, Ainslie J. Butler, Robyn M. Lucas, and Ruth Bonita. 2010. "Public health impact of global heating due to climate change: potential effects on chronic non-communicable diseases." *International Journal of Public Health* 55: 97–103.

Kuddus, Md Abdul, Emma S. McBryde, and Oyelola A. Adegboye. 2019. "Delay effect and burden of weather-related tuberculosis cases in Rajshahi province, Bangladesh, 2007–2012." *Nature* 9: 1–13.

Lal, N. 2016. *Indian Women Worst Hit by Water Crisis.* May 3. www.ipsnews.net/2015/07/poor-bearthe-.

Majumdar, P. P., and A. Basu. 2015. *A Genomic View of the Peopling and Population Structure of India.* Kalyani: National Institute of Biomedical Genomics/Cold Spring Harbor Laboratory Press.

Mash, Robert. 2010. "Chronic diseases, climate change and complexity: the hidden connections." *South African Family Practice* 52(5): 438–445.

McMichael, A. J., A. Nyong, and C. Corvalan. 2008. "Global environmental change and health: impacts, inequalities, and the health sector." *British Medical Journal* 336: 191–194.

McMichael, A. J., D. H. Campbell-Lendrum, C. F. Corvalán, K. L. Ebi, A. K. Githeko, J. D. Scheraga, and A. Woodward. 2003. *Climate Change and Human Health: Risks and Responses.* Geneva: World Health Organization.

McMichael, A. J., R. Lucas, A. L. Ponsonby, and S. J. Edwards. 2003. "Stratospheric ozone depletion, ultraviolet radiation and health." In *Climate Change and Human Health: Risks and Responses*, edited by A. J. McMichael, D. H. Campbell-Lendrum, C. F. Corvalán, K. L. Ebi, A. K. Githeko, J. D. Scheraga and A. Woodward, 159–180. Geneva: World Health Organization.

Morin, Cory W., Benjamin Stoner-Duncan, Kevin Winker, Matthew Scotch, John S. Meschke, Kristie L. Ebi, and Peter M. Rabinowitz. 2018. "Avian influenza virus ecology and evolution through a climatic lens." *Environment Internation* 119: 241–249.

Pandey, Pramod K., Philip H. Hass, Michelle L. Soupir, Sagor Biswas, and Vijay P. Singh. 2014. "Contamination of water resources by pathogenic bacteria." *AMB Express* 51(4): 1–16.

Patz, J. A., A. K. Githeko, J. P. McCarty, S. Hussein, U. Confalonieri, and N. de Wet. 2003. "Climate change and infectious diseases." In *Climate Change and Human Health: Risks and Responses*, edited by A. J. McMichael, D. H. Campbell-Lendrum, C. F. Corvalán, Kristine L. Ebi, A. K. Githeko, J. D. Scheraga and A. Woodward, 103–132. Geneva: World Health Organization.

Savolainen, K. 2016. *Stress and Cellular Aging – Associations Between Stress-Related Factors and Leukocyte Telomere Length.* Helsinki: Institute of Behavioral Sciences, University of Helsinki.

Semenza, Jan C., and Jonathan E. Suk. 2018. "Vector-borne diseases and climate change: a European perspective." *Federation of European Microbiological Societies* 365: 1–9.

Shammas, M. A. 2011. "Telomeres, lifestyle, cancer, and aging." *Current Opinion in Clinical Nutrition and Metabolism Care* 14(1): 28–34.

Timofeev, Vitalii, Irina Bahtejeva, Raisa Mironova, Galina Titareva, Igor Lev, David Christiani, Alexander Borzilov, Alexander Bogun, and Gilles Vergnaud. 2019. "Insights from *Bacillus anthracis* strains isolated from permafrost in the tundra zone of Russia." *PLoS One* e0209140.

Verbanas, Patti. 2020. *The Changes in the Environment and Biodiversity Brought on by Climate Change could be Responsible for Increases in Allergies, Autoimmune Diseases and Autism, According to a Rutgers Researcher.* August 5. Accessed October 29, 2020. www.rutgers.edu/news/how-climate-change-affects-allergies-immune-response-and-autism#:~:text=Climate%20change%20has%20worsened%20respiratory,the%20prevalence%20of%20immune%20diseases.

Walsh, Michael G., Allard W. deSmalen, and Siobhan M. Mor. 2018. Climatic influence on anthrax suitability in warming northern latitudes. *Nature* 8: 1–9.

Watts, Nick, D. Campbell-Lendrum, Marina Maiero, Lucia Fernandez Montoya, and Kelly Lao. 2015. *Strengthening Health Resilience to Climate Change.* Geneva: World Health Organization.

Wehner, M. F., J. R. Arnold, T. Knutson, K. E. Kunkel, and A. N. LeGrande. 2017. "Droughts, floods, and wildfire." In *Climate Science Special Report: Fourth National Climate Assessment*, edited by D. J. Wuebbles, D. H. Fahey, K. A. Hibbard, D. J. Dokken, B. C. Stewart and T. K. Maycock, 231–256. Washington D.C.: U.S. Global Change Research Program.

Zahran, S., J. G. Snodgrass, D. G. Maranon, C. Upadhyay, D. A. Granger, and S. M. Bailey. 2015. "Stress and telomere shortening among central Indian conservation refugees." *Proceedings of the National Academy of Sciences of the United States of America* E928–E936.

Unit II

Impact of Increasing Environmental Pollution on Human Health

3 Airborne *Staphylococcus aureus* and its Impact on Human Health
A Review in an Indian Context

Madhuri Singh*, Maneet Kumar Chakrawarti, Himani Kumari, Sonali Rajput and Kasturi Mukhopadhyay*

CONTENTS

* Corresponding authors: Madhuri Singh. chauhan.madhuri@gmail.com, Kasturi Mukhopadhyay. kastuim@mail.jnu.ac.in

DOI: 10.1201/9781003095422-3

3.1 INTRODUCTION

Staphylococcus aureus (*S. aureus*) is an opportunistic pathogen, which persistently colonizes the nares of 20% of the human population, while the rest of the population carries it intermittently throughout their lifetime (Van Kampen, Hoffmeyer et al. 2016). Persistent carriers of *S. aureus* are the potential source of spreading infections, particularly in hospitals. Therefore it is frequently isolated from the hospital environment, including air (Naruka, Gaur et al. 2014) and frequently touched surfaces (Price, Cole et al. 2017; Dancer, Adams et al. 2019). *S. aureus* infections are associated with high mortality and morbidity, particularly in patients with weaker immunity such as children, those in old age, having open wounds, or suffering from immunity disorders and cancer. Approximately 50% of *S. aureus* isolates from hospitals (Kang, Jung et al. 2016; Latha, Anil et al. 2019) as well as non-hospital environments are identified as methicillin-resistant *S. aureus* (MRSA) (David and Daum 2010; Lin, Lin et al. 2016; Lee, de Lencastre et al. 2018).

S. aureus strains developed resistance to penicillin G soon after its introduction in the 1940s by acquiring ß-lactamase plasmids harboring *blaZ* gene, which could neutralize the ß-lactam ring of penicillin (Hiramatsu, Katayama et al. 2014a). In 1959, methicillin was introduced to kill ß-lactamase/penicillinase-containing *S. aureus* strains. Soon after introduction, in 1961, the first clinical isolate of MRSA was reported from a hospital in UK, and by the 1990s it had disseminated in community settings (Jevons 1961). MRSA was derived from methicillin-sensitive *S. aureus* (MSSA) after acquiring *mecA* gene by horizontal gene transfer mediated by a mobile genetic element, staphylococcal cassette chromosome (SCC) (Ito, Katayama et al. 1999). The SCC element carries a *mecA* gene encoding for an altered cell wall-synthesizing enzyme called penicillin-binding protein 2a (PBP2a), and a *ccr* gene complex for the mobility of the entire *SCCmec* element. The *SCCmec* element is highly diverse and has been classified into several types based on the different combination of *mec* and *ccr* gene complexes and J region (Hiramatsu, Ito et al. 2013). So far, four homologues of *mec* gene have been identified among methicillin-resistant staphylococci (MRS); these are *mecA*, *mecB*, *mecC*, and *mecD* (Lakhundi and Zhang 2018). To date, the *SCCmec* elements have been classified into 13 different types (Lakhundi and Zhang 2018). *SCCmec* typing is highly prevalent all over the world for MRSA molecular typing and epidemiological and evolution studies (Zhang, McClure et al. 2012).

Most alarmingly, MRSA strains have rapidly acquired resistance to multiple agents from different groups, including vancomycin and other new antimicrobial agents against MRSA (Hiramatsu, Cui et al. 2001; Hiramatsu, Katayama et al. 2014b; Watkins, Holubar et al. 2019). Such multidrug-resistant *S. aureus* (MDR-SA) are invincible as regards existing antibiotics and the new antimicrobial approaches are the need of the hour (Hiramatsu, Katayama et al. 2014a; Shariati, Dadashi et al. 2020). Although MRSA treatment is decided by clinical indication, currently MRSA strains are treated with vancomycin, clindamycin, daptomycin, linezolid, tedizolid, dalvabancin, tigecycline, etc. (Turner, Sharma-Kuinkel et al. 2019). Among many novel antimicrobials that are in the pipeline to tackle rising antimicrobial resistance (AMR) in MRSA, the development of host-defense peptides as anti-MRSA agents is very promising (Hancock and Sahl 2006). Our lab has been engaged in the development of alpha-melanocyte-stimulating hormone (alpha-MSH) against MRSA for over a decade and we have successfully confirmed the anti-MRSA activity of alpha-MSH mainly through membrane pore formation (Madhuri, Tahsina et al. 2009; Singh and Mukhopadhyay 2011, 2014; Singh, Mumtaz et al. 2020).

Apart from the increasing AMR in MRSA the other physiological and epidemiological properties remain the same between MSSA and MRSA, therefore, all the research regarding the *S. aureus* transmission cycle between infection and health workers and the environment is also relevant to MRSA (Dancer 2008).

S. aureus and MRSA are majorly responsible for nosocomial infections such as hospital-acquired pneumonia (HAP), bacteremia, surgical site infections, and skin and soft-tissue infections (SSTIs) (Latha, Anil et al. 2019; Lounsbury, Reeber et al. 2019; Turner, Sharma-Kuinkel et al. 2019). The microbiological composition of air in an indoor setting plays a significant role in the spread of infectious diseases. Airborne particles originating from humans, animals, or plants that contain microorganisms or their byproducts are called bioaerosols. These bioaerosols play a major role in the spread of human pathogens, including bacteria, virus, and fungi, thereby causing serious health effects, from infectious diseases to respiratory problems (Kim, Kabir et al. 2018). According to recent reports, *S. aureus* has been identified as a predominating bacterium in airborne microbiomes collected from both hospital and other indoor environments (Nandalal and Somashekar 2007; Kumar and Goel 2016; Kozajda, Jeżak et al. 2019).

With increasing reports of health problems arising from exposure to *S. aureus* bioaerosols in both hospital and other settings, it is evident that not only direct contact by droplet infection but also the air play an important role in the transmission of *S. aureus* infections from a carrier to a susceptible host (Bos, Verstappen et al. 2016). Perhaps due to its thicker cell wall, *S. aureus* can survive in a dry environment for months (Dancer 2008), and can infect susceptible people not only in the immediate vicinity but also at distant sites through bioaerosols which can travel far due to their light weight (Lin, Lin et al. 2016). Since a third of the total population is always colonized with *S. aureus*, the possibility of aerosol transmission of *S. aureus* is greater in confined and crowded indoor environments.

The prevalence of both MSSA and MRSA has been identified in bioaerosols from various indoor and outdoor environmental settings, including hospitals and schools, libraries, residential buildings, public transport, metro stations, livestock farms, and so forth (Stepanović, Ćirković et al. 2008; Masclaux, Sakwinska et al. 2013; Moon, Huh et al. 2014; Solomon, Wadilo et al. 2017; Siddiqui and Whitten 2018; Kozajda, Jeżak et al. 2019). The airborne prevalence of MRSA in developing countries like India with a highly dense population, poor hygiene, and easy availability of antibiotics is expected to grow even higher. Very recently we have reported the occurrence of MRSA resistant to other conventional antibiotics in the indoor bioaerosols of Central Laboratory Animal Resources (CLAR) of Jawaharlal Nehru University, New Delhi, India (Kumari, Chakraborti et al. 2020). A strong correlation has been reported by other authors between airborne *S. aureus* strains and those isolated from infected patients in the same environmental setting (Boyce,

Potter-Bynoe et al. 1997; Sexton, Clarke et al. 2006; Gehanno, Louvel et al. 2009). However, the dynamics of airborne *S. aureus* transmission and its role in spreading infection to the vulnerable population is underestimated.

In this chapter, we will discuss the prevalence of MSSA and MRSA in the air collected from different settings in India only. Next, we will discuss in detail the various air sample collection methods, including passive and active techniques. Further, various metagenomic analyses to discriminate *S. aureus* from bioaerosol microbiome will be described. We will give an overview of the different possible transmission routes of *S. aureus* and its permissible exposure inocula in different environmental settings. Furthermore, the effect of environmental factors such as relative humidity (RH), temperature, aerodynamics of particles, seasons, and air change rate on *S. aureus* viability in the air will be discussed. Finally, different decontamination guidelines and strategies that are being followed in hospitals and general environments to tackle airborne MRSA will be outlined. We will conclude this chapter by providing our propositions regarding the containment of airborne MRSA infections in different settings.

3.2 PREVALENCE OF *S. AUREUS* AND MRSA IN THE INDOOR AIR OF INDIAN HOSPITALS

Air pollution has become a pressing global issue in the entire world. Biological aerosols (bioaerosols) are one of the important air pollutants. The dispersed phase of this colloidal system consists of microbes (bacteria, viruses, and their metabolites), plant pollen, plant debris, toxins, and suspended particles in air as small droplets (Mirhoseini, Nikaeen et al. 2016). These microbe-loaded aerosols are an important factor for the dispersal of contaminated air across different types of ecosystems. Bioaerosol-sensitive environments include walls, tables, and ceilings of indoor surfaces, animal and bird housing, composting and landfill sites, saw mills, hospitals, wastewater treatment plants, and manufacturing plants (Frankel, Bekö et al. 2012; Mentese, Rad et al. 2012).

Staphylococcus genus is one of the dominant genera among the bioaerosol flora. Here special attention has been given to genus *Staphylococcus* since the *S. aureus* species of this genus is most pathogenic and is frequently prevalent in the hospital indoor air and poses a great exposure risk to inpatients and medical staff (Faridi, Hassanvand et al. 2015; Mirhoseini, Nikaeen et al. 2016). Hospitals have complex environments which require proper ventilation for the convenience of patients and control of harmful emissions (Chuaybamroong, Choomseer et al. 2008). As per Centers for Disease Control (CDC), hospital environments are the main source of the spread of *S. aureus* (Centers for Disease Control and Prevention 2019). However, there are comparatively few Indian studies that demonstrate the prevalence of airborne *S. aureus* in hospital settings. Nandalal and Somashekar studied the predominance of *S. aureus* for two years in the indoor air of district hospital, Mandya, Bangalore. The highest load of *S. aureus* obtained was 95 CFU/m^3 in the pediatric ward. While this bacterial load in other parts of the hospital varied from 13 CFU/m^3 to 75 CFU/m^3. The samples collected from the outdoor environment did not contain any strains of *S. aureus*. Since no *S. aureus* was isolated from the outside environment, contamination might be due to the presence of crowd in the indoors of the hospital (Nandalal and Somashekar 2007). Tambekar et al. conducted an aerobiological study to analyze indoor and outdoor environments at 76 hospitals in Amravati, India. Of the total 670 air samples collected from indoor and outdoor environments of hospitals, *S. aureus* (29.59%) was the most dominant bacteria (Tambekar, Gulhane et al. 2007). Likewise, a very preliminary work reported 11.6% (34/292) *S. aureus* load in a tertiary care hospital, New Delhi. Out of a total of 34 *S. aureus* isolates, 18 were found to be MRSA. All these 18 MRSA also showed resistance to tetracycline, ciprofloxacin, and gentamicin. This study indicates the common prevalence of airborne MDR-SA strains in the critical premises of the tertiary care hospital (Tyagi and Mukhopadhyay 2012).

In a similar study by Taghizadeh et al., the largest proportion of isolated bacteria in Jehangir hospital, Pune, was of *S. aureus* (125 CFU/m^3), followed by *Micrococcus luteus* (*M. luteus*) (104 CFU/m^3) and coagulase-negative staphylococci (CNS) (106 CFU/m^3). In another hospital named Ruby Hall, again the most dominant bacteria in the hospital was *S. aureus* (90 CFU/m^3), followed by *M. luteus* (58 CFU/m^3) and CNS (78 CFU/m^3) (Taghizadeh, Delbari et al. 2014).

Kotgire et al. have reported a higher concentration of Gram-positive bacteria (GPB) than Gram-negative bacteria (GNB) in the air collected over three months from a tertiary care hospital in Jalna, Maharashtra. Among GPB, *S. aureus* was isolated from almost all the wards except for the medicine (male) ward (Kotgire, Akhtar et al. 2020). Similar findings were observed by Sudharsanam et al.; they also documented a higher concentration of GPB than GNB with the predominance of *S. aureus* in hospital settings (Sudharsanam, Srikanth et al. 2009). *S. aureus* was also found in all the wards of a tertiary care hospital in Jodhpur, Western Rajasthan, and its concentration ranged from 15% to 32% of total samples and these isolates also showed an MDR pattern. Notably, on the surgical ward, 100% *S. aureus* was found to be resistant to amoxyclav, ampicillin, and vancomycin (Rathore, Khatri et al. 2015). The prevalence of *S. aureus* was shown in the aeromicroflora of Kalyani hospital, West Bengal. The highest *S. aureus* concentration was found in the general and female ward while it was lowest in the operation theatre (Paul, Biswas et al. 2015). Other studies from tertiary care hospitals in Kolhapur (Chougale and Kumar 2019), Jaipur (Sabharwal and Sharma 2015), and three different hospitals in South Chennai (Sudharsanam, Srikanth et al. 2008) also reported the *S. aureus* prevalence in hospital bioaerosols.

3.3 PREVALENCE OF AIRBORNE *S. AUREUS* IN NON-HOSPITAL ENVIRONMENTS OF INDIA

Apart from hospitals, the predominance of airborne *S. aureus* in other general environments has been reported from all over India. A recent study was carried out in Agra (city of Taj), where the authors found the prevalence of *S. aureus* in the densely populated urban area including residential as well as office buildings

(Raghav, Shrivastava et al. 2020). We recently reported the prevalence of staphylococci spp. belonging to eight different species, including *S. aureus* in the indoor air of the Library and Animal house of Jawaharlal Nehru University in New Delhi (Kumari, Chakraborti et al. 2020). Yadav et al. have isolated *S. aureus* from air samples collected during the trade fair of Gwalior, India. Bacterial concentration was higher during a fair period compared to non-fair period. The authors obtained a total of 52 isolates which were resistant to oxacillin. Among these 52 isolates, eight strains (15%) were found to be positive for *mecA* gene and were called as MRS. However, only one isolate was confirmed as MRSA due to the presence of clfA (clumping factor A) (Yadav, Kumar et al. 2015). Public toilet rooms are heavily used and normally do not maintain proper hygiene, thus making them a major site for microbial growth and contamination. A study also identified isolates of *S. aureus* from the indoor air of a public toilet at Triplicane, Chennai (Anjum, Sivakumari et al. 2018). Further, the occurrence of *S. aureus* was confirmed in a dairy plant and slaughter house of Madras Veterinary College, Chennai (Vinayananda, Deepak et al. 2018).

Apart from crowded and heavily visited places, residential buildings are also equally contaminated with airborne *S. aureus*. In India, limited studies have been done on the prevalence of *S. aureus* in bioaerosols from residential buildings. A total of 14 residential houses were selected for indoor and outdoor bacterial aerosol sampling from Gwalior, Madhya Pradesh. The total staphylococcal concentration obtained in indoor and outdoor air was 5.9% and 4.6% of the total bacterial load, respectively. Among MRSs, 9.5% of the strains were isolated as *S. aureus* (Kumar and Goel 2016). *S. aureus* was the most commonly identified bacteria among the aeromicroflora of urban and rural houses of Pune, as reported by Roy et al. (Roy, Jan et al. 2020). However, in India very few studies have been done to determine the MDR pattern of airborne *S. aureus*, and this needs to be further explored.

3.4 TRANSMISSION OF *S. AUREUS* THROUGH AIR

Very shockingly, according to a recent study conducted in Japan, the nasal carriage rate of *S. aureus* was found to be as high as 90% in healthy adults. Of them, 69% had viable *S. aureus* (Lu, Sasaki et al. 2018). Furthermore, aerosolized *S. aureus* can endure harsh environmental conditions and remain alive for months to years in dry weather (Gehanno, Louvel et al. 2009; Moon, Huh et al. 2014; Kozajda, Jeżak et al. 2019). In this scenario, the role of air in spreading *S. aureus* from an infected person to a susceptible person is plausible. Most studies regarding the transmission of MRSA/MSSA through air have been restricted to hospitals (Boyce, Potter-Bynoe et al. 1997; Gehanno, Louvel et al. 2009; Creamer, Shore et al. 2014), livestock farms (Masclaux, Sakwinska et al. 2013; Bos, Verstappen et al. 2016), and poultry (Lin, Lin et al. 2016), where they have shown significant exposure risks to health workers and farm workers due to aerial dispersal of MRSA from infected patients and livestock, respectively.

Airborne transmission of pathogens is a matter of concern in indoor environments where people spend most of their time. Generally, aerial contamination of *S. aureus* anywhere indoors is attributed to the infected or colonized people present there, and the aerial burden of *S. aureus* keeps rising over time, particularly in settings with poor ventilation. A schematic presentation of various *S. aureus* transmission routes is shown in Figure 3.1; a person infected or colonized with *S. aureus* can discharge it in the surrounding environment as small-size (≤10 μM) contaminated aerosols or droplets produced during sneezing (Bischoff, Wallis et al. 2006), while comparatively large size (≥20 μM) bioaerosols are transmitted through shedding squamous skin (Ijaz, Zargar et al. 2016). Particle size distribution of MSSA/MRSA ranges from 2.1 μM to particle agglomerates (Li, Qi et al. 2011; Madsen, Kurdi et al. 2018; Kumari, Chakraborti et al. 2020), indicating that airborne *S. aureus* with particle size ≤10 μM can be inhaled by susceptible inpatients (Tellier, Li et al. 2019).

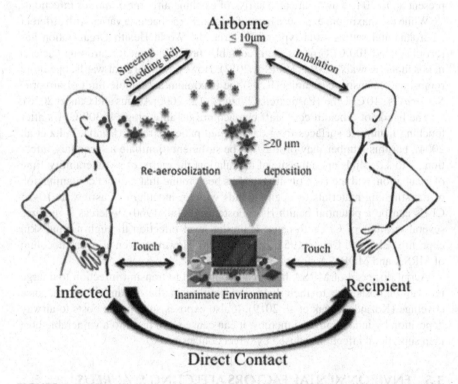

FIGURE 3.1 Transmission cycle of S. *aureus* including MRSA: Infected or colonized person discharges S. *aureus* containing aerosols or droplets of different sizes through sneezing or by shedding skin squamous. The droplets with diameter ≤10 μM becomes airborne and later can be inhaled by the recipient. Simultaneously, the air particles with diameter ≥20 μM containing S. *aureus*, especially those shedding from the skin are deposited on the environments surfaces, which become the secondary vehicle of S. *aureus*, disseminating it to the recipient through direct touching or through inhalation when they get re-aerosolized by various indoor activities. The particles with 10-20 μM diameter may either turned into airborne or deposited, depending upon the air turbulence. Alternatively, a direct or indirect (by touching the common surfaces) contact between infected and recipient may also spread the S. *aureus* infections.

Subsequently, the proportions of inhalable *S. aureus* can be deposited at various stages of the airways in decreasing order as we move from upper to lower respiratory tract (Hussain, Madl et al. 2011; Madsen, Kurdi et al. 2018). However, larger dust particles carrying *S. aureus* may settle on environmental surfaces in the vicinity of infected patients, and these may become the secondary vehicle of transmission through direct touching by recipients. Alternatively, this contaminated dust that has settled on inanimate surfaces can be re-aerosolized through various activities such as sweeping, flushing, and bed making, thereby leading to secondary dissemination (Creamer, Shore et al. 2014). A sneeze and cough can throw contaminated droplets up to 20 feet (Bischoff, Wallis et al. 2006), thus it is not only recipients who present in the immediate vicinity of an infected person are at risk of exposure, but those present up to 20 feet away are also at risk of catching airborne *S. aureus* infections.

While the maximum exposure limit of total airborne bacteria varies with different environmental settings and type of bacteria, the World Health Organization has recommended 100 CFU/m^3 as the acceptable threshold limit for airborne bacteria in hospitals (Kowalski 2011; US EPA 2013). However, in surgical wards, operating rooms, and intensive care units (ICUs) the maximum acceptable limit of airborne *S. aureus* is ≤10 CFU/m^3 (Pasquarella, Pitzurra et al. 2000; Adams and Dancer 2020).

The hands of a health care staff can acquire on an average 1–300 CFUs after touching inanimate surfaces from the infected patient's room (Bhalla, Pultz et al. 2004), but this number may or may not be sufficient to initiate a secondary infection, as this depends upon the site of inoculation, the recipient's vulnerability, time of incubation, and the type of strain. It has been found that a direct contamination of the stitching materials or open wounds with an inoculum of as few as 10–15 CFUs can be a potential health risk (Foster and Hutt 1960), whereas it requires several millions of CFUs to cause a similar level infection through normal skin exposure (Elek and Conen 1957; Dancer 2008). However, even a lesser inoculum of MRSA and MDR-SA strains can be lethal in the above cases.

Aerial dispersal of MRSA has greater potential to transmit infection to a large number of hosts due to their long survivability in the air and larger distance coverage (Kozajda, Jeżak et al. 2019). It also exposes susceptible hosts to airway deposition by inhalation, and thereby, it can cause more harm to a vulnerable host than superficial infections caused by direct contact.

3.5 ENVIRONMENTAL FACTORS AFFECTING *S. AUREUS* SURVIVABILITY IN THE AIR

S. aureus is a predominant pathogen in aerial microbiota and this could be due to its great adaptability to survive under harsh environmental conditions (Kowalski 2011). However, multiple abiotic factors such as temperature, RH, dryness, and air change rate influence its viability in aerosols. Usually, the optimal growth of *S. aureus* has been observed at a temperature range between 30°C and 37°C and at RH up to 70%. It has been seen that the number of soft-tissue infections grows during warm weather, suggesting that *S. aureus* concentration is positively correlated with temperature (Madsen, Moslehi-Jenabian et al. 2018). The prevalence of *S. aureus* in indoor air has been found to be highest during the monsoon season with high humidity; however in the outdoors it is maximum during summer (Kumari, Chakraborti et al. 2020).

Moon et al. have studied the correlation between the number of *S. aureus* in the indoor air with the seasons, and found that the aerial burden of *S. aureus* is highest during summer and lowest during winter (Moon, Huh et al. 2014). Furthermore, the air change rate has been shown to negatively affect the viability of *S. aureus* in the air (Madsen, Moslehi-Jenabian et al. 2018); this could be the reason why *S. aureus* concentration has been constantly found to be higher in indoor air than outdoors. Furthermore, the number of occupants indoors is directly correlated with the airborne concentration of *S. aureus* (Moon, Huh et al. 2014). Evidently, *S. aureus* can persist for several months in air suspensions, and can endure a wide range of RH, temperature, and sunlight exposure (Dancer 2008; Kozajda, Jeżak et al. 2019). It is extremely resistant to dry weather and thus can survive on dry inanimate surfaces for months (Kramer, Schwebke et al. 2006), and can be re-aerosolized again. *S. aureus* is the only bacteria which can persist at low humidity as well (Kramer, Schwebke et al. 2006).

A study was conducted to see the survivability of different microbes on the filter material used in respiratory masks. According to that, *S. aureus* showed the best survivability on filter fabrics with 40–200% moisture content (Majchrzycka, Okrasa et al. 2016). Overall, *S. aureus* is a robust bacterium and can survive under adverse environmental conditions, further increasing the exposure risks due to its aerosol transmission. Furthermore, not only live airborne MRSA cells, but also the aerosol transmission of dead MRSA carrying DNA encoding for antibiotic-resistant genes has the potential to spread AMR in the environmental susceptible counterparts through horizontal gene transfer (Liu, Chai et al. 2012).

3.6   HEALTH IMPACTS OF AIRBORNE *S. AUREUS* EXPOSURE

For many years, the prevalence of airborne infections particularly caused by *S. aureus* has been practically neglected. This is mainly due to the ability of this pathogen to infect patients via different routes (skin and respiratory system), thus making it difficult to establish any individual staphylococcal infection as airborne. Nevertheless, *S. aureus* remains viable and infective in dry aerosols and may therefore infect patients when the air is disturbed. Airborne MRSA is generally introduced into hospital environments via infected or colonized patients and health care workers. Within the institution, MRSA is transmitted from patients to other people via hand-to-hand contact and sneezing (Wilson, Huang et al. 2004). Besides health care sectors, *S. aureus* dispersal is also associated with community and livestock-acquired infections and thus the aerial exposure of resistant *S. aureus* – particularly MRSA – can cause occupational hazards among people working in animal husbandry like swine farms (Davis, Pisanic et al. 2018), pig and calf farms, and slaughterhouses (Masclaux, Sakwinska et al. 2013). While handling MRSA-infected patients in hospitals, and animals in farms, workers are colonized and thus become secondary MRSA carriers (Haamann, Dulon et al. 2011). Reports suggest that multidrug-resistant MRSA (MDR-MRSA) are also equally prevalent in the air of residences near these areas and thus people and children living there are affected (Hatcher, Rhodes et al. 2017).

S. aureus is normally colonized in the nose, ears, and throat and infection slowly spreads from the upper to lower respiratory tract, leading to complex situations such as pneumonia, bronchitis, and consecutive chronic obstructive pulmonary disease (David and Daum 2010). Particularly, there are a few groups of patients who are at high risk of MRSA infection and at higher risk of worsening clinical conditions such as SSTIs. These patients include individuals having lengthy hospitalization, admitted to nursing homes and ICUs, undergoing surgery, hemodialysis, or insertion of invasive devices, patients with burns or trauma, and individuals having serious illness such as muscle weakness, myopathy, or neuropathy (Vincent 2003; Rogers, Proczek et al. 2008; Lee, de Lencastre et al. 2018). In burnt patients, risk is associated with changes in the immune response and loss of skin, which is the first line of defense against microbes. MRSA infection leads to delayed wound healing causing longer duration of hospital stay which thus might enhance the rate of mortality (Rogers, Proczek et al. 2008).

MRSA is one of the endemic pathogens in many neonatal ICUs causing invasive disease and it can even lead to death. Neonates may acquire MRSA from silent reservoirs, possibly their parents. Medical device-related infections (MDRIs) are very rare, but can cause potentially severe infections and add an economic burden on patients. Moreover, *S. aureus* can remain at the implantation site by forming a biofilm which is completely recalcitrant to antibiotic action (Ferry, Uckay et al. 2010). Thus, the presence of antibiotic-resistant *S. aureus* in the air is a matter of serious concern for public health.

3.7 BIOAEROSOL COLLECTION METHODS FOR AIRBORNE *S. AUREUS*

Bioaerosol sampling is a prime step in the characterization of airborne *S. aureus*. Bioaerosol particles can be collected using passive or active air-sampling methodologies. Each sampling technique has its own merits as well as associated demerits. The selection of a bioaerosol sampler is based on sampler performance, expected bioaerosol concentration, and downstream bioaerosol analysis methods. Passive bioaerosol sampling through gravitational settling is a widely accepted method because of its user-friendliness and low cost. Airborne microorganisms passively settle on the exposed agar plate under the influence of gravity, thus bioaerosol collection is dependent on the size and shape of the particles and the surrounding air. Multiple bioaerosol samples can be collected simultaneously using multiple agar plates. However, volume of sampled air cannot be estimated in this passive sampling process, making it non-quantitative and not comparable to other sampling methods. Since only larger particle agglomerates readily settle on the agar plate, bacteria from inhalable particulate matters (PM_5 and PM_{10}) are also under-represented (Burge and Solomon 1987) in this method.

To overcome the limitation posed by passive air sampling, active bioaerosol-sampling techniques are employed. Active bioaerosol sampling may utilize impaction, impingement, or cyclone-based methods for bioaerosol collection. Popular air-sampling devices based on these three active sampling techniques are shown in Figure 3.2. In the impaction technique, airborne particles are separated from the air stream under the force of inertia and are deposited on solid or semi-solid collection medium (Macher and Hansson 1987; Li 1999; Yao and Mainelis 2007). The impaction of bioaerosol particles depends upon their inertial properties, e.g., density, diameter, and velocity, and also on the physical parameters of the impactors, e.g., dimensions of inlet nozzles and airflow pathways (Yao and Mainelis 2007). While in impingement, the air is aspirated horizontally, redirected downwards into a collection liquid. The inertial forces facilitate removal of bioaerosol particles from the air and they are finally collected into a liquid medium (Juozaitis, Willeke et al. 1994; Willeke, Lin et al. 1998).

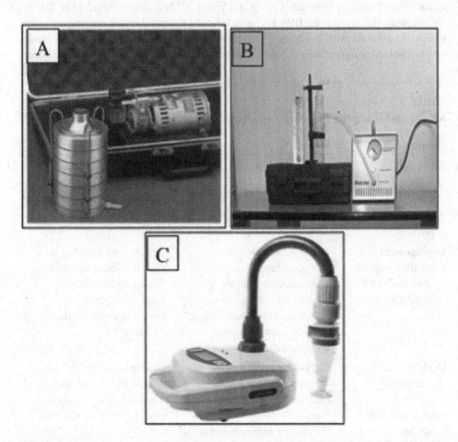

FIGURE 3.2   Air sampling devices representing each of the three active sampling techniques: A) Anderson six stage sampler is based on impaction technique, consists of six different stages correspond to six different particle size ranges, B) SKC sampler is based on impingement technique, C) Coriolis μ Air Sampler is based on cyclone technique.

However, in the cyclone method, the bioaerosol particles are captured into the liquid medium by swirling movement and centrifugal force. The collected bioaerosol particles (now hydrosol) are ready for downstream analysis using different culture or culture-independent methods (Chakrawarti, Singh et al. 2020). The merits and demerits of different air-sampling techniques are summarized in Table 3.1.

3.8 SELECTIVE GROWTH MEDIUM USED FOR ISOLATION OF *S. AUREUS* AND MRSA

Selective media is designed to allow the growth of specific microorganisms and inhibit the growth of other organisms (Schleifer and Krämer 1980). Baird Parker Agar (BPA) (Harding and Williams 1969) and mannitol salt agar (MSA) (Kateete, Kimani et al. 2010) are two important media that are frequently used for the enumeration of *S. aureus* from air (Chang and Wang 2015; Kozajda, Jeżak et al. 2019). The growth of *S. aureus* on BPA is characterized by typical black-colored colonies which are formed with the zone of lipid precipitation that is caused by secretion of glycerol ester hydrolases (lipase) (Zangerl and Asperger 2003). While tellurite

---

TABLE 3.1
Merits and demerits of active bioaerosol sampling

Sampler type	Merits	Demerits
Impaction (Anderson viable sampler) Airflow rate (28.3 litres/min)	Particle size discrimination is possible. Shorter post-sampling processing due to direct collection on agar plates	Suitable for culture-based analysis only. Overloading of agar plates may limit bioaerosol enumeration
Impingement (SKC BioSampler) Airflow rate (12.5 litres/min)	The liquid sample can be concentrated or diluted for downstream analysis. Suitable for culture-based as well as culture-independent downstream bioaerosol characterisation	Unfit for long sampling runs; causes violent bubbling resulting in the loss of collection liquid. Size fractionation is not possible
Cyclone (Coriolis μ air sampler) Airflow rate (100–300 litres/min)	The sampled liquid can be concentrated or diluted. Long sampling runs can be possible. Suitable for culture-based as well as culture-independent downstream bioaerosol characterisation	Evaporative loss of collection liquid during sampling. Experienced handling and maintenance are required

and lithium chloride are the other two ingredients of BPA that inhibit the growth of other microorganisms, glycine and pyruvate support the growth of *S. aureus* (Schleifer and Krämer 1980). Similarly, MSA with NaCl (7.5%) gives yellow-colored *S. aureus* colonies because of the fermentation of mannitol and the presence of high salt concentration prevents the growth of several other microorganisms (Chang and Wang 2015). To fasten the characterization process, many commercially available chromogenic media are also widely used to specifically detect *S. aureus*, thus saving time and reagent (Perry 2017). Some of the important media used for isolation of *S. aureus* are summarized in Table 3.2.

MRSA can also be isolated with the help of selective media such as BPA and MSA by adding oxacillin or methicillin (Karthy, Ranjitha et al. 2009) and other antibiotics (Rajput, Poudel et al. 2019), as mentioned in the Clinical and Laboratory Standards Institute (CSLI) guidelines (Wayne 2011). For the better screening of MRSA, MSA supplemented with cefoxitin (4 mg/L) and 3% NaCl has been proved to be better than MSA combined with oxacillin or methicillin (Smyth and Kahlmeter 2005). Apart from the above modifications in traditional media, the inclusion of oxacillin in chromogenic media provides selectivity for accurate enumeration of MRSA from air (Xu, Hou et al. 2016). The reliability of chromogenic media for MRSA had been contentious in very few studies but its sensitivity and specificity were verified to be outstanding when compared to many other modified media. More information on chromogenic medium used for MRSA isolation is given in Table 3.3.

3.9 CULTURE-INDEPENDENT IDENTIFICATION OF AIRBORNE *S. AUREUS*

Only 1% of total environmental bacterial communities can be cultured in the laboratory using traditional microbiological techniques (Hugenholtz 2002). Traditional culture-based methodologies fail to estimate the viable but not culturable (VBNC) air bacterial communities (Oliver 2010). Culture-independent DNA-based analytical methods can better determine the airborne bacterial concentration and composition in the sampled air. The culture-independent analysis using molecular marker genes, e.g., 16S rRNA gene, *hsp*60 gene and *rpo*B gene, are widely used techniques to analyze airborne *S. aureus*. The 16S rRNA gene is approximately 1.5 kb long and comprises different conserved as well as hypervariable regions (V1–V9). These hypervariable regions can accurately resolve the sequence diversity among the bacterial community up to genus level; however species level resolution is not accurate using 16S rRNA (Clarridge 2004). The V1 hypervariable region is best for the differentiation of *S. aureus* and coagulase-negative staphylococci (Chakravorty, Helb et al. 2007). This species level taxonomic identification of bacterial communities was made possible by using *hsp*60 gene as a novel genetic marker (Kwok, Su et al. 1999; Ishikawa, Sasaki et al. 2018). *hsp*60 gene encodes for 60 kDa heat-shock protein in all bacteria. A partial hsp60 gene sequence (600 bp) can be used to identify and differentiate between different *Staphylococcus*

TABLE 3.2
Selective growth media for isolation of *Staphylococcus aureus*

Medium	Selective agents	Diagnostic agents	Colony characteristics of *S. aureus*	Colony characteristics of coagulase-negative staphylococci	References
Baird Parker Agar	Lithium chloride, potassium tellurite, and glycine	Potassium tellurite and egg yolk	Black-colored colonies with formation of opaque zone around the colonies	Black-colored colonies without opaque zone formation around the colonies	Baird-Parker (1962); Chang and Wang (2015)
Mannitol salt agar	Sodium chloride	Mannitol phenol red	Yellow-colored colonies surrounded by yellow zone	Red-colored colonies	Chapman (1945); Sharp and Searcy (2006)
CHROM agar	Sodium chloride	Special chromogenic mixture	Mauve-colored colonies	White, beige, light blue, and navy blue-colored colonies	Kluytmans, Van Griethuysen et al.(2002); Hsiao, Chen et al. (2012)
***S. aureus* ID**	Not available	Not available	Green-colored colonies	White-colored colonies	Diederen, van Leest et al. (2006)

TABLE 3.3
Selective growth media for isolation of methicillin-resistant *Staphylococcus aureus* (MRSA)

Medium	Selective agents	Diagnostic agents	Colony characteristics of MRSA	Colony characteristics of coagulase-negative staphylococci.	References
Oxoid Brilliance MRSA	Selective mixture	Chromogenic enzymatic substrate	Blue-colored colonies	Pink, purple, or white-colored colonies	Verkade, Elberts et al. (2009); Xu, Hou et al. (2016)
ChromID MRSA	Cefoxitin	Chromogenic substrate for α-glycosidase enzyme	Green-colored colonies	Colonies do not grow	Diederen, van Leest et al. (2006); Xu, Hou et al. (2016)
MRSA Select	Antibiotics, antifungals, and salts	Chromogenic enzymatic substrate	Strong pink-colored colonies	Other than strong pink-colored colonies	Louie, Soares et al. (2006); Xu, Hou et al. (2016)
Spectra MRSA	Salt mixture and combination of antibacterial compounds	Chromogenic mixture that contains substrate for phosphatase enzyme	Denim blue-colored colonies	Colonies do not grow	Peterson, Riebe et al. (2010)

species (Kwok and Chow 2003). The *hsp*60 gene emerged as more accurate in species-specific identification in contrast to 16S rRNA gene-based identification in staphylococci. The *hsp*60 universal primers H279 and H280 differentiate different species of *Staphylococcus*. Very recently, the partial sequence of *rpo*B gene encoding the beta subunit of RNA polymerase has been used as a potential genetic marker to identify the *Staphylococcus* species (Drancourt and Raoult 2002).

. Currently, in addition to community identification up to species level, whole-genome sequencing (WGS) can be used for further functional characterization of bacteria such as virulence genes, metabolic pathways, and resistance markers (Price, Didelot et al. 2013; Price, Cole et al. 2017; Dancer, Adams et al. 2019). Proteomics study is also an emerging field which examines the proteins involved in the pathophysiology of *S. aureus* (Hecker, Mäder et al. 2018). Metabolome analysis investigates the metabolic processes linked to growth and virulence factor expression (Liebeke, Dörries et al. 2012). These high-throughput techniques emerged as a rapid identification tool for airborne *Staphylococcus* species and may help in infection control.

3.10 CURRENT AIR DECONTAMINATION AGAINST *S. AUREUS*

Airborne infectious agents settle on inanimate surfaces, and in turn are transferred to hands; thus airborne contamination and surface deposition of microbes are interrelated. Therefore, it is imperative to adopt an integral approach by including surface disinfection and hand hygiene to achieve a complete airborne disinfection (Kowalski 2011). For surface cleaning, apart from regular detergent-based disinfectants, currently hydrogen peroxide (H_2O_2)-based liquid cleaning reagents, a combination of H_2O_2 and peracetic acid, and electrolyzed water are some of the new surface-cleaning approaches that are being used to kill microbial pathogens settled on environmental surfaces in hospitals (Boyce 2016), while air decontamination technologies are very few and are seldom in use. Nevertheless, with the recognition of aerial dispersal as a significant transmission route of major human pathogens such as *S. aureus*, which is frequently prevalent in hospital settings (Kozajda, Jeżak et al. 2019), new techniques have been developed to decontaminate the indoor air (Ijaz, Zargar et al. 2016). For air disinfection, currently vaporized H_2O_2 systems and aerosolized H_2O_2 systems are in practice along with a few mobile devices that emit ultraviolet (UV) C light, which are available on the market to control airborne infections, although not all are effective against MRSA. Besides, various technologies based on oxygen reactive species (Choudhury, Portugal et al. 2018), UV irradiation (Chang, Li et al. 2013), high-efficiency particulate arrestor (HEPA) filtration, light-activated photosensitizers, and electrostatic particle ionization (EPI) (Alonso, Raynor et al. 2016) have been invented to overcome the airborne contamination of MSSA and MRSA in hospital settings (Alonso, Raynor et al. 2016; Boyce 2016; Ijaz, Zargar et al. 2016; Yates et al. 2016). There are many oxygen-based technologies available, as shown in Table 3.4; of them oxygen gas plasma, ozone generator, and vaporized hydrogen peroxide are potential candidates. Oxygen gas plasma is a mixture of highly reactive species including oxygen and ozone radicals; it is formed when oxygen is exposed to a high electric field (Yates et al. 2016). It can decontaminate a large number of airborne pathogens, including respiratory viruses and MRSA. A recent report has claimed that the ozone generated by a specifically designed plasma gas reactor could achieve a 5-log reduction in MRSA counts within 2 min (Choudhury, Portugal et al. 2018).

UV light with wavelength range from 200 to 280 nm is germicidal, as it can destabilize the double bond between the adjacent carbon atoms of various macromolecules such as DNA and RNA, resulting in the killing of microorganisms. UV at wavelength 254 nm is standardized to inactivate microorganisms including *S. aureus* (Chang, Li et al. 2013). Airborne disinfection of microbes can be achieved by placing UV-generating devices that continuously flow air in a confined indoor area (Yates et al. 2016). Various UV irradiation-based technologies are also listed in Table 3.4.

TABLE 3.4

Existing decontamination techniques for airborne *S aureus* and methicillin-resistant *S. aureus* (MRSA)

Technology	Decontamination agents	Inactivation of:
Oxygen-based		
Hydroxyl/Odorox	Hydroxyl radicals	MSSA and MRSA
Phocatox	Combination of O_3, hydroxyl radicals, HEPA, and UVC	MSSA and MRSA
TriAirT250	Hydroxyl radicals	All Gram-positive
Inov8AirDisinfection unit	Hydroxyl radicals	All pathogens
Ozone generator	Gaseous O_3	MSSA and MRSA
Oxygen cold gas	Mixture of O_3, O_2 radicals, H_2O_2	MSSA and MRSA
Vaporized H_2O_2	Utilizes 30% H_2O_2	MSSA and MRSA
UV irradiation-based		
UV germicidal irradiation	8 lamps emitting 254 nm UV-C	All pathogens
Microgenix air purification	Chemical coated UV-C light source	All pathogens
Pulsed-xenon device	Emits UV in 200–320 nm range	All pathogens
EPI	Causes ionization to reduce PM levels	Swine and zoonotic pathogens such as MRSA
Light-activated photosensitizers	UV-activated titanium dioxide, photocatalytic reaction to oxidize microbes	MSSA

HEPA, high-efficiency particulate arrestor; UVC, ultraviolet C; MSSA, methicillin-sensitive *S. aureus*; MRSA, methicillin-resistant *S. aureus*; EPI, electrostatic particle ionization; PM, particulate matter;

Adapted from Alonso, Raynor et al. (2016); Boyce (2016); Ijaz, Zargar et al. (2016); and Yates et al. (2016).

3.11   GUIDELINES TO REDUCE AIRBORNE *S. AUREUS* AND MRSA

The growing evidence on aerial transmission of potential nosocomial pathogens such as *S. aureus* and their increasing threat to human health has already been noticed by the US Environmental Protection Agency (US EPA), which set the guidelines for testing the efficacy of air sanitizers against airborne bacteria (US EPA 2013). According to the standards set by US EPA, an air-sanitizing device should be able to reduce the bacterial viable count by 3 $\log_{10}$ (99.9%) in enclosed air for each of the test bacteria within 5 min, compared to untreated air. Additionally, the device should be capable of measuring the settling rate of each of the test bacteria in the enclosed air of the test chamber and thereafter able to correct the total viability count of that test bacteria. More importantly, *S. aureus* (ATCC 6538) should be employed as test bacteria in the evaluation of products intended to be used in residential as well as in hospital environments as it is the most frequent and stable bacteria in indoor air (Ijaz, Zargar et al. 2016; Sattar and Ijaz 2016). The test enclosure to evaluate any air-sanitizing product should be a space the size of about a typical room (10 × 10 × 8 ft). In this context it is worth mentioning that Sattar et al. have designed an aerobiology chamber simulating the environmental conditions to monitor and decontaminate airborne pathogenic microbes and the study portable air decontamination device follows the standards set by the US EPA (Sattar, Kibbee et al. 2016).

In India, national airborne infection control (NAIC) guidelines were set in 2010 for the prevention of aerial transmission of infectious agents, particularly *Mycobacterium tuberculosis* (Directorate General of Health Services N.D.), however its implementation in health care facilities is still questionable (Parmar, Sachdeva et al. 2015). According to NAIC, the minimum environmental conditions such as proper natural ventilation should be maintained in health care facilities by regular measuring of airflow direction, air change rate, and air velocity. Moreover, infected patients should be isolated from non-infected ones in waiting areas. N95 masks and personal protective measures are recommended in high-risk settings such as TB wards, ICUs, and HIV wards. Regular monitoring of airborne bacterial counts in high-risk settings such as surgical wards and ICUs using the settle plate method is recommended. Overall, the aim of NAIC was to integrate airborne infection prevention guidelines into general infection control training and educational programs (Directorate General of Health Services N.D.). However, the airborne part is poorly represented in existing infection control modules, as reported by Parmar et al., who found poor implementation of NAIC guidelines in health care facilities in different states of India (Parmar, Sachdeva et al. 2015).

According to the revised health care infection control practice advisory committee (HICAP), USA, the role of bioaerosols and airborne transmission in spreading infections caused by newly evolving MDR organisms such as MRSA is a major health concern (Parmar, Sachdeva et al. 2015). Consequently, HICAP in 2007 revised the guidelines for preventing the transmission of infectious agents in health care facilities by suggesting that the health care professional should also adopt airborne infection control in addition to droplet and contact precautions in case of clinical conditions where MRSA, TB, SARS, and coronaviruses are potential etiological agents (Siegel, Rhinehart et al. 2007). As per the guidelines of the Infectious Disease Society of America (IDSA) and Centers for Disease Control and Prevention (CDC), in hospitals, decolonization of nasal and skin-associated MRSA should be done with mupirocin application twice daily, particularly for patients undergoing relatively high-risk surgery, or chlorhexidine wipes/wash prior to surgery. Additionally, a combination of environmental, hand, and surface hygiene should be implemented to manage the transmission of MRSA in high-risk zones (Liu, Bayer et al. 2011). MRSA falls in the biosafety level 2 category, and therefore it poses a moderate risk to laboratory workers. Nevertheless, the use of a biosafety cabinet is recommended to handle MRSA strains and all waste must be discarded after steam autoclaving. Due to hand-to-face contamination risk of MRSA infection a proper cleaning of hands and surfaces is recommended. Most importantly, a biohazard warning sign must be pasted on the doors of laboratories handling MRSA (Johnston, Eggett et al. 2014).

3.12 CONCLUSION

S. aureus is a ubiquitously present bacteria in the environment owing to its remarkable adaptability under extreme conditions (Kozajda, Jeżak et al. 2019). Although up to one-third of the human population is a carrier of *S. aureus*, it poses greater risk mainly to those with weaker immunity, including children, elderly people, and patients with HIV, cystic fibrosis, and cancer. It is spread by air as droplet infection and also through direct contact between infected and susceptible individuals (Ijaz, Zargar et al. 2016). The aerial transmission of *S. aureus*, particularly its MRSA strains in the hospital environment, can adversely affect the success of organ transplantation and other major surgeries (Creamer, Shore et al. 2014). MRSA is a pathogen that is frequently isolated in the air and on surfaces in hospital and other community settings (Madsen, Kurdi et al. 2018; Kobayashi, Nakaminami et al. 2020; Latha, Anil et al. 2019). Therefore, the airborne prevalence of MRSA is likely to contaminate environmental inanimate surfaces, which again become the secondary vehicle of dissemination, thereby multiplying exposure risks. Without the inclusion of aerial decontamination methods in existing infection control programs, it is difficult to achieve a pathogen-free environment (Directorate General of Health Services N.D.). Additionally, regular evaluation to check the effective cleaning of surfaces by utilizing reliable indicators of microbial contamination such as fluorescent gels is necessary, particularly in hospitals (Fernando, Gray et al. 2017). Likewise, a regular monitoring of airborne *S. aureus* in high-risk zones of hospitals is advisable. Furthermore, the use of aerial decontamination techniques such as UV light devices and H_2O_2 vapors can help to achieve the environmental eradication of MRSA (Fernando, Gray et al. 2017). Overall, the airborne transmission of MRSA should not be underestimated and the proper implementation of airborne infection control guidelines is indispensable to break this vicious cycle of MRSA transmission from environment to surface to hands to susceptible host.

REFERENCES

Adams, C. E. and S. J. Dancer (2020). "Dynamic transmission of *Staphylococcus aureus* in the intensive care unit." International Journal of Environmental Research and Public Health **17**(6): 2109.

Alonso, C., P. C. Raynor, P. R. Davies, R. B. Morrison and M. Torremorell (2016). "Evaluation of an electrostatic particle ionization technology for decreasing airborne pathogens in pigs." Aerobiologia **32**(3): 405–419.

Anjum, K. M. R., K. Sivakumari, K. Ashok and S. Rajesh (2018). "A pilot investigation into associations between various indoor airborne bacterial particles in Triplicane public toilet of Chennai, Tamil Nadu." European Journal of Biomedical **5**(5): 480–484.

Baird-Parker, A. C. (1962). "An improved diagnostic and selective medium for isolating coagulase positive staphylococci." Journal of Applied Bacteriology **25**(1): 12–19.

Bhalla, A., N. J. Pultz, D. M. Gries, A. J. Ray, E. C. Eckstein, D. C. Aron and C. J. Donskey (2004). "Acquisition of nosocomial pathogens on hands after contact with environmental surfaces near hospitalized patients." Infection Control & Hospital Epidemiology **25**(2): 164–167.

Bischoff, W. E., M. L. Wallis, B. K. Tucker, B. A. Reboussin, M. A. Pfaller, F. G. Hayden and R. J. Sherertz (2006). ""Gesundheit!" Sneezing, common colds, allergies, and *Staphylococcus aureus* dispersion." The Journal of Infectious Diseases **194**(8): 1119–1126.

Bos, M. E. H., K. M. Verstappen, B. A. G. L. Van Cleef, W. Dohmen, A. Dorado-García, H. Graveland, B. Duim, J. A. Wagenaar, J. A. J. W. Kluytmans and D. J. J. Heederik (2016). "Transmission through air as a possible route of exposure for MRSA." Journal of Exposure Science & Environmental Epidemiology **26**(3): 263–269.

Boyce, J. M. (2016). "Modern technologies for improving cleaning and disinfection of environmental surfaces in hospitals." Antimicrobial Resistance & Infection Control **5**(1): 1–10.

Boyce, J. M., G. Potter-Bynoe, C. Chenevert and T. King (1997). "Environmental contamination due to methicillin-resistant *Staphylococcus aureus* possible infection control implications." Infection Control & Hospital Epidemiology **18**(9): 622–627.

Burge, H. A. and W. R. Solomon (1987). "Sampling and analysis of biological aerosols." Atmospheric Environment (1967) **21**(2): 451–456.

Centers for Disease Control. (2019). Antibiotic resistance threats in the United States. Atlanta, GA: U.S. Department of Health and Human Services.

Chakravorty, S., D. Helb, M. Burday, N. Connell and D. Alland (2007). "A detailed analysis of 16S ribosomal RNA gene segments for the diagnosis of pathogenic bacteria." Journal of Microbiological Methods **69**(2): 330–339.

Chakrawarti, M. K., M. Singh, V. P. Yadav and K. Mukhopadhyay (2020). "Temporal dynamics of air bacterial communities in a university health centre using Illumina MiSeq sequencing." Aerosol and Air Quality Research **20**(5): 966–980.

Chang, C. W. and L. J. Wang (2015). "Impact of culture media and sampling methods on *Staphylococcus aureus* aerosols." Indoor Air **25**(5): 488–498.

Chang, C. W., S. Y. Li, S. H. Huang, C. K. Huang, Y. Y. Chen and C. C. Chen (2013). "Effects of ultraviolet germicidal irradiation and swirling motion on airborne *Staphylococcus aureus*, *Pseudomonas aeruginosa* and *Legionella pneumophila* under various relative humidities." Indoor Air **23**(1): 74–84.

Chapman, G. H. (1945). "The significance of sodium chloride in studies of staphylococci." Journal of Bacteriology **50**(2): 201.

Choudhury, B., S. Portugal, N. Mastanaiah, J. A. Johnson and S. Roy (2018). "Inactivation of *Pseudomonas aeruginosa* and methicillin-resistant *Staphylococcus aureus* in an open water system with ozone generated by a compact, atmospheric DBD plasma reactor." Scientific Reports **8**(1): 1–11.

Chougale, R. A. and P. A. Kumar (2019). "Aerobic microbiological surveillance of operation theatre from a tertiary care hospital, Kolhapur, India." International Journal of Current Microbiology and Applied Science **8**(10): 1210–1215.

Chuaybamroong, P., P. Choomseer and P. Sribenjalux (2008). "Comparison between hospital single air unit and central air unit for ventilation performances and airborne microbes." Aerosol and Air Quality Research **8**(1): 28–36.

Clarridge, J. E. (2004). "Impact of 16S rRNA gene sequence analysis for identification of bacteria on clinical microbiology and infectious diseases." Clinical Microbiology Reviews **17**(4): 840–862.

Creamer, E., A. C. Shore, E. C. Deasy, S. Galvin, A. Dolan, N. Walley, S. McHugh, D. Fitzgerald-Hughes, D. J. Sullivan and R. Cunney (2014). "Air and surface contamination patterns of meticillin-resistant *Staphylococcus aureus* on eight acute hospital wards." Journal of Hospital Infection **86**(3): 201–208.

Dancer, S. J. (2008). "Importance of the environment in meticillin-resistant *Staphylococcus aureus* acquisition: the case for hospital cleaning." The Lancet Infectious Diseases **8**(2): 101–113.

Dancer, S. J., C. E. Adams, J. Smith, B. Pichon, A. Kearns and D. Morrison (2019). "Tracking *Staphylococcus aureus* in the intensive care unit using whole-genome sequencing." Journal of Hospital Infection **103**(1): 13–20.

David, M. Z. and R. S. Daum (2010). "Community-associated methicillin-resistant *Staphylococcus aureus*: epidemiology and clinical consequences of an emerging epidemic." Clinical Microbiology Reviews **23**(3): 616–687.

Davis, M. F., N. Pisanic, S. M. Rhodes, A. Brown, H. Keller, M. Nadimpalli, A. Christ, S. Ludwig, C. Ordak and K. Spicer (2018). "Occurrence of *Staphylococcus aureus* in swine and swine workplace environments on industrial and antibiotic-free hog operations in North Carolina, USA: a One Health pilot study." Environmental Research **163**: 88–96.

Diederen, B. M. W., C. M. van Leest, I. van Duijn, P. Willemse, P. H. J. van Keulen and J. Kluytmans (2006). "Evaluation of *S. aureus* ID, a chromogenic agar medium for the detection of *Staphylococcus aureus*." Infection **34**(2): 95–97.

Directorate General of Health Services (N.D.). "Ministry of Health & Family Welfare, Nirman Bhawan; 2010. Guidelines on Airborne Infection Control in Healthcare and Other Settings – In the context of tuberculosis and other airborne infections" – April 2010 [Provisional]. www.tbcindia.nic.in.

Drancourt, M. and D. Raoult (2002). "rpoB gene sequence-based identification of *Staphylococcus* species." Journal of Clinical Microbiology **40**(4): 1333–1338.

Elek, S. D. and P. E. Conen (1957). "The virulence of *Staphylococcus pyogenes* for man. A study of the problems of wound infection." British Journal of Experimental Pathology **38**(6): 573.

Faridi, S., M. S. Hassanvand, K. Naddafi , M. Yunesian, R. Nabizadeh, M. H. Sowlat, H. Kashani, A. Gholampour, S. Niazi and A. Zare (2015). "Indoor/outdoor relationships of bioaerosol concentrations in a retirement home and a school dormitory." Environmental Science and Pollution Research **22**(11): 8190–8200.

Fernando, S. A., T. J. Gray and T. Gottlieb (2017). "Healthcare-acquired infections: prevention strategies." Internal Medicine Journal **47**(12): 1341–1351.

Ferry, T., I. Uckay, P. Vaudaux, P. Francois, J. Schrenzel, S. Harbarth, F. Laurent, L. Bernard, F. Vandenesch and J. Etienne (2010). "Risk factors for treatment failure in orthopedic device-related methicillin-resistant *Staphylococcus aureus* infection." European Journal of Clinical Microbiology & Infectious Diseases **29**(2): 171–180.

Foster, W. D. and M. S. R. Hutt (1960). "Experimental *Staphylococcus* infection in man." The Lancet **2**(7165): 1373–1376.

Frankel, M., G. Bekö, M. Timm, S. Gustavsen, E. W. Hansen and A. M. Madsen (2012). "Seasonal variations of indoor microbial exposures and their relation to temperature, relative humidity, and air exchange rate." Applied and Environmental Microbiology **78**(23): 8289–8297.

Gehanno, J. F., A. Louvel, M. Nouvellon, J. F. Caillard and M. Pestel-Caron (2009). "Aerial dispersal of meticillin-resistant *Staphylococcus aureus* in hospital rooms by infected or colonised patients." Journal of Hospital Infection **71**(3): 256–262.

Haamann, F., M. Dulon and A. Nienhaus (2011). "MRSA as an occupational disease: a case series." International Archives of Occupational and Environmental Health **84**(3): 259–266.

Hancock, R. E. W. and H.-G. Sahl (2006). "Antimicrobial and host-defense peptides as new anti-infective therapeutic strategies." Nature Biotechnology **24**(12): 1551–1557.

Harding, L. and R. E. O. Williams (1969). "Selection of *Staphylococcus aureus* in cultures from air samples." Epidemiology & Infection **67**(1): 35–39.

Hatcher, S. M., S. M. Rhodes, J. R. Stewart, E. Silbergeld, N. Pisanic, J. Larsen, S. Jiang, A. Krosche, D. Hall and K. C. Carroll (2017). "The prevalence of antibiotic-resistant *Staphylococcus aureus* nasal carriage among industrial hog operation workers, community residents, and children living in their households: North Carolina, USA." Environmental Health Perspectives **125**(4): 560–569.

Hecker, M., U. Mäder and U. Völker (2018). "From the genome sequence via the proteome to cell physiology – Pathoproteomics and pathophysiology of *Staphylococcus aureus*." International Journal of Medical Microbiology **308**(6): 545–557.

Hiramatsu, K., L. Cui, M. Kuroda and T. Ito (2001). "The emergence and evolution of methicillin-resistant *Staphylococcus aureus*." Trends in Microbiology **9**(10): 486–493.

Hiramatsu, K., T. Ito, S. Tsubakishita, T. Sasaki, F. Takeuchi, Y. Morimoto, Y. Katayama, M. Matsuo, K. Kuwahara-Arai and T. Hishinuma (2013). "Genomic basis for methicillin resistance in *Staphylococcus aureus*." Infection & Chemotherapy **45**(2): 117–136.

Hiramatsu, K., Y. Katayama, M. Matsuo, T. Sasaki, Y. Morimoto, A. Sekiguchi and T. Baba (2014a). "Multi-drug-resistant *Staphylococcus aureus* and future chemotherapy." Journal of Infection and Chemotherapy **20**(10): 593–601.

Hiramatsu, K., Y. Katayama, M. Matsuo, Y. Aiba, M. Saito, T. Hishinuma and A. Iwamoto (2014b). "Vancomycin-intermediate resistance in *Staphylococcus aureus*." Journal of Global Antimicrobial Resistance **2**(4): 213–224.

Hsiao, P.-K., W.-T. Chen, K.-C. Chang, Y.-J. Ke, C.-L. Kuo and C.-C. Tseng (2012). "Performance of CHROMagar *Staph aureus* and CHROMagar MRSA for detection of airborne methicillin-resistant and methicillin-sensitive *Staphylococcus aureus*." Aerosol Science and Technology **46**(3): 297–308.

Hugenholtz, P. (2002). "Exploring prokaryotic diversity in the genomic era." Genome Biology **3**(2): reviews0003. 0001.

Hussain, M., P. Madl and A. Khan (2011). "Lung deposition predictions of airborne particles and the emergence of contemporary diseases, Part-I." Health **2**(2): 51–59.

Ijaz, M. K., B. Zargar, K. E. Wright, J. R. Rubino and S. A. Sattar (2016). "Generic aspects of the airborne spread of human pathogens indoors and emerging air decontamination technologies." American Journal of Infection Control **44**(9): S109–S120.

Ishikawa, D., T. Sasaki, M. Takahashi, K. Kuwahara-Arai, K. Haga, S. Ito, K. Okahara, A. Nakajima, T. Shibuya and T. Osada (2018). "The microbial composition of Bacteroidetes species in ulcerative colitis is effectively improved by combination therapy with fecal microbiota transplantation and antibiotics." Inflammatory Bowel Diseases **24**(12): 2590–2598.

Ito, T., Y. Katayama and K. Hiramatsu (1999). "Cloning and nucleotide sequence determination of the entire mec DNA of pre-methicillin-resistant *Staphylococcus aureus* N315." Antimicrobial Agents and Chemotherapy **43**(6): 1449–1458.

Jevons, M. P. (1961). ""Celbenin"-resistant staphylococci." British Medical Journal **1**(5219): 124.

Johnston, J. D., D. Eggett, M. J. Johnson and J. C. Reading (2014). "The influence of risk perception on biosafety level-2 laboratory workers' hand-to-face contact behaviors." Journal of Occupational and Environmental Hygiene **11**(9): 625–632.

Juozaitis, A., K. Willeke, S. A. Grinshpun and J. Donnelly (1994). "Impaction onto a glass slide or agar versus impingement into a liquid for the collection and recovery of airborne microorganisms." Applied and Environmental Microbiology **60**(3): 861–870.

Kang, G. S., Y. H. Jung, H. S. Kim, Y. S. Lee, C. Park, K. J. Lee and J. O. Cha (2016). "Prevalence of major methicillin-resistant *Staphylococcus aureus* clones in Korea between 2001 and 2008." Annals of Laboratory Medicine **36**(6): 536–541.

Karthy, E. S., P. Ranjitha and A. Mohankumar (2009). "Performance of CHROM agar and oxacillin resistant screening agar base media for detection of methicillin resistant *Staphylococcus aureus* (MRSA) from chronic wound." Modern Applied Science **3**(5): 51–55.

Kateete, D. P., C. N. Kimani, F. A. Katabazi, A. Okeng, M. S. Okee, A. Nanteza, M. L. Joloba and F. C. Najjuka (2010). "Identification of *Staphylococcus aureus*: DNase and mannitol salt agar improve the efficiency of the tube coagulase test." Annals of Clinical Microbiology and Antimicrobials **9**(1): 1–7.

Kim, K.-H., E. Kabir and S. A. Jahan (2018). "Airborne bioaerosols and their impact on human health." Journal of Environmental Sciences **67**: 23–35.

Kluytmans, J., A. Van Griethuysen, P. Willemse and P. Van Keulen (2002). "Performance of CHROMagar selective medium and oxacillin resistance screening agar base for identifying *Staphylococcus aureus* and detecting methicillin resistance." Journal of Clinical Microbiology **40**(7): 2480–2482.

Kobayashi, T., H. Nakaminami, H. Ohtani, K. Yamada, Y. Nasu, S. Takadama, N. Noguchi, T. Fujii and T. Matsumoto (2020). "An outbreak of severe infectious diseases caused by methicillin-resistant *Staphylococcus aureus* USA300 clone among hospitalized patients and nursing staff in a tertiary care university hospital." Journal of Infection and Chemotherapy **26**(1): 76–81.

Kotgire, S., R. Akhtar, A. Damle, S. Siddiqui, H. Padekar and U. Afreen (2020). "Bioaerosol assessment of indoor air in hospital wards from a tertiary care hospital." Indian Journal of Microbiology Research **7**(1): 28–34.

Kowalski, W. (2011). Hospital airborne infection control. Boca Raton, FL: CRC Press.

Kozajda, A., K. Jeżak and A. Kapsa (2019). "Airborne *Staphylococcus aureus* in different environments – a review." Environmental Science and Pollution Research **26**(34): 1–13.

Kramer, A., I. Schwebke and G. Kampf (2006). "How long do nosocomial pathogens persist on inanimate surfaces? A systematic review." BMC Infectious Diseases 6(1): 130.

Kumar, P. and A. K. Goel (2016). "Prevalence of methicillin resistant staphylococcal bioaerosols in and around residential houses in an urban area in Central India." Journal of Pathogens 2016: 7163615.

Kumari, H., T. Chakraborti, M. Singh, M. K. Chakrawarti and K. Mukhopadhyay (2020). "Prevalence and antibiogram of coagulase negative staphylococci in bioaerosols from different indoors of a university in India." BMC Microbiology 20(1): 1–14.

Kwok, A. Y. C. and A. W. Chow (2003). "Phylogenetic study of Staphylococcus and Macrococcus species based on partial hsp60 gene sequences." International Journal of Systematic and Evolutionary Microbiology 53(1): 87–92.

Kwok, A. Y. C., S.-C. Su, R. P. Reynolds, S. J. Bay, Y. Av-Gay, N. J. Dovichi and A. W. Chow (1999). "Species identification and phylogenetic relationships based on partial HSP60 gene sequences within the genus Staphylococcus." International Journal of Systematic and Evolutionary Microbiology 49(3): 1181–1192.

Lakhundi, S. and K. Zhang (2018). "Methicillin-resistant Staphylococcus aureus: molecular characterization, evolution, and epidemiology." Clinical Microbiology Reviews 31(4): e00020-18.

Latha, T., B. Anil, H. Manjunatha, M. Chiranjay, D. Elsa, N. Baby and G. Anice (2019). "MRSA: the leading pathogen of orthopedic infection in a tertiary care hospital, South India." African Health Sciences 19(1): 1393–1401.

Lee, A. S., H. de Lencastre, J. Garau, J. Kluytmans, S. Malhotra-Kumar, A. Peschel and S. Harbarth (2018). "Methicillin-resistant Staphylococcus aureus." Nature Reviews Disease Primers 4(1): 1–23.

Li, C.-S. (1999). "Sampling performance of impactors for bacterial bioaerosols." Aerosol Science & Technology 30(3): 280–287.

Li, M., J. Qi, H. Zhang, S. Huang, L. Li and D. Gao (2011). "Concentration and size distribution of bioaerosols in an outdoor environment in the Qingdao coastal region." Science of the Total Environment 409(19): 3812–3819.

Liebeke, M., K. Dörries, H. Meyer and M. Lalk (2012). Metabolome analysis of Gram-positive bacteria such as Staphylococcus aureus by GC-MS and LC-MS. In: Functional Genomics. Springer, New York, NY, pp. 377–398.

Lin, J., D. Lin, P. Xu, T. Zhang , Q. Ou, C. Bai and Z. Yao (2016). "Non-hospital environment contamination with Staphylococcus aureus and methicillin-resistant Staphylococcus aureus: proportion meta-analysis and features of antibiotic resistance and molecular genetics." Environmental Research 150: 528–540.

Liu, C., A. Bayer, S. E. Cosgrove, R. S. Daum, S. K. Fridkin, R. J. Gorwitz, S. L. Kaplan, A. W. Karchmer, D. P. Levine and B. E. Murray (2011). "Clinical practice guidelines by the Infectious Diseases Society of America for the treatment of methicillin-resistant Staphylococcus aureus infections in adults and children." Clinical Infectious Diseases 52(3): e18–e55.

Liu, D., T. Chai, X. Xia, Y. Gao, Y. Cai, X. Li, Z. Miao, L. Sun, H. Hao and U. Roesler (2012). "Formation and transmission of Staphylococcus aureus (including MRSA) aerosols carrying antibiotic-resistant genes in a poultry farming environment." Science of the Total Environment 426: 139–145.

Louie, L., D. Soares, H. Meaney, M. Vearncombe and A. E. Simor (2006). "Evaluation of a new chromogenic medium, MRSA Select, for detection of methicillin-resistant Staphylococcus aureus." Journal of Clinical Microbiology 44(12): 4561–4563.

Lounsbury, N., M. G. Reeber, G. Mina and C. Chbib (2019). "A mini-review on ceftaroline in bacteremia patients with methicillin-resistant *Staphylococcus aureus* (MRSA) infections." Antibiotics **8**(1): 30.

Lu, Y. J., T. Sasaki, K. Kuwahara-Arai, Y. Uehara and K. Hiramatsu (2018). "Development of a new application for comprehensive viability analysis based on microbiome analysis by next-generation sequencing: insights into staphylococcal carriage in human nasal cavities." Applied and Environmental Microbiology **84**(11).

Macher, J. M. and H.-C. Hansson (1987). "Personal size-separating impactor for sampling microbiological aerosols." American Industrial Hygiene Association Journal **48**(7): 652–655.

Madhuri, M. S., Tahsina, S. K. Venugopal, D. Ghosh, R. Gadepalli, B. Dhawan and K. Mukhopadhyay (2009). "In vitro antimicrobial activity of alpha-melanocyte stimulating hormone against major human pathogen *Staphylococcus aureus*." Peptides **30**(9): 1627–1635.

Madsen, A. M., I. Kurdi, L. Feld and K. Tendal (2018). "Airborne MRSA and total *Staphylococcus aureus* as associated with particles of different sizes on pig farms." Annals of Work Exposures and Health **62**(8): 966–977.

Madsen, A. M., S. Moslehi-Jenabian, M. Z. Islam, M. Frankel, M. Spilak and M. W. Frederiksen (2018). "Concentrations of *Staphylococcus* species in indoor air as associated with other bacteria, season, relative humidity, air change rate, and *S. aureus*-positive occupants." Environmental Research **160**: 282–291.

Majchrzycka, K., M. Okrasa, J. Skóra and B. Gutarowska (2016). "Evaluation of the survivability of microorganisms deposited on filtering respiratory protective devices under varying conditions of humidity." International Journal of Environmental Research and Public Health **13**(1): 98.

Masclaux, F. G., O. Sakwinska, N. Charrière, E. Semaani and A. Oppliger (2013). "Concentration of airborne *Staphylococcus aureus* (MRSA and MSSA), total bacteria, and endotoxins in pig farms." Annals of Occupational Hygiene **57**(5): 550–557.

Mentese, S., A. Y. Rad, M. Arısoy and G. Güllü (2012). "Seasonal and spatial variations of bioaerosols in indoor urban environments, Ankara, Turkey." Indoor and Built Environment **21**(6): 797–810.

Mirhoseini, S. H., M. Nikaeen, K. Satoh and K. Makimur (2016). "Assessment of airborne particles in indoor environments: Applicability of particle counting for prediction of bioaerosol concentrations." Aerosol and Air Quality Research **16**(8): 1903–1910.

Moon, K. W., E. H. Huh and H. C. Jeong (2014). "Seasonal evaluation of bioaerosols from indoor air of residential apartments within the metropolitan area in South Korea." Environmental Monitoring and Assessment **186**(4): 2111–2120.

Nandalal, P. and R. K. Somashekar (2007). "Prevalence of *Staphylococcus aureus* and *Pseudomonas aeruginosa* in indoor air flora of a district hospital, Mandya, Karnataka." Journal of Environmental Biology **28**(2): 197–200.

Naruka, K., J. Gaur and R. Charaya (2014). "Bioaerosols in healthcare settings: a brief review." International Journal of Geology, Earth & Environmental Science **4**(3): 59–64.

Oliver, J. D. (2010). "Recent findings on the viable but nonculturable state in pathogenic bacteria." FEMS Microbiology Reviews **34**(4): 415–425.

Parmar, M. M., K. S. Sachdeva, K. Rade, M. Ghedia, A. Bansal, S. B. Nagaraja, M. D. Willis, D. P. Misquitta, S. A. Nair and P. K. Moonan (2015). "Airborne infection control in India: baseline assessment of health facilities." Indian Journal of Tuberculosis 62(4): 211–217.

Pasquarella, C., O. Pitzurra and A. Savino (2000). "The index of microbial air contamination." Journal of Hospital Infection 46(4): 241–256.

Paul, D., K. Biswas, C. Sengupta and S. N. Sinha (2015). "Studies on environmental monitoring of aeromicroflora in a hospital at Kalyani, West Bengal, India." Frontiers in Environmental Microbiology 1: 47–50.

Perry, J. D. (2017). "A decade of development of chromogenic culture media for clinical microbiology in an era of molecular diagnostics." Clinical Microbiology Reviews 30(2): 449–479.

Peterson, J. F., K. M. Riebe, G. S. Hall, D. Wilson, S. Whittier, E. Palavecino and N. A. Ledeboer (2010). "Spectra MRSA, a new chromogenic agar medium to screen for methicillin-resistant Staphylococcus aureus." Journal of Clinical Microbiology 48(1): 215–219.

Price, J. R., K. Cole, A. Bexley, V. Kostiou, D. W. Eyre, T. Golubchik, D. J. Wilson, D. W. Crook, A. S. Walker and T. E. A. Peto (2017). "Transmission of Staphylococcus aureus between health-care workers, the environment, and patients in an intensive care unit: a longitudinal cohort study based on whole-genome sequencing." The Lancet Infectious Diseases 17(2): 207–214.

Price, J. R., X. Didelot, D. W. Crook, M. J. Llewelyn and J. Paul (2013). "Whole genome sequencing in the prevention and control of Staphylococcus aureus infection." Journal of Hospital Infection 83(1): 14–21.

Raghav, N., J. N. Shrivastava, G. P. Satsangi and R. Kumar (2020). "Enumeration and characterization of airborne microbial communities in an outdoor environment of the city of Taj, India." Urban Climate 32: 100596.

Rajput, A., S. Poudel, H. Tsunemoto, M. Meehan, R. Szubin, C. A. Olson, A. Lamsa, Y. Seif, N. Dillon and A. Vrbanac (2019). "Profiling the effect of nafcillin on HA-MRSA D712 using bacteriological and physiological media." Scientific Data 6(1): 1–6.

Rathore, L., P. K. Khatri, A. Chandora, S. Meena, A. Bora, V. Maurya, N. Sharma and S. Khullar (2015). "Microbial profile and antibiogram of air contamination in hospital wards of a tertiary care hospital, western Rajasthan, India." International Journal of Current Microbiology and Applied Science 4(8): 40–46.

Rogers, S. N., K. Proczek, R. A. Sen, J. Hughes, P. Banks and D. Lowe (2008). "Which patients are most at risk of methicillin resistant Staphylococcus aureus: a review of admissions to a regional maxillofacial ward between 2001 and 2005." British Journal of Oral and Maxillofacial Surgery 46(6): 439–444.

Roy, R., R. Jan, U. Joshi, R. Bhor, K. Pai and P. G. Satsangi (2020). "Characterization, pro-inflammatory response and cytotoxic profile of bioaerosols from urban and rural residential settings in Pune, India." Environmental Pollution 114698.

Sabharwal, E. R. and R. Sharma (2015). "Estimation of microbial air contamination by settle plate method: are we within acceptable limits?" Scholars Academic Journal of Biosciences 3(8): 703–707.

Sattar, S. A. and M. K. Ijaz (2016). "The role of indoor air as a vehicle for human pathogens: summary of presentations, knowledge gaps, and directions for the future." American Journal of Infection Control 44(9): S144–S146.

Sattar, S. A., R. J. Kibbee, B. Zargar, K. E. Wright, J. R. Rubino and M. K. Ijaz (2016). "Decontamination of indoor air to reduce the risk of airborne infections: studies on survival and inactivation of airborne pathogens using an aerobiology chamber." American Journal of Infection Control **44**(10): e177–e182.

Schleifer, K.-H. and E. Krämer (1980). "Selective medium for isolating staphylococci." Zentralblatt für Bakteriologie: I. Abt. Originale C: Allgemeine, angewandte und ökologische Mikrobiologie **1**(3): 270–280.

Sexton, T., P. Clarke, E. O'Neill, T. Dillane and H. Humphreys (2006). "Environmental reservoirs of methicillin-resistant *Staphylococcus aureus* in isolation rooms: correlation with patient isolates and implications for hospital hygiene." Journal of Hospital Infection **62**(2): 187–194.

Shariati, A., M. Dadashi, Z. Chegini, A. van Belkum, M. Mirzaii, S. S. Khoramrooz and D. Darban-Sarokhalil (2020). "The global prevalence of daptomycin, tigecycline, quinupristin/dalfopristin, and linezolid-resistant *Staphylococcus aureus* and coagulase-negative staphylococci strains: a systematic review and meta-analysis." Antimicrobial Resistance & Infection Control **9**: 1–20.

Sharp, S. E. and C. Searcy (2006). "Comparison of mannitol salt agar and blood agar plates for identification and susceptibility testing of *Staphylococcus aureus* in specimens from cystic fibrosis patients." Journal of Clinical Microbiology **44**(12): 4545–4546.

Siddiqui, A. H. and R. A. Whitten (2018). Methicillin resistant *Staphylococcus aureus* (MRSA). Treasure Island, FL: StatPearls.

Siegel, J. D., E. Rhinehart, M. Jackson, L. Chiarello and the Healthcare Infection Control Practices Advisory Committee (2007). "2007 guideline for isolation precautions: preventing transmission of infectious agents in health care settings." American Journal of Infection Control **35**(10): S65.

Singh, J., S. Mumtaz, S. Joshi and K. Mukhopadhyay (2020). "In vitro and ex vivo efficacy of novel Trp-Arg rich analogue of α-MSH against *Staphylococcus aureus*." ACS Omega **5**(7): 3258–3270.

Singh, M. and K. Mukhopadhyay (2011). "C-terminal amino acids of alpha-melanocyte-stimulating hormone are requisite for its antibacterial activity against *Staphylococcus aureus*." Antimicrobial Agents and Chemotherapy **55**(5): 1920–1929.

Singh, M. and K. Mukhopadhyay (2014). "Alpha-melanocyte stimulating hormone: an emerging anti-inflammatory antimicrobial peptide." BioMed Research International 2014.

Smyth, R. W. and G. Kahlmeter (2005). "Mannitol salt agar-cefoxitin combination as a screening medium for methicillin-resistant *Staphylococcus aureus*." Journal of Clinical Microbiology **43**(8): 3797–3799.

Solomon, F. B., F. W. Wadilo, A. A. Arota and Y. L. Abraham (2017). "Antibiotic resistant airborne bacteria and their multidrug resistance pattern at university teaching referral hospital in South Ethiopia." Annals of Clinical Microbiology and Antimicrobials **16**(1): 29.

Stepanović, S., I. Ćirković, S. Djukić, D. Vuković and M. Švabić-Vlahović (2008). "Public transport as a reservoir of methicillin-resistant staphylococci." Letters in Applied Microbiology **47**(4): 339–341.

Sudharsanam, S., P. Srikanth, S. Krishnamurthy and R. Steinberg (2009). "Microorganisms in bioaerosols in indoor air of hospital and non-hospital settings." Sri Ramachandra Journal of Medicine **2**: 52.

Sudharsanam, S., P. Srikanth, M. Sheela and R. Steinberg (2008). "Study of the indoor air quality in hospitals in South Chennai, India – microbial profile." Indoor and Built Environment **17**(5): 435–441.

Taghizadeh, G., A. S. Delbari and D. K. Kulkarni (2014). "Assessment of airborne pathogens & non pathogens and fungi in healthcare settings Pune India." American Journal of Pharmtech Research 4(6): 1–13.

Tambekar, D. H., P. B. Gulhane and D. D. Bhokare (2007). "Studies on environmental monitoring of microbial air flora in the hospitals." Journal of Medical Science 7(1): 67–72.

Tellier, R., Y. Li, B. J. Cowling and J. W. Tang (2019). "Recognition of aerosol transmission of infectious agents: a commentary." BMC Infectious Diseases 19(1): 101.

Turner, N. A., B. K. Sharma-Kuinkel, S. A. Maskarinec, E. M. Eichenberger, P. P. Shah, M. Carugati, T. L. Holland and V. G. Fowler (2019). "Methicillin-resistant Staphylococcus aureus: an overview of basic and clinical research." Nature Reviews Microbiology 17(4): 203–218.

Tyagi, P. and K. Mukhopadhyay (2012). "Assessment of bio aerosols in rooms of tertiary care hospital in New Delhi, India." Iasta Bulletin 20(1): 461.

US EPA (2013). "Air sanitizers–efficacy data recommendations." Test Guideline No. #OCSPP 810.2500-Air Sanitizers -2013- 03-12[EPA 730-C-11-003]. Available from: www.noticeandcomment.com/-ocspp-810-2500-air-sanitizers-2013-03-12-epa-730-c-11-003-fn-24288.aspx. Accessed December 4, 2015.

Van Kampen, V., F. Hoffmeyer, A. Deckert, B. Kendzia, S. Casjens, H. D. Neumann, M. Buxtrup, E. Willer, C. Felten and R. Schöneich (2016). "Effects of bioaerosol exposure on respiratory health in compost workers: a 13-year follow-up study." Occupational and Environmental Medicine: oemed-2016-103692.

Verkade, E., S. Elberts, C. Verhulst and J. Kluytmans (2009). "Performance of Oxoid Brilliance™ MRSA medium for detection of methicillin-resistant Staphylococcus aureus: an in vitro study." European Journal of Clinical Microbiology & Infectious Diseases 28(12): 1443.

Vinayananda, C. O., S. J. Deepak, A. Rongsensusang, K. Porteen, V. Apparao and B. Dhanalakshmi (2018). "Analysis of microbial quality of the air in meat and dairy plants by impaction technique." Bulletin of Environmental and Pharmacological Life Science 7: 7–13.

Vincent, J.-L. (2003). "Nosocomial infections in adult intensive-care units." The Lancet 361(9374): 2068–2077.

Watkins, R. R., M. Holubar and M. Z. David (2019). "Antimicrobial resistance in methicillin-resistant Staphylococcus aureus to newer antimicrobial agents." Antimicrobial Agents and Chemotherapy 63(12).

Wayne, P. A. (2011). Performance standards for antimicrobial susceptibility testing. Twenty-fourth informational supplement. Wayne, PA: Clinical and Laboratory Standards Institute.

Willeke, K., X. Lin and S. A. Grinshpun (1998). "Improved aerosol collection by combined impaction and centrifugal motion." Aerosol Science and Technology 28(5): 439–456.

Wilson, R. D., S. J. Huang and A. S. McLean (2004). "The correlation between airborne methicillin-resistant Staphylococcus aureus with the presence of MRSA colonized patients in a general intensive care unit." Anaesthesia and Intensive Care 32(2): 202–209.

Xu, Z., Y. Hou, B. M. Peters, D. Chen, B. Li, L. Li and M. E. Shirtliff (2016). "Chromogenic media for MRSA diagnostics." Molecular Biology Reports 43(11): 1205–1212.

Yadav, J., A. Kumar, P. Mahor, A. K. Goel, H. S. Chaudhary, P. K. Yadava, H. Yadav and P. Kumar (2015). "Distribution of airborne microbes and antibiotic susceptibility pattern of bacteria during Gwalior trade fair, Central India." Journal of the Formosan Medical Association **114**(7): 639–646.

Yao, M. and G. Mainelis (2007). "Use of portable microbial samplers for estimating inhalation exposure to viable biological agents." Journal of Exposure Science & Environmental Epidemiology **17**(1): 31–38.

Yates, M. V., Nakatsu, C. H., Miller, R. V. and Pillai, S. D. (2016). Manual of environmental microbiology. Washington, DC: ASM Press.

Zangerl, P. and H. Asperger (2003). Media used in the detection and enumeration of *Staphylococcus aureus*. Progress in Industrial Microbiology **37**: 91–110.

Zhang, K., J.-A. McClure and J. M. Conly (2012). "Enhanced multiplex PCR assay for typing of staphylococcal cassette chromosome mec types I to V in methicillin-resistant *Staphylococcus aureus*." Molecular and Cellular Probes **26**(5): 218–221.

4 Time Series Analysis of Coliform Bacterial Density in the River Ganges as a Potential Indicator of Water Contamination and Associated Risks to Human Health

Pritam Mukherjee*, Sufia Zaman and Abhijit Mitra

CONTENTS

* Corresponding author: Pritam Mukherjee. mukherjee.pritam14@gmail.com

DOI: 10.1201/9781003095422-4

4.1   INTRODUCTION

Over the past few decades, increased anthropogenic activities have caused rapid
environmental alterations associated with adverse impacts on aquatic ecosystems
around the globe and the mighty River Ganges (or Ganga) flowing through India
is no exception. This river (2,525 km long) primarily originates in the Gangotri
glacier (~7,010 m above average sea level) located in the western Himalayan range
of the Indian hilly state of Uttarakhand. It flows down towards the southeast along
the Gangetic Plains of India and Bangladesh, and eventually divides into several
dis/tributaries including Hooghly (in India) and Padma (in Bangladesh) before it
empties into the Bay of Bengal, forming one of the largest estuaries (Hooghly
estuary in the Indian Sundarbans) of the world.

Among the several perennial rivers of India, the River Ganges is considered
one of the most significant as it flows through some of the most densely-populated
cities or regions of India. Like many other metropolitan cities of the world, the
city of Kolkata (the former capital of British India and the present capital of the
eastern maritime state of West Bengal, India) lies on the bank of the mighty River
Ganges or Hooghly as the river is known in this region of the country. The River
Ganges provides lifeline support (including water for irrigation, domestic usage,
and drinking) to several millions of people inhabiting along its course of flow. It
is regarded as a sacred river by the Hindus and worshiped by religious devotees
as goddess Ganga according to Hinduism. However, over the past several decades
the River Ganges has been threatened by severe pollution mostly owing to rapid
urbanization, industrialization, and many other increased anthropogenic activities,
including but not limited to tourism and fishing. Practice of various religious rituals (such as immersion of painted mud idols of Hindu gods and goddesses during
the festival seasons, cremation of dead bodies, religious offerings of burnt ashes of
the deceased/dead bodies, fruit and flowers, bathing activities, etc.) is carried out
throughout the year by several thousands of worshippers/pilgrims along its banks,
which together with daily rituals including laundry (by domestic and launderer's

communities), ferry and freight services, fishing ventures, and touristic activities severely contaminate the river water and surrounding sediments with various organic and inorganic pollutants, including detergents, heavy metals, and hydrocarbons [such as polycyclic aromatic hydrocarbons (PAHs)] (Goswami and Mazumdar 2016; Paul 2017; Srivastava et al. 2017; Kumar et al. 2018; Rakshit and Sarkar 2018). Moreover, numerous industries (including brick kilns, jute mills, tanneries, battery industries, fertilizers and soap factories, oil refineries, thermal power plants, fishery and shrimp farming units) lining this river along with untreated/semi-treated sewage discharge from the several sewage canals connected with this river are additional point sources of organic/inorganic pollutants and coliform bacteria, which eventually contaminate the river and estuarine water of coastal West Bengal (Mitra 1998; Mitra 2013; Biswas et al. 2015; Haritash et al. 2016) (Figure 4.1).

Together, these toxic river water pollutants pose a serious threat not only to humans, but also to endemic faunal communities as the River Ganges is home and breeding ground to ~140 species of fishes and ~90 species of amphibians. The river water also harbors several species of mammals and reptiles, including South Asian river dolphins and critically endangered species like gharials. In addition, the overall health of the river water has a significant influence on the aquatic microflora since the microbes derive their nutrition from the dissolved solids present in

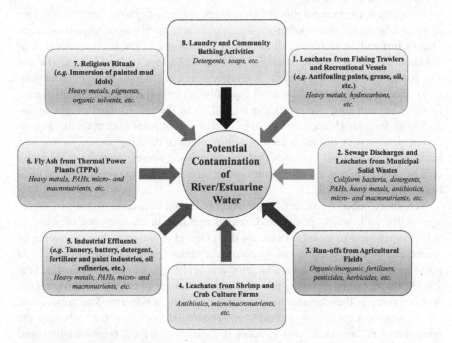

FIGURE 4.1 An overview of the potential point/non-point sources of organic/inorganic pollutants of various anthropogenic origins responsible for river and estuarine water contamination. PAHs, polycyclic aromatic hydrocarbons.

the ambient water and sediments, and the presence of pollutants stimulates microbial growth and proliferation. The load of fecal coliform bacteria originating from human feces in sewage waste in certain locations of the river is a hundred times higher than the Indian Government's official permissible limit. The Ganga Action Plan, an environmental initiative of the Government of India to clean up/purify the river water, is yet to see the light of success for various reasons, including inadequate technical expertise, poor environmental planning, and lack of awareness amongst the people about the numerous ecosystem services provided by this mighty river of the Indian sub-continent.

Various industrial effluents enriched with toxic heavy metals and PAHs, discharge of untreated sewage water containing waste organic matter, run-offs from agricultural fields carrying inorganic fertilizers, pesticides, herbicides, and insecticides, and several other miscellaneous inorganic and organic waste materials are constantly added to this river ecosystem; together they serve as dissolved nutrients for the indigenous microbial communities, thereby promoting their growth and multiplication. A special group of microbes known as coliform bacteria is routinely used as a bioindicator of water contamination/water quality and the associated threats to human health in terms of ensuing diseases, especially of the rural and urban populations whose lives orient around the aquatic or river ecosystems on a day-to-day basis.

Coliform bacteria are a group of rod-shaped, Gram-negative, aerobic and facultative anaerobic, non-spore-forming, motile/non-motile microorganisms capable of fermenting lactose (a disaccharide carbon source) with the formation of acid and gas as end products within 48 hours when kept under 35–37°C (Li and Liu 2018). Besides being present in the environment (such as in soil and vegetation), this special group of bacteria typically inhabits the intestine of all warm-blooded animals and comprises the microflora of the fecal matter of mammals, including humans (Martin et al. 2016). Although coliform bacteria generally do not cause illness or diseases, their presence either in drinking water (ground and surface water) or food indicates that the water/food sources may be at potential risk of contamination by other pathogenic (disease-causing) organisms of fecal origin (Li and Liu 2018).[1]

The entire coliform bacterial population is known as total coliform (TC) (present in the soil, water, plants, and animal and human excreta) out of which a subset is referred to as fecal coliform (FC) (found in the intestines and feces of mammals) and *Escherichia coli* comprises a major fraction of this FC bacterial population (that does not naturally grow and proliferate in the environment) (Pal 2014).[2] Interestingly, *E. coli* is the only known member of the TC bacterial group, which thrives in the mammalian gut, including that of humans. The presence of TC in aquatic ecosystems indicates environmental contamination whereas the presence of FC and/or *E. coli* in water is indicative of fecal contamination, and this may suggest the possible occurrence of other deleterious pathogens like bacteria, fungal/protozoan parasites, and viruses. Hence, among the coliform bacteria FC and *E. coli* are the best bioindicators of fecal contamination and the possible

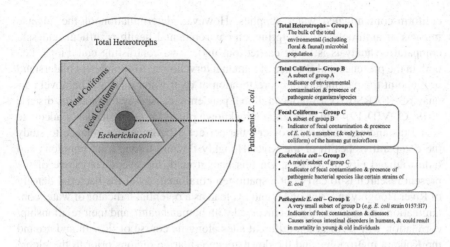

FIGURE 4.2 An overview of the general classification of coliform bacteria in aquatic ecosystems.

occurrence of pathogenic strains. Although most strains of *E. coli* are regarded as harmless, certain rare strains of this bacterial species (particularly *E. coli* strain O157:H7) may cause severe illness (Hamner et al. 2007; Pal 2014).[3] An overview of the general classification of coliform bacteria in aquatic environments is schematically represented in Figure 4.2.

Although recent disease outbreaks due to *E. coli* strain O157:H7 have generated considerable public concern regarding this organism, reports of human cases with *E. coli* O157:H7-mediated disease from contaminated drinking water supplies have been rare since the strain has been mostly associated with poultry and livestock, and most of the reported human cases are because of eating/consumption of undercooked meat (Ameer et al. 2020).

Interestingly, most of the transmissible diseases in the world (about 80%) are waterborne in nature. Based on an estimation by the World Health Organization (WHO), about 80% of water pollution in developing nations like India results from domestic waste and about 70% of the waterbodies in India is severely contaminated. This results in around 75% of disease cases and 80% of the total incidence of child mortality. The ill management of the aquatic ecosystems may give rise to serious problems in the quality of water together with their availability for drinking. Moreover, most bacterial pathogens accountable for waterborne diseases are mainly spread through the fecal–oral/orofecal route where water seems to play an intermediate role (Pal 2014).

In lieu of the current scenario, the present paper addresses the pertinent issue of increased pollutant load in the river and estuarine water as total dissolved solid (TDS), which acts as a nutrient/nutritional boost for the coliforms, thereby causing a hike in their population densities. Hence their proper and timely detection would help to estimate the potential human health hazards associated with using such coliform-contaminated water supplies. However, determination of the adverse impacts of anthropogenic footprints on environmental health is difficult unless a comparative analysis is being carried out under two contrasting conditions, i.e., both in the presence and absence of human interventions, to completely understand or pinpoint the parameters of ecorestoration of river water quality. The novel coronavirus (SARS-CoV-2)-induced global pandemic caused by coronavirus disease 2019 (COVID-19)[4] and concomitant lockdown phase for maintenance of adequate social distancing measures provided the perfect experimental ambience to study the comparative health of the River Hooghly flowing through the populous and industrialized city of Kolkata. On this background, the overall objective of the present research is to carry out a spatio-temporal analysis of the bacterial density of River Hooghly in terms of TC and FC load as a potential indicator of water contamination and associated risks involved with human health, and their relationship/ correlation with TDS at ten different sites along its course of flow in and around the Kolkata metropolis, and the downstream estuarine regions prior to the global COVID-19 pandemic (May 2015–2019) and during the COVID-19-induced lockdown period (May 2020).

4.2   MATERIALS AND METHODS

4.2.1   Sampling of River and Estuarine Water

Water samples from the Hooghly River and estuary were collected periodically in sterilized glass containers using aseptic techniques on a yearly basis with utmost care and caution from ten selected stations located along either the River Hooghly flowing through Kolkata and Howrah districts of West Bengal, India or the Hooghly estuarine region near the fringes of Indian Sundarbans for a period of six years during 2015–2020 in the premonsoon season (i.e., in the middle of the month of May). The selected stations are Ramkrishna Ghat (station 1; 22°34'19.8"N; 88°20'17.0"E), Shibpur Ghat (station 2; 22°33'41.2"N; 88°19'40.4"E), Princep Ghat (station 3; 22°33'30.9"N; 88°19'52.5"E), Botanical Garden (station 4; 22°33'06.4"N; 88°18'06.6"E), Babughat (station 5; 22°34'10.3"N; 88°20'28.5"E), Second Hooghly Bridge (station 6; 22°33'31.4"N; 88°19'38.5"E), Diamond Harbour (station 7; 22°11'04.2"N; 88°11'22.2"E), Namkhana (station 8; 21°45'53.7"N; 88°13'51.5"E), Kakdwip (station 9; 21°52'26.5"N; 88°08'04.5"E), Bakkhali (station 10; 21°34'22.8"N; 88°17'52.1"E), and these have been tabulated in Table 4.1.

The map depicting the selected study sites is shown in Figure 4.3. Interestingly, the time period of water sample collection covers both the pre-COVID-19 pandemic phase and the COVID-19-induced lockdown phase. The collected water samples were quickly transferred to portable ice boxes equipped with airtight lids, and brought to the research laboratory for physico-chemical and microbiological analysis.

TABLE 4.1

The selected study sites along the Hooghly River and estuary with their geographical coordinates

Stations with name and no.	Latitude	Longitude
Ramkrishna Ghat (Station 1)	22°34'19.8"N	88°20'17.0"E
Shibpur Ghat (Station 2)	22°33'41.2"N	88°19'40.4"E
Princep Ghat (Station 3)	22°33'30.9"N	88°19'52.5"E
Botanical Garden (Station 4)	22°33'06.4"N	88°18'06.6"E
Babughat (Station 5)	22°34'10.3"N	88°20'28.5"E
Second Hooghly Bridge (Station 6)	22°33'31.4"N	88°19'38.5"E
Diamond Harbour (Station 7)	22°11'04.2"N	88°11'22.2"E
Namkhana (Station 8)	21°45'53.7"N	88°13'51.5"E
Kakdwip (Station 9)	21°52'26.5"N	88°08'04.5"E
Bakkhali (Station 10)	21°34'22.8"N	88°17'52.1"E

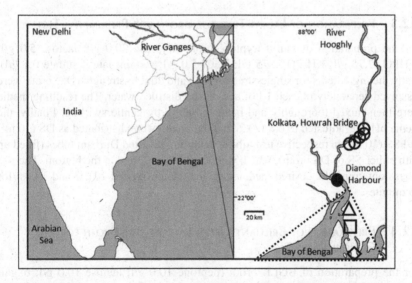

FIGURE 4.3 Map of the study area with selected study sites. The schematic image shows the Hooghly River and estuarine region of coastal West Bengal (a maritime state of India) including Indian Sundarbans with ten selected stations: Ramkrishna Ghat, Shibpur Ghat, Princep Ghat, Botanical Garden, Babughat, Second Hooghly Bridge (stations 1–6, respectively, which lie along the bank of Hooghly River; indicated with open circles), Diamond Harbour, Namkhana, Kakdwip and Bakkhali (stations 7–10, respectively, which lie in the Hooghly estuarine region; indicated with closed circle, open triangle, open square and open rhombus, respectively). The Hooghly estuarine belt is demarcated with dotted lines (modified after Batabyal et al. 2014).

4.2.2 Determination of Total Coliform and Fecal Coliform from Water Samples

The TC and FC loads of the water samples were determined by a multiple-tube fermentation technique (APHA 1998), which comprises a three-stage procedure where the results are expressed statistically in terms of most probable number (MPN).[5] The technique involves inoculating the sampled water in a liquid culture medium of lauryl tryptose broth; this is a selective medium used for the identification of coli-aerogenes bacteria present in water (Corry et al. 2003). After incubation, the tubes were assessed for bacterial growth as well as acid and gas production by the coliforms. This is known as a presumptive test. Since bacteria other than the coliforms can also produce acid and gas, all positive tubes from the presumptive test were further subjected to a confirmatory test. The bacterial density was estimated based on the combination of positive and negative tubes. The results obtained were finally expressed in MPN/100 ml (APHA 1998; Surendran et al. 2006). The TC and FC were determined using lauryl tryptose broth, brilliant green lactose bile (BGLB) broth, and *Escherichia coli* (EC) broth.

4.2.3 Preparation of Lauryl Tryptose Broth for Presumptive Test

For the preparation of lauryl tryptose broth (tryptose 20.0 g/l; lactose 5.0 g/l; K_2HPO_4 2.75 g/l; KH_2PO_4 2.75 g/l; NaCl 5.0 g/l; sodium lauryl sulfate 0.1 g/l), firstly the ingredients for single-strength (SS) and double-strength (DS) broth were dissolved separately in each 1 l of autoclaved distilled water. The resulting media were then mixed thoroughly and heated slightly by gentle swirling. Finally, the media pH was adjusted to 6.8 ± 0.2, and the media were distributed as DS (10 ml) and SS (10 ml) in respective test tubes containing inverted Durham tubes (filled up with either SS or DS broth), which were carefully inserted at the bottom. The test tubes containing the desired media were then autoclaved at 121°C and 15 psi for 15 minutes.

4.2.4 Preparation of Brilliant Green Lactose Bile Broth for Confirmatory Test

For the preparation of BGLB broth (peptone 10.0 g/l; lactose 10.0 g/l; oxgall 20.0 g/l; brilliant green 0.0133 g/l), firstly the ingredients were dissolved in 1 l of sterilized distilled water, and then the following medium was mixed thoroughly and heated slightly by gentle swirling. The pH of the medium was then adjusted to 6.8 ± 0.2. Finally, 10 ml of broth was distributed in each of the test tubes with an inverted Durham tube (filled up with the same medium) placed at the bottom, and the test tubes were sterilized in the autoclave at 121°C and 15 psi for 15 minutes.

4.2.5 PREPARATION OF EC BROTH FOR FECAL COLIFORM

For the preparation of EC broth (tryptose 20.0 g/l; lactose 5.0 g/l; bile salts 1.5 g/l; K_2HPO_4 4.0 g/l; KH_2PO_4 1.5 g/l), at first the ingredients were dissolved in 1 l of sterile distilled water by thorough mixing and slight heating with occasional swirling. The pH of the medium was then adjusted to 6.8 ± 0.2, after which the broth was distributed in test tubes (10 ml each) with inverted Durham tubes filled up with the same medium. The tubes were then sterilized at 121°C and 15 psi for 15 minutes.

4.2.6 PRESUMPTIVE TEST FOR THE DETECTION OF TOTAL COLIFORM IN WATER SAMPLES

For presumptive test of TC, lauryl tryptose broth was used as the culture medium. For analysis of sampled water, three sets of five test tubes with each set containing 10 ml, 1 ml, and 0.1 ml of sample were used for the presumptive test. The first set consists of five tubes each with 10 ml DS broth. The second and third sets contain ten tubes, each with 10 ml SS broth. Each tube in a set of five containing 10 ml, 1 ml, and 0.1 ml of water samples was inoculated into the first, second, and third sets of media tubes, respectively, and mixed thoroughly. In each case, a control set was also run in parallel. The inoculated test tubes were then incubated at 36 ± 1°C. After 24 hours of incubation, the tubes were examined for bacterial growth, acid and gas production. In the absence of acid and gas production, the tubes were further incubated and examined again after 48 hours. Within each tube, an inverted Durham tube (filled up with the respective medium) was placed at the bottom to demonstrate bacterial growth with emission of gas. Bacterial growth with production of acid and trapped gas bubbles within the Durham tubes within 48 hours of incubation constitutes a presumptive reaction. After 48 hours, the numbers of positive tubes were counted and finally proceeded for the confirmatory test.

4.2.7 CONFIRMATORY TEST FOR THE DETECTION OF TOTAL COLIFORM IN WATER SAMPLES

For confirmatory test of TC, the culture medium used was BGLB broth. The positive presumptive test tubes were gently shaken, and a loop full of culture was taken with a sterile inoculation loop (3.0–3.5 mm in diameter) and transferred to test tubes containing 10 ml BGLB broth with inverted Durham tubes (each filled up with the same medium) placed at the bottom. After inoculation, the culture tubes were incubated at 36 ± 1°C. Formation of gas bubbles with bacterial growth within 48 hours of incubation constitutes a confirmatory test. The results were obtained by comparing with a standard MPN table and expressed in MPN/100 ml.

4.2.8 Determination of Fecal Coliform from Water Samples

For enumeration of FC, inocula from 24-hour positive presumptive test tubes were transferred aseptically to tubes containing EC broth. These culture tubes were incubated overnight at $44.0 \pm 0.5°C$ and finally examined for the presence of bacterial growth along with production of gas. Results were expressed in MPN/100 ml.

4.2.9 Determination of Total Dissolved Solid from Water Samples

TDS from river and estuarine water samples was determined by filtering a measured volume of water samples through standard glass fiber filters. The filtrates were then transferred to pre-weighed glass/ceramic containers placed on a drying oven set at 103–105°C. High temperature results in rapid evaporation of the filtered water samples and eventually complete drying of the solid residues on the containers. The increase in weight of the containers represents the TDS of the water samples.

4.2.10 Statistical Analysis

Analyses of water samples for the determination of TDS, TC, and FC were done in triplicates. Two-way analysis of variance (ANOVA) was performed to assess whether the different hydrological parameters, namely TC, FC, and TDS, varied significantly between stations and years. p value < 0.01 is considered to be statistically significant. Correlation coefficients were performed to determine the interrelationship between bacterial load (TC and FC) and TDS. The graphs were generated using GraphPad Prism Software 7 (San Diego, CA, USA). All statistical analyses were carried out using SPSS software version 21.0 for Windows (SPSS Inc., USA).

4.3 RESULTS

4.3.1 Spatio-Temporal Analyses of Total Coliform, Fecal Coliform, and Total Dissolved Solid Load

The river and estuarine water samples were aseptically collected from ten different study sites/stations (station 1–station 10) during the premonsoon season from May 2015 to May 2020 for comparative/spatio-temporal analyses of TC, FC, and TDS load in the River Ganges/Hooghly (flowing through the metropolitan city of Kolkata and Howrah) and the Hooghly estuary. The results obtained are represented graphically in Figures 4.4–4.6.

The temporal variations in the average TC and FC matrices (in × 10^3 MPN/ 100 ml) between ten stations during the pre-COVID-19 pandemic period (i.e., May 2015–May 2019) and COVID-19-induced lockdown phase (i.e., May 2020) exhibited the order 2019 (TC = 14.44 ± 6.45; FC = 7.69 ± 2.68) > 2018 (TC = 12.35 ± 5.27; FC = 7.31 ± 2.59) > 2016 (TC = 10.93 ± 5.04; FC = 6.91 ± 2.53) > 2017 (TC = 10.19 ± 4.34; FC = 6.67 ± 2.43) > 2015 (TC = 9.67 ± 4.06;

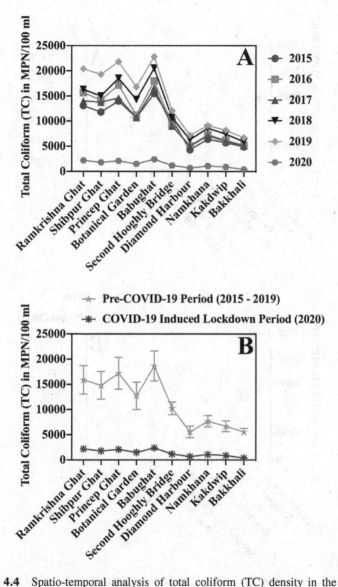

FIGURE 4.4 Spatio-temporal analysis of total coliform (TC) density in the Hooghly River and estuarine water during premonsoon season. (A) TC load during the period of 2015–2020 at ten different study sites. (B) Comparison of TC load during the pre-COVID-19 pandemic period and COVID-19-induced lockdown phase. Each symbol represents the mean of triplicate values. Error bars represent the standard deviation from the mean value of five years (2015–2019) irrespective of the study sites.

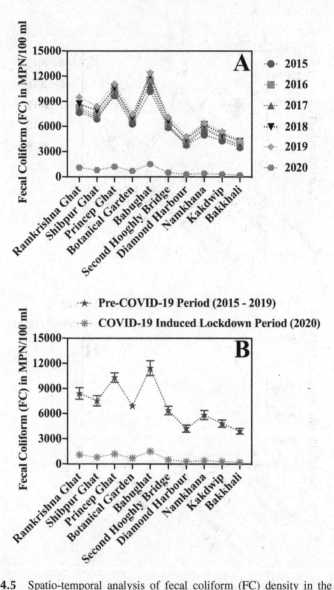

FIGURE 4.5 Spatio-temporal analysis of fecal coliform (FC) density in the Hooghly River and estuarine water during premonsoon season. (A) FC load during the period of 2015–2020 at ten different study sites. (B) Comparison of FC load during the pre-COVID-19 pandemic period and COVID-19-induced lockdown phase. Each symbol represents the mean of triplicate values. Error bars represent the standard deviation from the mean value of five years (2015–2019) irrespective of the study sites.

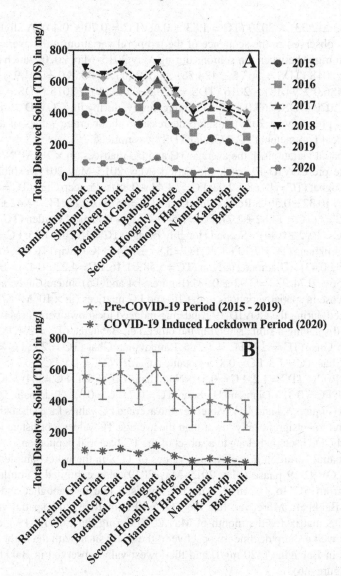

FIGURE 4.6 Spatio-temporal analysis of total dissolved solid (TDS) content in the Hooghly River and estuarine water during premonsoon season. (A) TDS content during 2015–2020 at ten different study sites. (B) Comparison of TDS content during the pre-COVID-19 pandemic period and COVID-19-induced lockdown phase. Each symbol represents the mean of triplicate values. Error bars represent the standard deviation from the mean value of five years (2015–2019) irrespective of the study sites.

FC = 6.33 ± 2.33) > 2020 (TC = 1.43 ± 0.68; FC = 0.70 ± 0.44). A slight alteration was observed in the sequence of the temporal variation in the average TDS
matrix (in mg/l) between ten stations during May 2015–May 2020, which follows
the order 2018 (TDS = 563.5 ± 128.56) > 2019 (TDS = 558.0 ± 101.93) > 2017
(TDS = 486.0 ± 94.13) > 2016 (TDS = 420.5 ± 112.88) > 2015 (TDS = 307.5 ±
95.69) > 2020 (TDS = 63.0 ± 35.45). Interestingly, during the COVID-19-induced
lockdown phase (May 2020), a sharp decrease in the average values of all three
hydrological parameters (TC, FC, and TDS) was noticed.

The spatial variations in the average TC and FC matrices (in × 10^3 MPN/100 ml)
during the pre-COVID-19 pandemic period (May 2015–May 2019) exhibited the
order Babughat (TC = 18.68 ± 2.97; FC = 11.44 ± 0.88) > Princep Ghat (TC = 17.22 ±
3.16; FC = 10.32 ± 0.56) > Ramkrishna Ghat (TC = 15.90 ± 2.82; FC = 8.42 ± 0.70) >
Shibpur Ghat (TC = 14.82 ± 2.77; FC = 7.54 ± 0.61) > Botanical Garden (TC = 12.74
± 2.72; FC = 6.92 ± 0.44) > Second Hooghly Bridge (TC = 10.26 ± 1.25; FC = 6.38 ±
0.51) > Namkhana (TC = 7.70 ± 1.12; FC = 5.84 ± 0.54) > Kakdwip (TC = 6.70 ± 1.06;
FC = 4.82 ± 0.43) > Diamond Harbour (TC = 5.58 ± 1.16; FC = 4.22 ± 0.42) > Bakkhali
(TC = 5.56 ± 0.74; FC = 3.92 ± 0.33) (Figures 4.4 and 4.5). Interestingly, a significant decrease in spatial variations in the TC and FC matrices (in × 10^3 MPN/100 ml)
was noticed during the COVID-19 pandemic-induced lockdown period (May 2020),
although displaying a similar trend in the order, i.e., Babughat (TC = 2.4; FC = 1.5)
> Princep Ghat (TC = 2.1; FC = 1.2) > Ramkrishna Ghat (TC = 2.2; FC = 1.1) >
Shibpur Ghat (TC = 1.8; FC = 0.8) > Botanical Garden (TC = 1.5; FC = 0.7) > Second
Hooghly Bridge (TC = 1.2; FC = 0.5) > Namkhana (TC = 1.1; FC = 0.4) > Kakdwip
(TC = 0.9; FC = 0.3) > Diamond Harbour (TC = 0.7; FC = 0.3) > Bakkhali (TC = 0.4;
FC = 0.2) (Figures 4.4 and 4.5). Moreover, the average FC values for each station/year
were found to be significantly lower than the average TC values, consistent with the
fact that the FC bacteria belong to a subset of the TC bacterial population.

The spatial variation in the average values of TDS in the water samples during
the pre-COVID-19 phase (May 2015–May 2019) also exhibited a similar trend
ranging from 612 to 316 mg/l, with the highest value in Babughat and lowest
value in Bakkhali. Moreover, like the TC and FC matrices, the spatial variation
in the TDS matrix for the month of May 2020 during the COVID-19 lockdown
phase showed a sharp decline irrespective of the study sites, with the highest value
observed in Babughat (120 mg/l) and the lowest value observed in Bakkhali (15
mg/l) (Figure 4.6).

4.3.2 ANOVA Showing Spatio-Temporal Variations in the Selected Hydrological Parameters

ANOVA results show significant spatio-temporal variations of TC, FC, and TDS
load in the Hooghly River/estuarine water with a p value < 0.0001, as shown in
Table 4.2, which may have been attributed to the different anthropogenic activities to which the selected stations are exposed, thereby conferring a differential
pollution level to each station under study.

TABLE 4.2
Analysis of variance (ANOVA) showing the variations of total coliform (TC), fecal coliform (FC), and total dissolved solid (TDS) load between stations and years in the Hooghly River and estuarine water collected during the premonsoon season of 2015–2020

Factor	Variable	F_{cal}	F_{crit}	p value
TC load (in water samples)	Between stations	26.86863695	2.095755094	$p < 0.0001$
	Between years	48.59844723	2.422085466	$p < 0.0001$
FC load (in water samples)	Between stations	37.5564211	2.095755094	$p < 0.0001$
	Between years	90.86868462	2.422085466	$p < 0.0001$
TDS load (in water samples)	Between stations	49.18070535	2.095755094	$p < 0.0001$
	Between years	333.9803444	2.422085466	$p < 0.0001$

$p < 0.0001$ = statistically significant

4.3.3 CORRELATION BETWEEN THE SELECTED HYDROLOGICAL PARAMETERS

Furthermore, the TC and FC values between stations at each given year showed a direct/positive correlation with the respective TDS values, as depicted in Table 4.3, thereby confirming the regulatory roles of waste materials and dissolved solids on coliform bacterial counts in the water samples of the study sites.

4.4 DISCUSSION

The River Hooghly, a tributary of the River Ganges (which has its origin in the Gangotri glacier in the northwestern part of India), flows through Kolkata, the capital city of the maritime Indian state of West Bengal, and empties in the Bay of Bengal through the Hooghly estuary. It forms an integral part of the city's urban population, and several industries (including aquaculture sectors) and domestic lives are heavily dependent on this perennial freshwater source. However, various anthropogenic inputs, like untreated industrial effluents, sewage discharge, agricultural run-offs, remnants of religious rituals, and tourism, not only contaminate the river water with toxic heavy metals, pesticides/insecticides, herbicides, inorganic fertilizers, antibiotics, and PAHs, but also increase the overall TDS or nutrient level of the water, thereby facilitating/promoting microbial growth including that of the coliform group of bacteria (Mitra 2019). The estuarine region of the River Hooghly, which provides a perfect habitat (i.e., brackish water ecosystem) and breeding ground for several commercially important variety of finfish, shellfish, and edible crustaceans, is also burdened with uncontrolled fishing activities from India and Bangladesh alike. The numerous fishing trawlers and vessels that operate

TABLE 4.3
The results of correlation coefficient analysis between total coliform (TC), fecal coliform (FC), and total dissolved solid (TDS) in the Hooghly River and estuarine water samples collected during the premonsoon season of 2015–2020

Year	Combination	r value	p value
2015	TC × TDS	0.990553	$p < 0.001$
	FC × TDS	0.974273	$p < 0.001$
	TC × FC	0.963983	$p < 0.001$
2016	TC × TDS	0.983788	$p < 0.001$
	FC × TDS	0.970604	$p < 0.001$
	TC × FC	0.961395	$p < 0.001$
2017	TC × TDS	0.975244	$p < 0.001$
	FC × TDS	0.969596	$p < 0.001$
	TC × FC	0.952910	$p < 0.001$
2018	TC × TDS	0.986235	$p < 0.001$
	FC × TDS	0.939471	$p < 0.001$
	TC × FC	0.970800	$p < 0.001$
2019	TC × TDS	0.991264	$p < 0.001$
	FC × TDS	0.964457	$p < 0.001$
	TC × FC	0.951077	$p < 0.001$
2020	TC × TDS	0.984626	$p < 0.001$
	FC × TDS	0.978118	$p < 0.001$
	TC × FC	0.968158	$p < 0.001$

$p < 0.001$ = statistically significant

in this area add significant amounts of heavy metals, namely zinc (Zn), copper (Cu), and lead (Pb), mainly due to the heavy-metal-rich antifouling paints, which are used to coat the bottom of these wooden vessels.

Although the gradual rise of industries and human interventions has an adverse effect on the overall health of aquatic ecosystems, it is congenial for the growth and proliferation of microbial communities as the latter obtain various types of nutrition from these industrial and sewage discharges. Moreover, in developing nations like India where sewage wastes are mostly discharged without adequate/proper treatment, the river water upon receiving the untreated/semi-treated sewage water from the canals [e.g., the dry weather flow (DWF) and storm weather flow (SWF) canals running through the city of Kolkata] that are connected with the river is contaminated with human fecal matter as well (Strauss 1996). Literature on the growth and proliferation of microbes in the context of increasing pollution is available worldwide, and the present study area with a massive quantum of solid and liquid waste materials is a suitable experimental bed for rapid microbial growth and proliferation [especially the coliform group of bacteria (i.e., the TCs and FCs) and the bacterial pathogens of fecal origin like certain strains of *E. coli*]. Consistent with this idea, we found a direct correlation of TC and FC load with TDS in the present study area.

In addition, a small subset of FC is *E. coli*, some strains of which are even known human pathogens like *E. coli* serotype O157:H7 and which could cause intestinal disorders (including hemorrhagic colitis and hemolytic-uremic syndrome (HUS), characterized by bloody diarrhea) associated with mortality in young and elderly individuals (Nataro and Kaper 1998; Ameer et al. 2020). It is noteworthy that one such strain was isolated from River Ganges by Hamner et al. (2007). Although drinking water or food contaminated with coliform bacteria does not necessarily cause an illness, if pathogenic bacterial strains of *E. coli* are present, the most common symptoms could include gastrointestinal problems and general flu-like symptoms such as fever, abdominal cramps, and diarrhea.

The spatial variations in TDS and the coliform bacterial load (i.e., TC and FC) may be attributed to the uneven distribution of industries, sewage disposal, tourism, ferry services, fishing ventures, bathing activities, and practice of religious rituals along the course of the River Hooghly. The study stations situated near the city of Kolkata with huge industrial and other anthropogenic pressure have more TDS load while those which are away from the city (i.e., the stations in the estuarine region) have comparatively much less TDS load, which in turn dictates and is reflected in the relative abundance of TC and FC bacterial densities in these stations under investigation. Moreover, the relatively high TDS, TC, and FC values at Namkhana and Kakdwip may be attributed to the large-scale fish landing activities in these stations.

The global pandemic caused by the novel coronavirus-mediated COVID-19 had led to a worldwide lockdown, starting in March 2020 in India. The Indian metropolis including Kolkata was no exception. Interestingly, the global pandemic-induced lockdown had a positive impact on overall environmental health. Monitoring of the temporal variations in hydrological parameters such as the TC, FC, and TDS load over a period of six years (2015–2020) revealed that the COVID-19-induced lockdown phase during May 2020 greatly improved the quality of the Hooghly River and estuarine water. The sharp decline in TDS content, and subsequent reduction in the TC and FC load, in the water of the Hooghly River and Hooghly estuary during the lockdown phase may be a direct consequence of reduced/non-functioning of various industrial units, water traffic, and tourism along with reduction in industrial/household waste disposal, fishing maneuvers, community bathing, and religious rituals along the banks of the River Hooghly and the estuarine belts, which together limit/minimize the influx of additional nutrient supplies for these coliform bacterial communities.

Taken together, the overall findings of the present research study have shed light on the significance of lockdown-induced reduction in human interventions of the surrounding aquatic environments (i.e., the Hooghly River and estuary in this case), thereby drastically improving river and estuarine water quality in terms of dissolved solids/nutrients (i.e., waste materials) and microbial densities.

4.5   CONCLUSIONS

Over the past few decades, increased anthropogenic activities including unplanned urbanization, industrialization, and tourism have caused rapid changes in river water ecosystems around the globe. In this context, the present research work documents a spatio-temporal analysis of coliform bacterial density in the Hooghly River/estuary in India for a span of six years during the premonsoon season as a potential bioindicator of water contamination and the associated risks to human health, especially of the tribal, rural, and urban populace whose lives orient around the freshwater and brackish water ecosystems. The present study has led to a few important findings, as listed here:

1.   We found that spatial variations in the TC and FC matrices exhibited the order Babughat > Princep Ghat > Ramkrishna Ghat > Shibpur Ghat > Botanical Garden > Second Hooghly Bridge > Namkhana > Kakdwip > Diamond Harbour > Bakkhali.
2.   The TDS also displayed a similar trend, which confirms the regulatory roles of waste materials and dissolved solids on the bacterial densities in the water of the study sites, thereby establishing a direct correlation of TDS with TC and FC.
3.   The elevated TC and FC load in some of the stations under study may have direct implications for human health as a subset of the FCs could be pathogenic in nature, and therefore, could cause enteric diseases in humans.
4.   The sudden drop in TDS, TC, and FC values during May 2020 coincides with the coronavirus-mediated global pandemic and the subsequent COVID-19-induced lockdown period irrespective of the ten stations under study.

4.6   PROPOSED MITIGATING MEASURES

We propose a few mitigating measures that could be undertaken at private, public, and/or government level(s) to control the contamination of the River Ganges water and potential human health hazards, which include: (1) release of treated industrial waste; (2) appropriate treatment of sewage wastes before their discharge into the river water; (3) prohibition of community or public bathing; (4) regulation of religious ritual activities in river water; (5) controlled anthropogenic ventures like fishing, ferrying, water freight, water sports, etc.; (6) routine monitoring of water quality with respect to several physico-chemical parameters, including temperature, pH, salinity, dissolved oxygen, TDS, etc.; (7) periodic microbial analysis (overall coliform load) of river water; (8) occasional monitoring of the microbio-logical health of edible aquatic organisms like freshwater/brackish water fishes, shrimps, oysters, and crabs; (9) prevention of excessive run-off of rain water carrying nutrients that are rich in nitrates and phosphates from nearby agricultural fields; and (10) introduction of coliphages (bacteriophages that could kill coliform bacteria such as *E. coli*) with in-depth environmental impact assessment, although such bacteria-eating viruses have already been found in plenty in the Ganges water.

4.7 CHALLENGES AND FUTURE PERSPECTIVES

Funding from the government, public, and/or private sectors is required to undertake the River Ganges clean-up project(s) and their proper execution in a coordinated and timely fashion. Tracking and identifying the point and non-point sources of river water contamination, and sanctioning funds for establishing infrastructure of sewage treatment plants are the need of the hour. More research with special emphasis on the analysis of microbiological health of the river/estuarine water and associated edible aquatic fauna should be done to track, document, and spread awareness among the public who are daily more exposed to coliform bacteria-contaminated water and food, since some pathogenic species of *E. coli* can result in fatal outcomes in humans. In addition, the presence of heavy metals and antibiotics in polluted water can cause the emergence of novel multi-drug-resistant and mul-tiple heavy-metal-resistant bacterial strains, which would pose serious challenges in future disease therapeutics. However, in a densely populated and developing nation like India, where out of around 130 crore people only about 74% are literate, spreading public awareness and their proper execution, and practice of personal hygiene measures/restoration of environmental health seem to be a far-fetched idea without developing stringent laws and policies, and the involvement of strict regu-latory bodies, environmentalists, researchers, and policy makers.

NOTES

1   www.health.ny.gov/environmental/water/drinking/coliform_bacteria.htm.
2   www.health.ny.gov/environmental/water/drinking/coliform_bacteria.htm.
3   www.health.ny.gov/environmental/water/drinking/coliform_bacteria.htm.
4   www.who.int/emergencies/diseases/novel-coronavirus-2019.
5   www.epa.gov/sites/production/files/2015-12/documents/9131.

REFERENCES

Ameer, M. A., Wasey, A., and P. Salen. 2020. *Escherichia coli* (*E. coli* O157 H7). StatPearls, NCBI Bookshelf. www.ncbi.nlm.nih.gov/books/NBK507845/ (October 30, 2020).
APHA. 1998. *Standard methods for the examination of water and wastewater*. Washington, DC: American Public Health Association, American Water Works Association and Water Environmental Federation.
Batabyal, P., Einsporn, M. H., Mookerjee, S., Palit, A., Neogi, S. B., Nair, G. B., and R. J. Lara. 2014. Influence of hydrologic and anthropogenic factors on the abundance

variability of enteropathogens in the Ganges estuary, a cholera endemic region. *Sci. Total Environ.* 472: 154–161.

Biswas, K., Paul, D., and S. N. Sinha. 2015. Prevalence of multiple antibiotic-resistant coliform bacteria in the water of river Ganga. *Front. Environ. Microbiol.* 1:44–6.

Corry, J. E. L., Curtis, G. D. W., and R. M. Baird. (Eds.) 2003. Lauryl tryptose broth. In *Progress in industrial microbiology, Handbook of culture media for food microbiology*, 499–500. Amsterdam: Elsevier Science.

Goswami, K., and I. Mazumdar. 2016. How idol immersion is polluting the Ganga River in Kolkata, West Bengal: An overview. *Ind. J. Appl. Res.* 6(10): 460–462.

Hamner, S., Broadaway, S. C., Mishra, V. B. et al. 2007. Isolation of potentially pathogenic *Escherichia coli* O157: H7 from the Ganges River. *Appl. Environ. Microbiol.* 73(7): 2369–2372.

Haritash, A. K., Gaur, S., and S. Garg. 2016. Assessment of water quality and suitability analysis of River Ganga in Rishikesh, India. *Appl. Water Sci.* 6(4): 383–392.

Kumar, V., Kumar, S., Srivastava, S., Singh, J., and P. Kumar. 2018. Water quality of River Ganga with reference to physico-chemical and microbiological characteristics during Kanwar Mela 2017, at Haridwar, India: A case study. *Arch. Agric. Environ. Sci.* 3(1): 58–63.

Li, D., and S. Liu. 2018. *Water quality monitoring and management: Basis, technology and case studies*. Cambridge: Academic Press.

Martin, N. H., Trmčić, A., Hsieh, T. H., Boor, K. J., and M. Wiedmann. 2016. The evolving role of coliforms as indicators of unhygienic processing conditions in dairy foods. *Front. Microbiol.* 7:1–8.

Mitra, A. 1998. Status of coastal pollution in West Bengal with special reference to heavy metals. *J. Ind. Ocean Studies* 5(2): 135–138.

Mitra, A. 2013. *Sensitivity of mangrove ecosystem to changing climate*. New Delhi: Springer India.

Mitra, A. 2019. *Estuarine pollution in the Lower Gangetic Delta: Threats and management*. Cham: Springer International Publishing.

Nataro, J. P., and J. B. Kaper. 1998. Diarrheagenic *Escherichia coli*. *Clin. Microbiol. Rev.* 11: 142–201.

Pal, P. 2014. Detection of coliforms in drinking water and its effect on human health – A review. *Int. Lett. Nat. Sci.* 17: 122–131.

Paul, D. 2017. Research on heavy metal pollution of river Ganga: A review. *Ann. Agrar. Sci.* 15(2): 278–286.

Rakshit, D., and S. K. Sarkar. 2018. Idol immersion and its adverse impact on water quality and plankton community in Hooghly (Ganges) River Estuary, India: Implications for conservation management. *Ind. J. Mar. Sci.* 47(09): 1870–1879.

Srivastava, P., Sreekrishnan, T. R., and A. K. Nema. 2017. Human health risk assessment and PAHs in a stretch of river Ganges near Kanpur. *Environ. Monit. Assess.* 189(9): 445.

Strauss, M. 1996. Health (pathogen) considerations regarding the use of human waste in aquaculture. *Environ. Res. Forum* 5(6): 83–98.

Surendran, P., Thampuran, K. N., Narayanannambiar, V., and K. V. Lalitha. 2006. *Laboratory manual on microbiological examination of seafood*. Cochin: Central Institute of Fisheries Technology (CIFT).

5 Evaluation of Health Quality in Two Studied Groups of School Children from an Arsenic-Exposed Area of West Bengal, India

*Antara Das, Madhurima Joardar,
Nilanjana Roy Chowdhury and
Tarit Roychowdhury**

CONTENTS

* Corresponding author: Tarit Roychowdhury. rctarit@yahoo.com; tarit.roychowdhury@ jadavpuruniversity.in

DOI: 10.1201/9781003095422-5

5.1 INTRODUCTION

Groundwater arsenic (As) contamination is a prolonged indelible threat to the population of Ganga Meghna Brahmaputra (GMB) plain, especially West Bengal, India. For years, several districts like Malda, Murshidabad, Nadia, North and South 24 Paraganas have been suffering from As poisoning: an area of approximately 38,861 km^2 is highly As-contaminated (Santra et al., 2013). The contamination mainly originates from the release of As from natural geological sources into aquifers by redox reactions with As-containing minerals or alluvial sediments at various hydro-geochemical conditions (Nickson et al., 2000). With time, it is understood that people are being exposed to As toxicity from As-contaminated foodstuffs along with contaminated drinking water (Roychowdhury et al., 2002, 2003; Roychowdhury, 2008). A huge amount of As is accumulated in rice grains and vegetables in As-endemic areas from contaminated irrigational water (Bhattacharya et al., 2010; Chowdhury et al., 2018a, 2018b). Prolonged consumption of As-contaminated rice can bring a serious health risk in the future, as has been reported in many recent articles (Chowdhury et al., 2020; Joardar et al., 2021).

It is widely known that being a group I carcinogen, chronic As exposure causes serious health problems, including cancer. In highly endemic areas, every year numerous patients who have been identified as having been exposed to As have had skin carcinoma (Chowdhury et al., 2000; Mazumder et al., 1998). Continuous intake of As for a short period of time may cause abdominal pain, diarrhea, or vomiting, while the most familiar manifestations of chronic As exposure are lung dysfunction, persistent cough, obstetric problems, thickening of the skin, hyperpigmentation, keratosis, and melanosis (Rahman et al., 2009; Ratnaike, 2003).

It is not only adults who are affected; reports say that, worldwide, children, infants, and young adults are also facing a future health risk of cancer due to consumption of contaminated drinking water (Baig et al., 2016; Brahman et al., 2016; Singh and Ghosh, 2012). Even a low level of As exposure can prove to be a health risk in children with many disorders (Biswas et al., 2018). Recently, children of endemic areas of West Bengal (Gaighata, North 24 Paraganas district) have been sub-clinically affected and have a substantial future cancer risk (Joardar et al., 2021). Earlier, children aged <9 years from South 24 Paraganas, West Bengal, India were reported with skin pigmentation and keratosis after As exposure, although to a lower degree compared to adults (Mazumder et al., 1998). Children from Bangladesh (age: 4–15 years) were also reported with dermatological symptoms due to consumption of As-contaminated drinking water (Rahman et al., 2001; Watanabe et al., 2007). The effects of acute or chronic As exposure on children throughout the world include slow growth rate, weight loss, impaired intelligence, and loss of memory due to (Calderon et al., 2001; Wasserman et al., 2004, 2007, 2011, 2018; Wright et al., 2006). As exposure may also have affected the cognitive function of children aged 68 years in Mexico (Rosado et al., 2007). Children with prenatal and early-life As exposure (> 500 µg/l in drinking water) were observed to have pulmonary difficulties in Bangladesh (Smith et al., 2013). In utero As exposure also caused a reduction in the thymic development of children with increasing morbidity in Bangladesh (Raqib et al., 2009). Enhanced mortality due to different forms of malignancy was also reported in young adults with in utero and childhood As exposure in Chile (Smith et al., 2012). In addition, in developing and under-developed countries, malnutrition of children influences As toxicity and reduces their quality of health (Calderon et al., 2001; Milton et al., 2004; Rahman et al., 2001).

In human systems, the mechanism of As in terms of toxicity is still the subject of research. However, it is reported that inorganic As is more toxic than its other metabolites; methylarsonic acid (MMA), dimethylarsinic acid (DMA), and the methylated forms of As are more readily excreted than inorganic As (Concha et al., 1998). The metabolism system results in elimination of half of ingested As in the urine in 3–5 days. DMA is the dominant urinary metabolite (60–70%) in comparison to MMA while a small amount of inorganic As is also excreted directly (Hopenhaynrich et al., 1993; Ratnaike 2003). Another report says that approximately 60–90% of soluble inorganic As components is absorbed through the gastrointestinal tract (Hall, 2002). Around 50–70% of absorbed As is eliminated by the kidneys by methylation and the rest accumulates in hair, nail, and other tissues (Nielsen, 2001).

While urinary As is a good biomarker for recent exposure (Nermell et al., 2008; Vahter, 1994), evaluation of As in hair and nail tissues is the best way to measure chronic As exposure (Brima et al., 2006; Rahman et al., 2001; Samanta et al., 2004). Hair tissues accumulate considerably greater amounts of As than other biological samples due to keratin proteins which constitute sulfur-containing amino acids (Byrne et al., 2010; Gault et al., 2008). Therefore, in children where skin manifestation from As toxicity is obscure, sub-acute or sub-clinical toxicity is assessed through the biomarkers.

The present study aims to estimate the current health status of two different age groups of school children from an As-affected area in the Nadia district of West Bengal. On the basis of As concentration in drinking water and rice grain, the daily dietary intake of As in children will be evaluated in comparison to the provisional tolerable daily intake (PTDI) value. The health exposure will be investigated by examining the As concentration in their biological samples (hair, nail, and urine) and the corresponding interrelations with As intake. Consequently, the lifetime cancer and non-cancer risk of the children will be assessed to make a note of awareness for the young generation of the study area. The focus of the study lies in the extent of As exposure in the school children and whether it has any impact on age. To the best of our knowledge, this type of comparative study on two different age groups of children in a single zone will be a new attempt of work in Nadia.

5.2 MATERIALS AND METHODS

5.2.1 STUDY AREA

The study area of the work has been selected from an As-affected zone under Haringhata Municipality, located in the Nadia district of West Bengal. Our earlier report had already stated that groundwater from all 17 blocks of Nadia district is

As-contaminated, which corroborated other previous findings (Das et al., 2020; Rahman et al., 2014; Roychowdhury et al., 2008). A water quality index (WQI) study by Das et al. (2020) has also informed that approximately 66% of the groundwater sample of this district is not recommended for drinking and other domestic purposes. Haringhata (latitude: 22.95°N, longitude: 88.57°E), a municipal town under Haringhata block, Nadia, has a total population of 3,989 (Census of India, 2011). It is important to mention that Haringhata block is one of the most As-affected community development blocks in the whole district: around 58.4% of a groundwater sample was found to have a higher As concentration than the permissible limit, 10 µg/l (Rahman et al., 2014). Apart from drinking water, crops and vegetables are also As-affected (Biswas et al., 2012; Roychowdhury et al., 2008; Sarkar et al., 2016). Two different age groups of school children (9–10 years, Laupala Kalpataru Primary School and 14–15 years, Laupala Kalpataru High School respectively) from the same locality were chosen as the subject of the study.

5.2.2 Sample Collection, Preparation, and Preservation

Initially the drinking water samples from the two schools were collected from the hand tube wells of the school premises. The next work was carried out with collection of the domestic drinking water, raw rice grain, and respective biological samples (urine, scalp hair, and nail) from the children ($n = 100$) of the selected age groups. Water samples were collected in sterile polyethylene containers and preserved by adding 0.1% (v/v) concentrated nitric acid, placed in an icebox, transported to the laboratory, and finally stored in a refrigerator at 4°C prior to the analysis of As (Roychowdhury, 2008, 2010). Raw rice grain samples of the children's daily diets were collected in sterilized zip-lock packets, which are brought by individual children. Individual urine samples were collected in sterilized polyethylene containers without adding any chemical for preservation and stored at –20°C until analysis. Respective scalp hair and nail samples were directly collected and preserved individually in sealed polyethylene zip-lock packets at room temperature.

Once these samples had been brought to the laboratory, the hair and nail samples were washed thoroughly with double-distilled water, followed by acetone using a magnetic stirrer (REMI Elektrotechnik Ltd, India, Model 2 ML) to remove external As from the surface. Samples were placed in glass beakers separately and allowed to dry at 50°C overnight in a hot-air oven. The urine samples were diluted in 1:1 ratio using double-distilled water and filtered before estimation of As to eradicate colloidal particles and reduce matrix effects. Detailed information on sample collection, preservation, and preparation has been described earlier (Chowdhury et al., 2018a; Joardar et al., 2021; Roychowdhury, 2010).

5.2.3 Chemicals and Reagents

All the chemicals used in the present study were of analytical grade. Double-distilled water was used throughout the analytical work. For digestion of solid samples, concentrated nitric acid (HNO_3) and 30% (v/v) hydrogen peroxide (H_2O_2)

were used, procured from Merck (Mumbai, India). About 10% of potassium iodide (KI) solution and 8% of concentrated hydrochloric acid (HCl) were added during preparation of the samples; the final volume (5–10 ml) was made and kept for 45 min before analysis. A solution of 0.6% sodium borohydride (NaBH$_4$) in 0.5% sodium hydroxide (NaOH) and 5–10 M hydrochloric acid (both from Merck, Mumbai, India) was used for estimation of As with the flow injection–hydride generation–atomic absorption spectrometry (FI–HG–AAS) method.

5.2.4 DIGESTION

No digestion protocol was followed for As estimation in water and urine samples. All the solid samples (hair, nail, and rice grain) were digested in a Teflon bomb for 6 h at 120°C by adding a mixture solution of concentrated HNO$_3$ and 30% (v/v) H$_2$O$_2$ in a 2:1 ratio and digested samples were evaporated on a hot plate at 90°C for 1 h. The evaporated samples were made up to a final volume of 2–5 ml with double-distilled water and passed through a suction filter of 0.45-μm diameter. Details of the sample digestion process have been mentioned earlier (Joardar et al., 2021).

5.2.5 ANALYSIS

As concentrations of all the digested solid and liquid samples were estimated in an atomic absorption spectrophotometer (Varian AA140, USA) coupled with vapor generation accessory (VGA-77, Agilent Technologies, Malaysia) with software version 5.1 (Chowdhury et al., 2018a, 2018b; Roychowdhury, 2008).

5.2.6 DATA ANALYSIS

All the statistical analysis performed for the evaluation and better understanding of the research work was done with Excel 2016 (Microsoft Office). A risk assessment study was done following the model established by the US Environmental Protection Agency (USEPA, 1986).

5.2.7 QUALITY CONTROL AND QUALITY ASSURANCE

The quality of the work was maintained by digesting 20–30% of the solid samples using a hot plate digestion method. The procedure for hot plate digestion was similar to that of Teflon bomb digestion (Joardar et al., 2021). To validate the results of analysis, the As concentration of a standard reference material (SRM) was also examined by both digestion methods. In this study, the SRM samples used were 'human hair ERM-DB001' (European Commission, JRC, IRMM, Retieseweg, Geel, Belgium) and 'rice flour 1568a' (NBS, Gaithersburg, MD, USA). Analysis of As concentration in these two SRMs showed good recovery against their certified values. Quality control experiments were also done by analyzing duplicates, blank measurements, spiking some digested samples, and inter-laboratory testing.

5.3 RESULTS AND DISCUSSION

5.3.1 DRINKING WATER As CONTAMINATION STATUS

Our study began when drinking water samples of the 15 schools of Haringhata town were analyzed and showed an As concentration in the range 60.2–366 µg/l with a mean value of 136 ± 79 µg/l. Previous research by Rahman et al. (2014) in Tehatta II block of Nadia district showed that 87.5% of drinking water samples of school premises (total sample n = 96) was beyond recommendations with a maximum of 254 µg/l. In the present study, two school tube wells (depth: 250 and 400 ft, respectively), which have the highest As concentration among others, were selected. The drinking water source of the primary school (latitude: N: 22°57'32.99", longitude: S: 88°33'28.76") showed an As concentration of 216 µg/l. This source is being used by approximately 280 persons every day whereas that from the high school (latitude: N: 22°57'33.24", longitude: S: 88°33'24.76") was 366 µg/l and is being used by around 850 persons daily. This observation pushed us to undertake the present study, i.e., evaluation of health exposure in selected children of the two selected schools distinguished by two different age groups (9–10 and 14–15 years).

Besides drinking As-contaminated water during school time, analysis of domestic drinking water samples of the two groups of children showed that they were still consuming As-contaminated water knowingly or unknowingly at home. As described earlier, Nadia being an As-affected district, several mitigation strategies have been undertaken. Still, the ill effects of As-contaminated drinking water and the suffering of those poor affected people are unbearable in Nadia (Chakraborti et al., 2013; Rahman et al., 2014). Mean As concentrations in domestic drinking water of the two groups of children are observed to be 25.4 ± 26 and 45.5 ± 53.6 µg/l (range: 3–101 µg/l; n = 45 and range: 3–210 µg/l; n = 50), respectively (Table 5.1).

5.3.2 RICE GRAIN As CONTAMINATION STATUS

Rice is a staple food in West Bengal, and contributes 73% of an individual's total calorie intake (Ninno and Dorosh, 2001). But, with time it has been systematically proven that rice is a major route of As exposure to mankind. Paddy plant is a huge accumulator of As and consequently rice grain is a serious health risk factor to be taken into consideration (Chowdhury et al., 2018a, 2020). Paddy cultivated in the fields of Nadia district is sufficiently As-contaminated to cause a future health risk (Mondal and Polya, 2008; Roychowdhury, 2008). Rice grain cultivated in Chakdaha block, Nadia showed As accumulation of 950, 790, 600, 470, and 290 µg/kg in Gosai, Satabdi, Banskathi, Kunti, and Ranjit varieties, respectively (Upadhyay et al., 2019). The present study analyzed As concentration in the rice grain samples consumed by the children on a daily basis (Table 5.2). It showed that the range of As concentration in the younger children was 89–354 µg/kg (n = 45) while that in the older group was 39–650 µg/kg (n = 45), though mean As concentration was quite similar in both cases (186 ± 78 and 180 ± 122 µg/kg). RICE grain

TABLE 5.1

Status of domestic drinking water and rice grain in children

Age group: 9–10 years

	No. of samples (*n*)	Mean	Median	sd	Range
Domestic drinking water (µg/l)	45	25.4	14.9	26	3–101
Rice grain (µg/kg)	45	186	168	78	89–354
Age group: 14–15 years					
Domestic drinking water (µg/l)	50	45.5	18.5	53.6	3–210
Rice grain (µg/kg)	45	180	160	122	39–650

As concentration is higher than permissible As concentration in rice, i.e., 100 µg/kg of As-endemic sites (Meharg et al., 2006).

5.3.3 DAILY DIETARY INTAKE OF AS

Daily dietary intake of As is calculated on the basis of the daily consumption of rice and water for the studied groups of children as, in the Bengal delta, people mostly rely on rice and vegetables. Raw rice, parboiled rice, and different types of rice byproducts are As-contaminated at a level that will cause a health risk for the population residing in the As-exposed area (Chowdhury et al., 2018b; Islam et al., 2017). Groundwater used for drinking and rice grain both contain ample amounts of inorganic As and, more importantly, above 80% of the total As content of food is reflected from inorganic As (Huq and Naidu, 2003; Roychowdhury, 2008, 2010; Signes-Pastor et al., 2008). Presently, the PTDI value of inorganic As is considered to be 3.0 µg/kg bw/day, based on a range of 2–7 µg/kg bw/day (WHO, 2011). Our study reveals that, in the present study area, the daily dietary intake of both studied groups of children is much higher than recommended (Table 5.2). Dietary intake of As for the older group of children is 8.58 µg/kg bw/day, which is higher than in the other group of children (9–10 years), 7.23 µg/kg bw/day. It is noticeable that the greatest contribution towards daily As intake among the three sources (3.6 and 4.6 µg/kg bw/day, respectively) is from the As concentration in drinking water from the school tube well..

5.3.4 BIOMARKERS: HEALTH EXPOSURE

The health exposure study of the children analyzes their biological samples, i.e., urine, hair, and nail, elaborated in Table 5.3. Urine is the measurement of acute exposure as As is primarily metabolized in liver and most of its species are excreted

TABLE 5.2
Dietary intake of arsenic (As) per day in the two studied groups of children

Source	Consumption rate per day*		As concentration (ppb)		As consumption per day (μg)		Daily dietary intake of As per day (μg/kg bw/day)**	
	9–10 years	14–15 years	9–10 years	14–15 years	9–10 years	14–15 years	9–10 years	14–15 years
School tube well drinking water	0.51	0.51	216	366	108	183	3.6	4.6
Domestic tube well drinking water	1.51	21	25.4	45.5	38.1	91	1.27	2.27
Rice grain consumed in home	0.38 kg	0.38 kg	186	180	70.9	68.6	2.36	1.71
Total	-	-	-	-	217	342	7.23	8.58

*Joardar et al. (2021).
**$BW_{(9-10)} = 30$ kg, $BW_{(14-15)} = 40$ kg.

TABLE 5.3
Status of biological samples in children

| Parameters | Biomarkers | | | | | |
| | Urine As (µg/l) | | Scalp hair As (µg/kg) | | Nail As (µg/kg) | |
	9–10 years	14–15 years	9–10 years	14–15 years	9–10 years	14–15 years
No. of samples (n)	45	40	45	43	45	44
Mean	3.98	5.49	1520	1240	2400	2400
Median	3	4.3	1160	300	1850	1540
SD	1.85	3.26	1480	2550	1690	2140
Range	<3–11.2	<3–18.5	90–5930	40–13,200	410–8230	120–9300

through this pathway (Buchet al., 1981; National Research Council, 1999; Orloff et al., 2009). Urine As concentration in the children studied (9–10 years: 3.98 µg/l, and 14–15 years: 5.49 µg/l) is found to be strictly within the normal range, i.e., 3–26 µg/l (Joardar et al., 2021). Moreover, reports say that individuals not exposed to As may have urine As below 100 µg/l (ATSDR, 2007; Chakraborti et al., 2016). After urine As excretion in the first one or two days of direct exposure, As slowly accumulates in hair. Therefore, hair As can reveal long-term or past exposure as it reflects accumulation growing with age (Orloff et al., 2009). The normal range of hair As concentration is 80–250 µg/kg (Arnold et al., 1990) while 20–200 µg/kg is the usual As concentration range in the hair of people with no As exposure (National Research Council, 1999). Hair As is mostly arsenite [As(III)], though a few researchers have mentioned the existence of DMA in hair (Lin et al., 1998; Yamato, 1988). The present studied population has seemingly higher As concentration in hair, which shows that they have been exposed to As for a prolonged period of time (Table 5.3). The scalp hair As concentration range in the older children is 40–13,200 µg/kg (n = 45) while that in the younger aged children is 90–5,930 µg/kg (n = 43).

Fingernails and toenails are intermittently used as biomarkers for As exposure as they grow at a slower rate than hair (Orloff et al., 2009). According to the National Research Council, the normal range of As in nails of people who have had no As exposure is 20–500 µg/kg (National Research Council, 1999, 2001) while its referred range is stated to be 430–1080 µg/kg by Ioanid et al. (1961). Nail As concentration range in the present studied population has also crossed referred limits: 120–9300 µg/kg in the older group of children and 410–8230 µg/kg in the younger one.

5.3.5 CONTRIBUTION OF INTAKE AS ON BIOMARKERS

The As excreted through biomarkers is directly dependent on the As consumed daily through drinking water and rice grain, which is expressed through the regression relation (Figure 5.1: 9–10 years) and (Figure 5.2: 14–15 years). In the younger

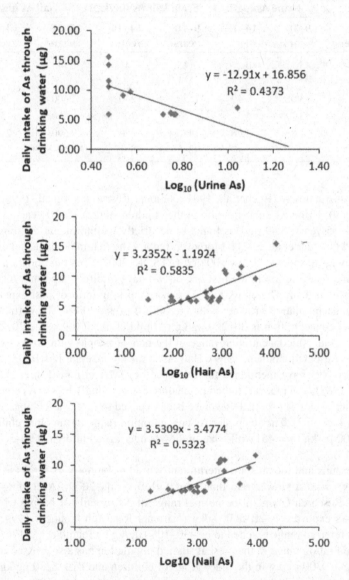

FIGURE 5.1 Relation between excreted arsenic (As) and intake As in children aged 9–10 years. (a) Drinking water–urine; (b) drinking water–hair; (c) drinking water–nail; (d) rice grain–urine; (e) rice grain–hair; (f) rice grain–nail ($\log_{10}$ value is taken for As concentrations in biological samples).

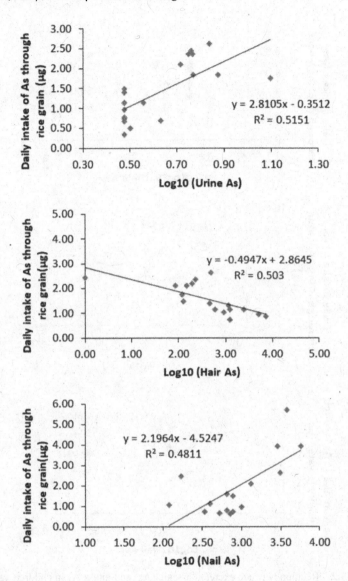

FIGURE 5.1 Continued

children, the effect of drinking water As is more closely related with As excreted through urine ($R^2 = 0.437$, Figure 5.1a), hair ($R^2 = 0.583$, Figure 5.1b) and nail ($R^2 = 0.532$, Figure 5.1c) respectively compared to that of the older children ($R^2 = 0.348$, Figure 5.2a; $R^2 = 0.437$, Figure 5.2b; $R^2 = 0.512$, Figure 5.2c). Baig et al. (2016) and Brahman et al. (2016) also showed similarly good correlation between drinking water As concentration and scalp hair As concentration among children aged 6–15 years. Rice grain As is also shown to contribute significantly towards excreted As in both groups of children in the present study. In the younger group, the effect of

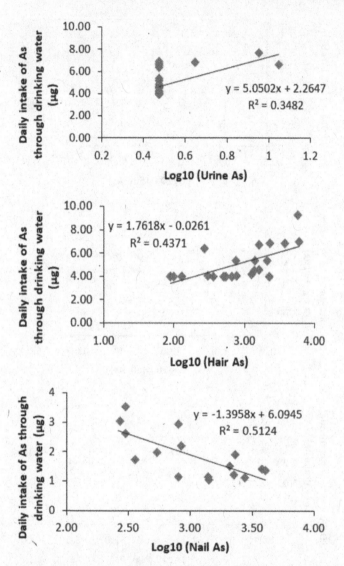

FIGURE 5.2 Relation between excreted arsenic (As) and intake As in children aged 14–15 years. (a) Drinking water–urine; (b) drinking water–hair; (c) drinking water–nail; (d) rice grain–urine; (e) rice grain–hair; (f) rice grain–nail ($\log_{10}$ value is taken for As concentrations in biological samples).

consumed As through rice grain is more prominent in urine ($R^2= 0.515$, Figure 5.1d) and hair ($R^2= 0.503$, Figure 5.1e) than nail ($R^2= 0.481$, Figure 5.1e), while the same effect is pronounced to be greatest in nails in the older group of children ($R^2= 0.771$, Figure 5.2f). In this age group of subjects, the effect of As through rice grain is comparatively moderate on hair tissues ($R^2= 0.393$, Figure 5.2e).

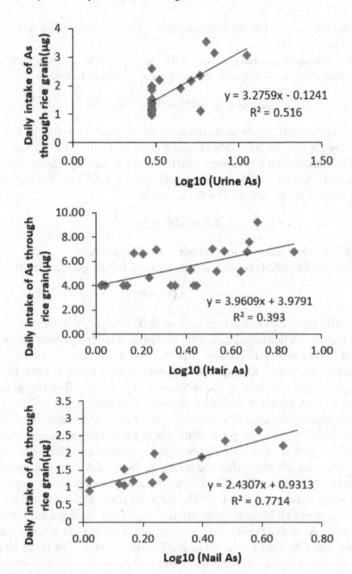

FIGURE 5.2 Continued

5.3.6 HEALTH RISK ASSESSMENT

Health risk assessment is a very important and necessary study towards the estimation of the extent of exposure and future health hazard. Risk of As-induced diseases increases with increasing toxicity in body system, and increasing As intake. In an As-exposed and endemic area like Haringhata, it is mandatory to evaluate the health risk of children who are apparently consuming As a daily basis. Health risk is calculated related to the lifetime cancer and non-cancer risk model set by USEPA (1986, 2001).

At first, the average daily dose (ADD) of As due to consumption of As-contaminated drinking water and rice grain is calculated as follows:

$$ADD = (C*IR*ED*EF)/(BW*AT) \tag{1}$$

where C = As concentration in respective item; IR = ingestion rate (l/day for drinking water, g/day for rice grain); ED = exposure duration (years); EF = exposure frequency (365 days/year); BW = body weight 30 and 40 kg respectively for the two age groups of children; and AT = average life time (365*65 = 23,725 days).

Cancer risk (CR) is estimated by the equation:

$$CR = ADD*CSF \tag{2}$$

where CSF is cancer slope factor (1.5 per mg/kg/day for As).

Non-cancer risk (NCR) is calculated in terms of hazard quotient (HQ).

$$HQ = ADD/RfD \tag{3}$$

where RfD represents oral reference dose (0.0003 mg/kg/day for As).

In the present studied population, both groups of children face substantial future health risk. The elder children have a greater risk than the younger ones, probably because they have had longer As exposure in their lifetime. Drinking water contributes a significant cancer and non-cancer risk compared to rice grain. The health risk for both groups of children is figuratively explained in Figure 5.3. Cancer risk for the older group of children is $1.58*10^{-3}$–$5.04*10^{-3}$ for drinking water and $1.27*10^{-4}$–$2.06*10^{-3}$ for rice grain while that for the younger group of children is $8.22*10^{-4}$–$1.89*10^{-3}$ and $2.47*10^{-4}$–$9.83*10^{-4}$ respectively. The mean values of cancer risk are clearly more than the threshold value of As-induced cancer risk, 10^{-6} (Das et al., 2020; USEPA, 2005). The mean total cancer risk (summation of drinking water and rice grain) is $1.58*10^{-3}$ for 9–10-year-oldchildren and $2.87*10^{-3}$ for 14–15-year-old children respectively (Figure 5.3a). The apparent non-cancer risk caused by As is also beyond the permitted rate in the present study because the HQ values are all beyond 1 (Das et al., 2020; USEPA, 2005). The mean total non-cancer risk (summing up drinking water and rice grain) is 3.5 for 9–10-year-old children and 6.38 for 14–15-year-old children respectively (Figure 5.3b). The range of HQ for drinking water and rice grain is 1.82–4.21 and 0.6–2.18 in younger-aged children while that in the older group of children is 3.51–11.2 and 0.28–4.6.

5.4 CONCLUSION

The Laupala Kalpataru school children of Haringhata, Nadia in West Bengal are at a high risk of As exposure through the consumption of contaminated drinking water. The risk is aggravated by daily intake of As-contaminated rice grain. Apparently, the older children (14–15 years) are at greater risk because of a longer period of

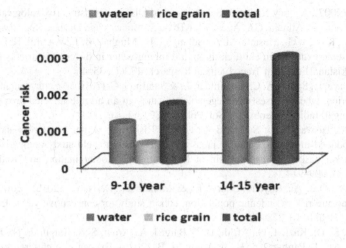

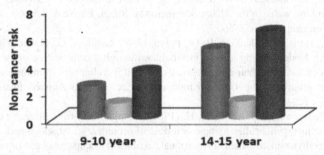

FIGURE 5.3 (a and b) Health risk assessment in the children studied.

exposure than the younger children (9–10 years). The dietary intake of the children is visibly more than twice greater than the recommended limit of the Joint FAO/WHO Expert Committee on Food Additives. Urine As concentration is higher in the older group of children compared to the younger group of children. Evidently, both scalp hair and nail are indicators of As exposure with significant correlation with As intake through daily diets. Although no skin manifestations are observed in these children, they are clearly sub-clinically affected. Hence, to reduce As exposure, the children are immediately advised not to consume drinking water from the school premises. They are also advised to find alternative As-free drinking water sources for their domestic purposes to diminish the health risk in future. In addition, to combat As toxicity, nutritious foods with antitoxic components should be provided to the children.

REFERENCES

Arnold, H. L., Odam, R. B., & James, W. D. (1990). Disease of the skin. Clinical dermatology. Philadelphia: W.B. Saunders, pp. 121–122.

ATSDR. (2007). Agency for Toxic Substances and Disease Registry. Toxicological profile for arsenic. Atlanta, GA: Agency for Toxic Substances and Disease Registry.

Baig, J. A., Kazi, T. G., Mustafa, M. A., Solangi, I. B., Mughal, M. J., & Afridi, H. I. (2016). Arsenic exposure in children through drinking water in different districts of Sindh, Pakistan. Biological Trace Element Research, 173(1), 35–46.

Bhattacharya, P., Samal, A. C., Majumdar, J., & Santra, S. C. (2010). Arsenic contamination in rice, wheat, pulses, and vegetables: a study in an arsenic affected area of West Bengal, India. Water, Air, & Soil Pollution, 213(1–4), 3–13.

Biswas, A., Biswas, S., & Santra, S. C. (2012). Risk from winter vegetables and pulses produced in arsenic endemic areas of Nadia District: field study comparison with market basket survey. Bulletin of Environmental Contamination and Toxicology, 88(6), 909–914.

Biswas, A., Das, A., Roychowdhury, T., & Mazumder, D. N. G. (2018). Low arsenic exposure risk in endemic population, cohort study for consecutive years. Exposure and Health, 10, 273–286.

Brahman, K. D., Kazi, T. G., Afridi, H. I., Baig, J. A., Arain, S. S., Talpur, F. N., Kazi, A. G., Ali, J., Panhwar, A. H., & Arain, M. B. (2016). Exposure of children to arsenic in drinking water in the Tharparkar region of Sindh, Pakistan. Science of the Total Environment, 544, 653–660.

Brima, E. I., Haris, P. I., Jenkins, R. O., Polya, D. A., Gault, A. G., & Harrington, C. F. (2006). Understanding arsenic metabolism through a comparative study of arsenic levels in the urine, hair and fingernails of healthy volunteers from three unexposed ethnic groups in the United Kingdom. Toxicology and Applied Pharmacology, 216(1), 122–130.

Buchet, J. P., Lauwerys, R., & Roels, H. (1981). Comparison of the urinary excretion of arsenic metabolites after a single oral dose of sodium arsenite, monomethylarsonate, or dimethylarsinate in man. International Archives of Occupational and Environmental Health, 48, 71–79.

Byrne, S., Amarasiriwardena, D., Bandak, B., Bartkus, L., Kane, J., Jones, J., Yanes, J., Arriaza, B., & Cornejo, L. (2010). Were Chinchorros exposed to arsenic? Arsenic determination in Chinchorro mummies' hair by laser ablation inductively coupled plasma-mass spectrometry (LA-ICP-MS). Microchemical Journal, 94(1), 28–35.

Calderon, J., Navarro, M. E., Jimenez-Capdeville, M. E., Santos-Diaz, M. A., Golden, A., Rodriguez-Leyva, I., Borja-Aburto, V. & Diaz-Barriga, F. (2001). Exposure to arsenic and lead and neuropsychological development in Mexican children. Environmental Research, 85(2), 69–76.

Census of India. (2011). Series-20 Part XII-B District Census Handbook Nadia, Directorate of Census Operations West Bengal. https://censusindia.gov.in/2011census/dchb/1910_PART_B_DCHB_NADIA.pdf.

Chakraborti, D., Rahman, M. M., Das, B., Nayak, B., Pal, A., Sengupta, M. K., Hossain, M. A., Ahamed, S., Sahu, M., Saha, K. C., Mukherjee, S. C., Pati, S., Dutta., R. N., & Quamruzzaman, Q. (2013). Groundwater arsenic contamination in Ganga–Meghna–Brahmaputra plain, its health effects and an approach for mitigation. Environmental Earth Sciences, 70(5), 1993–2008.

Chakraborti, D., Rahman, M. M., Ahamed, S., Dutta, R. N., Pati, S., & Mukherjee, S. C. (2016). Arsenic groundwater contamination and its health effects in Patna district (capital of Bihar) in the middle Ganga plain, India. Chemosphere, 152, 520–529.

Chowdhury, U. K., Biswas, B. K., Chowdhury, T. R., Samanta, G., Mandal, B. K., Basu, G. C., Chanda, C. R., Lodh, D., Saha, K. C., Mukherjee, S. K., Roy, S., Kabir, S., Quamruzzaman, Q., & Chakraborti, D. (2000). Groundwater arsenic contamination in Bangladesh and West Bengal, India. Environmental Health Perspectives, 108(5), 393–397.

Chowdhury, N. R., Das, R., Joardar, M., Ghosh, S., Bhowmick, S., & Roychowdhury, T. (2018a). Arsenic accumulation in paddy plants at different phases of pre-monsoon cultivation. Chemosphere, 210, 987–997.

Chowdhury, N. R., Ghosh, S., Joardar, M., Kar, D., & Roychowdhury, T. (2018b). Impact of arsenic contaminated groundwater used during domestic scale post harvesting of paddy crop in West Bengal: arsenic partitioning in raw and parboiled whole grain. Chemosphere, 211, 173–184.

Chowdhury, N. R., Das, A., Joardar, M., De, A., Mridha, D., Das, R., Rahman, M. M., & Roychowdhury, T. (2020). Flow of arsenic between rice grain and water: Its interaction, accumulation and distribution in different fractions of cooked rice. Science of the Total Environment, 731, 138937. https://doi.org/10.1016/j.scitotenv.2020.138937.

Concha, G., Nermell, B., & Vahter, M. V. (1998). Metabolism of inorganic arsenic in children with chronic high arsenic exposure in northern Argentina. Environmental Health Perspectives, 106(6), 355–359.

Das, A., Das, S. S., Chowdhury, N. R., Joardar, M., Ghosh, B., & Roychowdhury, T. (2020). Quality and health risk evaluation for groundwater in Nadia district, West Bengal: an approach on its suitability for drinking and domestic purpose. Groundwater for Sustainable Development, 10, 100351.

Gault, A. G., Rowland, H. A., Charnock, J. M., Wogelius, R. A., Gomez-Morilla, I., Vong, S., Leng, M., Samreth, S., Sampson, M. L., & Polya, D. A. (2008). Arsenic in hair and nails of individuals exposed to arsenic-rich groundwaters in Kandal province, Cambodia. Science of the Total Environment, 393(1), 168–176.

Hall, A. H. (2002). Chronic arsenic poisoning. Toxicology Letters, 128(1–3), 69–72.

Hopenhaynrich, C., Smith, A. H., & Goeden, H. M. (1993). Human studies do not support the methylation threshold hypothesis for the toxicity of inorganic arsenic. Environmental Research, 60(2), 161–177.

Huq, S. I., & Naidu, R. (2003). Arsenic in groundwater of Bangladesh: contamination in the food chain. In: Ahmed, M. F. (Ed.) Arsenic contamination: Bangladesh perspective. Dhaka: ITN-Bangladesh, Bangladesh University of Engineering and Technology, 203–226.

Ioanid, N., Bors, G., & Popa, I. (1961) Beiträgezur Kenntnis des normalen Arsengehaltesron Nägeln und des Gehaltes in den Fällen von Arsenpolyneuritis. International Journal of Legal Medicine, 52(1), 90–94.

Islam, S., Rahman, M. M., Rahman, M. A., & Naidu, R. (2017). Inorganic arsenic in rice and rice-based diets: health risk assessment. Food Control, 82, 196–202.

Joardar, M., Das, A., Mridha, D., De, A., Chowdhury, N. R., & Roychowdhury, T. (2021). Evaluation of acute and chronic arsenic exposure on school children from exposed and apparently control areas of West Bengal, India. Exposure and Health 13: 33–50. https://doi.org/10.1007/s12403-020-00360-x.

Lin, T. H., Huang, Y. L., & Wang, M. Y. (1998). Arsenic species in drinking water, hair, fingernails, and urine of patients with black foot disease. Journal of Toxicology and Environmental Health Part A, 53, 85–93.

Mazumder, D. N. G., Haque, R., Ghosh, N., De, B. K., Santra, A., Chakraborty, D., & Smith, A. H. (1998). Arsenic levels in drinking water and the prevalence of skin lesions in West Bengal, India. International Journal of Epidemiology, 27(5), 871–877.

Meharg, A. A., Adomaco, E., Lawgali, Y., Deacon, C., & Williams, P. (2006). Food Standards Agency Contract C101045: levels of arsenic in rice: literature review. www.food.gov. uk/sites /default/files /169-1-605.

Milton, A. H., Hasan, Z., Shahidullah, S. M., Sharmin, S., Jakariya, M. D., Rahman, M., Dear, K., & Smith, W. (2004). Association between nutritional status and arsenicosis due to chronic arsenic exposure in Bangladesh. International Journal of Environmental Health Research, 14(2), 99–108.

Mondal, D., & Polya, D. A. (2008). Rice is a major exposure route for arsenic in Chakdaha block, Nadia district, West Bengal, India: a probabilistic risk assessment. Applied Geochemistry, 23(11), 2987–2998.

National Research Council. (1999). Arsenic in drinking water. Washington, DC: National Academies Press.

National Research Council. (2001) Arsenic in drinking water: 2001 update, Subcommittee on arsenic in drinking water. Washington, DC: National Academic Press.

Nermell, B., Lindberg, A. L., Rahman, M., Berglund, M., Persson, L. Å., El Arifeen, S., & Vahter, M. (2008). Urinary arsenic concentration adjustment factors and malnutrition. Environmental Research, 106(2), 212–218.

Nickson, R. T., McArthur, J. M., Ravenscroft, P., Burgess, W. G., & Ahmed, K. M. (2000). Mechanism of arsenic release to groundwater, Bangladesh and West Bengal. Applied Geochemistry, 15(4), 403–413.

Nielsen, F. H. (2001). Trace minerals. Nutrition in health and sickness, 9th edn. Mexico City: McGraw-Hill, 328–331.

Ninno, C. D., & Dorosh, P. A. (2001). Averting a food crisis: private imports and public targeted distribution in Bangladesh after the 1998 flood. Agricultural Economics, 25(2–3), 337–346.

Orloff, K., Mistry, K., & Metcalf, S. (2009). Biomonitoring for environmental exposures to arsenic. Journal of Toxicology and Environmental Health, Part B, 12(7), 509–524.

Rahman, M. M., Chowdhury, U. K., Mukherjee, S. C., Mondal, B. K., Paul, K., Lodh, D., Biswas, B. K., Chanda, C. R., Basu, G. K., Saha, K. C., Roy, S., Das, R., Palit, S. K., Quamruzzaman, Q., & Chakraborti, D. (2001). Chronic arsenic toxicity in Bangladesh and West Bengal, India – a review and commentary. Journal of Toxicology: Clinical Toxicology, 39(7), 683–700.

Rahman, M. M., Ng, J. C., & Naidu, R. (2009). Chronic exposure of arsenic via drinking water and its adverse health impacts on humans. Environmental Geochemistry and Health, 31(1), 189–200.

Rahman, M. M., Mondal, D., Das, B., Sengupta, M. K., Ahamed, S., Hossain, M. A., Samal, A. C., Saha, K. C., Mukherjee, S. C., Dutta, R. N., & Chakraborti, D. (2014). Status of groundwater arsenic contamination in all 17 blocks of Nadia district in the state of West Bengal, India: a 23-year study report. Journal of Hydrology, 518, 363–372.

Raqib, R., Ahmed, S., Sultana, R., Wagatsuma, Y., Mondal, D., Hoque, A. W., Nermell, B., Yunus, M., Roy, S., Persson, L. A., Arifeen, S. E., Moore, S., & Vahter, M. (2009). Effects of in utero arsenic exposure on child immunity and morbidity in rural Bangladesh. Toxicology Letters, 185(3), 197–202.

Ratnaike, R. N. (2003). Acute and chronic arsenic toxicity. Postgraduate Medical Journal, 79(933), 391–396.

Rosado, J. L., Ronquillo, D., Kordas, K., Rojas, O., Alatorre, J., Lopez, P., Garcia-Vargas, G., Caamano, M. D. C., Cebrian, M. E., & Stoltzfus, R. J. (2007). Arsenic exposure and cognitive performance in Mexican schoolchildren. Environmental Health Perspectives, 115(9), 1371–1375.

Roychowdhury, T. (2008). Impact of sedimentary arsenic through irrigated groundwater on soil, plant, crops and human continuum from Bengal delta: special reference to raw and cooked rice. Food and Chemical Toxicology, 46 (8), 2856–2864. https://doi.org/10.1016/j.fct.2008.05.019.

Roychowdhury, T. (2010). Groundwater arsenic contamination in one of the 107 arsenic-affected blocks in West Bengal, India: Status, distribution, health effects and factors responsible for arsenic poisoning. International Journal of Hygiene and Environmental Health, 213(6), 414–427.

Roychowdhury, T., Uchino, T., Tokunaga, H., & Ando, M. (2002). Survey of arsenic in food composites from an arsenic-affected area of West Bengal, India. Food and Chemical Toxicology, 40(11), 1611–1621.

Roychowdhury, T., Tokunaga, H., & Ando, M. (2003). Survey of arsenic and other heavy metals in food composites and drinking water and estimation of dietary intake by the villagers from an arsenic-affected area of West Bengal, India. Science of the Total Environment, 308(1–3), 15–35.

Roychowdhury, T., Uchino, T., & Tokunaga, H. (2008). Effect of arsenic on soil, plant and foodstuffs by using irrigated ground water and pond water from Nadia district, West Bengal. International Journal of Environmental Pollution, 33(2/3), 218–234.

Samanta, G., Sharma, R., Roychowdhury T., & Chakraborti, D. (2004). Arsenic and other elements in hair, nails, and skin-scales of arsenic victims in West Bengal, India. Science of the Total Environment, 326(1–3), 33–47.

Santra, S. C., Samal, A. C., Bhattacharya, P., Banerjee, S., Biswas, A., & Majumdar, J. (2013). Arsenic in food chain and community health risk: a study in Gangetic West Bengal. Procedia Environmental Sciences, 18, 2–13.

Sarkar, P., Ray, P. R., Ghatak, P. K., & Sen, M. (2016). Arsenic concentration in water, rice straw and cow milk – a micro level study at Chakdaha and Haringhata block of West Bengal. Indian Journal of Dairy Sciences, 69, 6.

Signes-Pastor, A. J., Mitra, K., Sarkhel, S., Hobbes, M., Burló, F., De Groot, W. T., & Carbonell-Barrachina, A. A. (2008). Arsenic speciation in food and estimation of the dietary intake of inorganic arsenic in a rural village of West Bengal. Journal of Agricultural and Food Chemistry, 56(20), 9469–9474.

Singh, S. K., & Ghosh, A. K. (2012). Health risk assessment due to groundwater arsenic contamination: children are at high risk. Human and Ecological Risk Assessment: An International Journal, 18(4), 751–766.

Smith, A. H., Marshall, G., Liaw, J., Yuan, Y., Ferreccio, C., & Steinmaus, C. (2012). Mortality in young adults following in utero and childhood exposure to arsenic in drinking water. Environmental Health Perspectives, 120(11), 1527–1531.

Smith, A. H., Yunus, M., Khan, A. F., Ercumen, A., Yuan, Y., Smith, M. H., Liaw, J., Balmes, J., Ehrenstein, O. V., Raqib, R., Kalman, D., Alam, D. S., Streatfield, P. K., & Steinmaus, C. (2013). Chronic respiratory symptoms in children following in utero and early life exposure to arsenic in drinking water in Bangladesh. International Journal of Epidemiology, 42(4), 1077–1086.

Upadhyay, M. K., Majumdar, A., Barla, A., Bose, S., & Srivastava, S. (2019). An assessment of arsenic hazard in groundwater–soil–rice system in two villages of Nadia district, West Bengal, India. Environmental Geochemistry and Health, 41(6), 2381–2395.

USEPA. (1986). Guidelines for carcinogenic risk assessment. Federal Register CFR 2984, 51(185), 33992–34003.

USEPA. (2001). Integrated Risk Information System (IRIS). Washington, DC: National Centre for Environmental Assessment, Office of Research and Development.

USEPA. (2005). Guidelines for carcinogen risk assessment. Washington, DC: Risk Assessment Forum, United States Environmental Protection Agency. EPA/630/P-03/001F

Vahter, M. (1994). Species differences in the metabolism of arsenic compounds. Applied Organometallic Chemistry, 8(3), 175–182.

Wasserman, G. A., Liu, X., Parvez, F., Ahsan, H., Factor-Litvak, P., van Geen, A., Slavkovich, V., Lolacono, N. J., Cheng, Z., Hussain, I., Momotaj, H., & Graziano, J. H. (2004). Water arsenic exposure and children's intellectual function in Araihazar, Bangladesh. Environmental Health Perspectives, 112(13), 1329–1333.

Wasserman, G. A., Liu, X., Parvez, F., Ahsan, H., Factor-Litvak, P., Kline, J., van Geen, A., Slavkovich, V., Lolacono, N. J., Levy, D., Cheng, Z., & Cheng, Z. (2007). Water arsenic exposure and intellectual function in 6-year-old children in Araihazar, Bangladesh. Environmental Health Perspectives, 115(2), 285–289.

Wasserman, G. A., Liu, X., Parvez, F., Factor-Litvak, P., Ahsan, H., Levy, D., Kline, J., van Geen, A., Mey, J., Slavkovich, V., Siddique, A. B., Islam, T., & Graziano, J. H. (2011). Arsenic and manganese exposure and children's intellectual function. Neurotoxicology, 32(4), 450–457.

Wasserman, G. A., Liu, X., Parvez, F., Chen, Y., Factor-Litvak, P., LoIacono, N. J., Levy, D., Shahriar, H., Uddin, M. N., Islam, T., Lomx, A., Saxena, R., Gibson, E. A., Kioumourtzoglou, M., Balac, O., Sanchez, T., Kline, J. K., Santiago, D., Ellis, T., van Geen, A., & Graziano, J. H. (2018). A cross-sectional study of water arsenic exposure and intellectual function in adolescence in Araihazar, Bangladesh. Environment International, 118, 304–313.

Watanabe, C., Matsui, T., Inaoka, T., Kadono, T., Miyazaki, K., Bae, M. J., Ono, T., Ohtsuka, R., & Mozammel Haque Bokul, A. T. M. (2007). Dermatological and nutritional/growth effects among children living in arsenic-contaminated communities in rural Bangladesh. Journal of Environmental Science and Health, part A, 42(12), 1835–1841.

WHO. (2011). Evaluation of certain contaminants in food. Seventy second report of the joint FOA/WHO expert committee on food additives. WHO technical report series no. 959. Geneva: World Health Organization (WHO).

Wright, R. O., Amarasiriwardena, C., Woolf, A. D., Jim, R., & Bellinger, D. C. (2006) Neuropsychological correlates of hair arsenic, manganese, and cadmium levels in school-age children residing near a hazardous waste site. Neurotoxicology, 27(2), 210–216.

Yamato, N. (1988). Concentrations and chemical species of arsenic in human urine and hair. Bulletin of Environmental Contamination and Toxicology, 40, 633–640.

6 Evaluation of Health Effects and Risk Assessment of Arsenic on an Unexposed Population from an Arsenic-Exposed Zone of West Bengal, India

Madhurima Joardar, Nilanjana Roy Chowdhury, Antara Das and Tarit Roychowdhury*

CONTENTS

* Corresponding author: Tarit Roychowdhury. rctarit@yahoo.com; tarit.roychowdhury@
jadavpuruniversity.in

DOI: 10.1201/9781003095422-6

6.1   INTRODUCTION

Arsenic (As) is well known as an environmental pollutant which is toxic and carcinogenic. Globally As is recognized as a class I carcinogen for causing cancer due to its long-term exposure (ATSDR, 2007; International Agency for Research on Cancer (IARC), 2012). Human exposure to toxic heavy metals has the tendency to occur for a lifetime, due to long-term exposure through water, food consumption, soil, and air (EFSA, 2009; Carlin et al., 2016; Rebelo and Caldas, 2016). For a long time; millions of people have been exposed to As toxicity through ingesting contaminated drinking water (Chakraborti et al., 2009, 2013). As being a slow poison, it increases the toxicity burden in the human body through consumption of contaminated foodstuffs (Roychowdhury et al., 2002; Roychowdhury, 2010). The use of As-contaminated groundwater paved the way for As to enter the food chain during agricultural practices and food preparation (Zhao et al., 2010; Halder et al., 2014). Adults are more prone to As toxicity than children (Goswami et al., 2020). Children (aged between 12 and 15 years) are sub-clinically affected by As toxicity (Joardar et al., 2021). Various studies have shown the possibility of maternal to fetal contaminant (As) transfer (Vahter, 2009; Gürbay et al., 2012). Starting from an early stage, exposure to toxic metals through consumption of contaminated water and foodstuffs is continued throughout life (Rebelo and Caldas, 2016). Depending on the rate of exposure worldwide, the presence of toxic metals has been categorized in human milk (Chao et al., 2014; Ettinger et al., 2014; Rebelo and Caldas, 2016).

This chapter focuses on a survey performed on an unexposed population of mothers and infants from a severely As-prone area. This chapter highlights the present scenario of As exposure of the population through drinking water, foodstuffs, and baby food products. On a particular note, the level of toxicity has been analyzed through As biomarkers justifying the acute and chronic exposure rate of the mother and infant population. Statistical interpretation was performed to study the interrelations between As intakes and excretion of the population. Furthermore, a health risk assessment was evaluated to put forward the carcinogenic and non-carcinogenic risk of the unexposed population.

6.2 MATERIALS AND METHODS

6.2.1 STUDY AREA

A group of mothers (aged between 23 and 31 years old) and infants (aged between 7 months and 4 years old) was selected from an As-exposed area for this study. The As-exposed zone selected was Madhusudankati village (22°53´53.82"N, 88°46´38.33"E), located in Sutia gram panchayat of Gaighata block, North 24 Parganas district. Sutia is considered to be one of the severely As-affected gram panchayats in Gaighata block (Roychowdhury, 2010).

6.2.2 SAMPLE COLLECTION AND PRESERVATION

A detailed study was performed on the unexposed population (mothers and infants) of an As-exposed area. Dietary intake, namely drinking water, cooked rice grain (parboiled), baby food products (commercial and homemade), breast milk, and cow's milk were collected from ten families in the studied area. Drinking water samples were collected in sterile containers with 0.1% (v/v) concentrated nitric acid, which is used as a preservative. No preservative was used during the collection of milk samples. All these liquid samples were placed in an ice cooled box during transportation and stored at 4°C prior to As estimation (Das et al., 2020; Joardar et al., 2021). The cooked rice grain (parboiled) and baby food product samples were collected and stored in sterile zip-locks and further processed for acid diges-tion prior to As analysis.

Biomarkers of As, namely urine, scalp hair, and nail samples, were collected from the unexposed (mother and infant) population. Spot urine samples were collected in sterile containers, preserved without any chemical treatment, and stored at –20°C until As analysis. The scalp hair and fingernail clippings were dir-ectly collected and stored in sterile zip-locks at room temperature respectively. Detailed information on the above-mentioned sample collection, preservation, storage, and preparation has been given in our earlier publications (Roychowdhury, 2010; Chowdhury et al., 2020a; Joardar et al., 2021).

6.2.3 CHEMICALS AND REAGENTS

To perform the experimental analysis, double-distilled water was used. All ana-lytical graded chemicals and reagents were used at the time of analytical work. Chemicals, namely concentrated nitric acid (HNO_3) (69%) and hydrogen peroxide (H_2O_2) (30% v/v), were used for acid digestion of the samples. For As estimation using the hydride generation-atomic absorption spectrometry (HG-AAS) method, 0.6% $NaBH_4$ mixed with 0.5% NaOH and 5–10 M HCl were used. During sample preparation an aqueous solution (10% of KI) and concentrated HCl (8%) were added to the samples and kept for 45 min prior to As estimation (Chowdhury et al., 2020b; Joardar et al., 2021).

6.2.4 SAMPLE DIGESTION AND ANALYSIS

No acid digestion was performed for the liquid samples (water and urine). The solid samples (cooked rice, baby food products, scalp hair, and nail) were digested using Teflon bomb digestion protocol. The Teflon bomb digestion was carried out at 120°C for 6 h by adding concentrated nitric acid (69%) and hydrogen peroxide (30% v/v) in the ratio of 2:1 to the samples. The volume of digested samples was reduced using a hot plate at 90°C for 1 h. The final volume of the evaporated samples was made up to 2–5 ml using double-distilled water and stored after filtration (suction filter: Millipore 0.45 µm). The details of the digestion method for the solid samples have been given earlier (Roychowdhury, 2010; Chowdhury et al., 2020a; Joardar et al., 2021). Total concentration of As was quantified using the HG-AAS system (model: Varian AA140, USA) coupled with vapor generation accessory (VGA-77: software version 5.1) (Chowdhury et al., 2020b; Joardar et al., 2021).

6.2.5 QUALITY CONTROL AND QUALITY ASSURANCE

Quality control analysis was performed by analyzing blank, duplicate samples, and calculating the recovery of spiked digested samples. The accuracy and precision of the analytical work were validated through examination of standard reference material (SRM) samples using the two methods of digestion. The SRM samples used in this study were rice flour 1568a (NBS, Gaithersburg, MD, USA) and human hair ERM-DB001 (European Commission, JRC, IRMM, Retieseweg, Geel, Belgium). A good percentage of recoveries were observed for the SRM samples against their certified values (0.29 and 0.044 µg/g, respectively). Detailed information on the digestion procedure and As recovery in SRM samples has been given in our earlier publications (Chowdhury et al., 2018a; Joardar et al., 2021).

6.2.6 HEALTH RISK ASSESSMENT

Health risk depiction was performed to evaluate the carcinogenic and non-carcinogenic effects on the mother and infant through their dietary intakes (drinking water, cooked rice, breast milk, cow's milk, commercial food (Cerelac), and home-made food mixture) from the studied area (Chattopadhyay et al., 2020). USEPA (2001) describes the different models to evaluate cancer and non-cancer risk measurement depending on the ingestion rate of inorganic As.

6.2.6.1 Carcinogenic Health Risk Assessment

Carcinogenic risk factor analysis estimates the possibility of mothers and infants being exposed to As toxicity through intake of drinking water and cooked rice. The intake rate of As through drinking water and cooked rice for both the mother and infant population was determined by estimating the daily intake of As (DIA) equation, as given by Chattopadhyay et al. (2020):

$$DIA = [C * IR * ED * EF] / [BW * AT]$$

where C = concentration of drinking water and cooked rice As (mg/l or mg/kg); IR = ingestion rate (1 or g per day); ED = exposure duration (years); EF = exposure frequency (365 days/year); BW = body weight (kg); and AT = average lifetime (365*60 days).

The carcinogenic risk (CR) due to As exposure was calculated following the equation:

$$CR = ADD * SF$$

where ADD represents average daily dose; and SF represents the slope factor of As for ingestion, i.e., 1.5 (per mg/kg/day).

6.2.6.2 Non-Carcinogenic Health Risk Assessment

The non-carcinogenic risk analysis due to As exposure was observed using the following equation:

$$Hazard\ quotient\ (HQ) = (ADD / RfD)$$

where RfD represents the oral reference dose for As ingestion, i.e., 0.0003 mg/kg bw/day.

6.3   RESULTS AND DISCUSSION

6.3.1   Arsenic Contamination Scenario of the Exposed Zone

6.3.1.1   Groundwater Arsenic Scenario

In West Bengal, Gaighata is well known as an As-affected block in North 24 Parganas district (Roychowdhury, 2010; Joardar et al., 2021). Among 13 gram panchayats of Gaighata block, in Sutia gram panchayat a village named Madhusudankati (22°53´53.18"N, 88°46´38.55"E) has been targeted in our study. The distribution of As concentrations in drinking water collected from the unexposed families of the studied area is shown in Figure 6.1. The As concentration in the water ($n = 10$) collected from the unexposed families which is used for drinking, cooking, and household purposes ranged from 3 to 7.95 μg/l with an average concentration of 3.92 ± 1.76 μg/l. The study that reported on the water samples (mean = 49 μg/l, $n = 83$) collected from Sutia gram panchayat showed that the As concentration was higher than the World Health Organization (WHO)-recommended value of 10 μg/ l (Joardar et al., 2021). Water As concentration of the studied population revealed that they are presently consuming As-free groundwater.

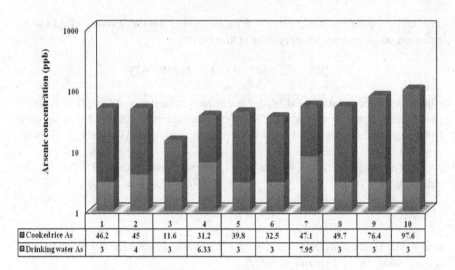

	1	2	3	4	5	6	7	8	9	10
▣ Cooked rice As	46.2	45	11.6	31.2	39.8	32.5	47.1	49.7	76.4	97.6
▣ Drinking water As	3	4	3	6.33	3	3	7.95	3	3	3

FIGURE 6.1   Distribution of arsenic (As) concentrations in drinking water and cooked rice collected from the families of the exposed area.

6.3.1.2   Arsenic in Cooked Rice

Rice grain is well known as the staple food crop which has paved a pathway to human health exposure through its consumption on a daily basis globally (Kumarathilaka et al., 2019) as well as for the rural population residing in West Bengal (Chowdhury et al., 2020a). Use of As-contaminated groundwater during cultivation practices (Chowdhury et al., 2018a) and at the time of the parboiling process to obtain parboiled rice grain (Chowdhury et al., 2018b) leads to food chain contamination. The mean As concentration in the parboiled rice grain collected from the studied (mother and infant) population was 356 µg/kg (range: 189–628 µg/kg, $n = 10$). The maximum tolerable level of As is 100 µg/kg for infants in food and 200 µg/kg for adults in rice-based products (European Commission, 2015). Several reports have highlighted that populations are exposed to nearly 90% of the total As concentration that accounts for the inorganic form in parboiled rice grain (Biswas et al., 2019; Chowdhury et al., 2020a).

In rural Bengal, parboiled rice grain is consumed in the form of cooked rice as a dietary intake on a daily basis. Locally grown rice grains when consumed in the form of cooked rice pose a health risk to populations from rural Bengal (Halder et al., 2012, 2014; Chowdhury et al., 2020a). Distribution of As concentrations in cooked rice collected from unexposed families of the studied area has been shown in Figure 6.1. At domestic level, the parboiled rice grains were cooked in the ratio of 1:3 (rice to water) using domestic water for both drinking and cooking. The mean As concentration in the cooked rice grain collected from the studied population ($n = 10$) was 47.7 µg/kg, ranging from 11.6 to 97.6 µg/kg. In rural Bengal, cooking of parboiled rice grain in low As-contaminated water showed a decreasing trend of As accumulation in cooked rice compared to parboiled rice grain (Chowdhury et al., 2020a). As accumulation in cooked rice varies depending on its geographical area, variety, cooking water, and cooking process (Pal et al., 2009; Mondal et al., 2010; Chowdhury et al., 2020a). This study shows that the use of As-free cooking water during the cooking process results in low accumulation of As in cooked rice.

Presently, in our survey the studied population is exposed to As-free drinking water, hence the cooked rice grain contributes as a major dietary source of As intake. Earlier studies have reported that As intake through rice grain plays a vital role for the population exposed to As-free water (Chatterjee et al., 2010; Biswas et al., 2019).

6.3.1.3 Accumulation of Arsenic in Dietary Baby Food Products

In rural Bengal, infants consume breast milk, cow's milk, commercial baby food (Cerelac), and homemade mixture baby food on a daily basis in their diet. As concentrations in the daily diets for the studied populations are shown in Table 6.1. In this study, the mean As concentration observed in breast milk, cow's milk was 6.35 ± 5.06 µg/l, and 17.4 ± 8.59 µg/l respectively. Several reports found that the breast milk contributes least amount of As (Carignan et al., 2015; Rebelo and Caldas, 2016).

A rice-based diet among the rural population is mainly responsible for exposure to As toxicity. In a similar way, commercial baby food (Cerelac) and homemade food mixtures showed an average As concentration of 79.8 ± 16.7 µg/kg, and 207 ± 78.8 µg/kg, respectively. In India, a large population is dependent on rice and its derivatives through their daily dietary intake (Chowdhury et al., 2018b; Rahman

---

TABLE 6.1
Arsenic concentrations in daily diets for the studied populations

Groups	Samples	No. of samples (*n*)	Mean	SD	Range
Mother	Drinking water (µg/l)	10	3.93	1.76	3–7.95
	Cooked rice (µg/kg)	10	47.7	24	11.6–97.6
Infant	Drinking water (µg/l)	11	4.29	2.06	3–7.95
	Cooked rice (µg/kg)	11	47.6	22.7	11.6–97.6
	Breast milk (µg/l)	2	6.35	5.06	2.76–9.93
	Cow's milk (µg/l)	3	17.4	8.59	11.3–27.2
	Commercial food (Cerelac) (µg/kg)	3	79.8	16.7	60.6–90.5
	Homemade food mixture (µg/kg)	3	207	78.8	125–282

et al., 2008). Several studies have reported that rice byproducts accumulate high concentrations of As compared to rice grain (Sun et al., 2009; Chowdhury et al., 2018b). This study reflects that the As accumulation in rice-based products is high compared to milk products from the studied population as the rice-based products are prepared from As-contaminated rice grains which were locally cultivated in the As-exposed areas.

6.3.2 OBSERVED DAILY DIETARY INTAKE RATE OF ARSENIC FOR MOTHER AND INFANT THROUGH DRINKING WATER AND COOKED RICE

As content (µg) distribution as a percentage in the daily dietary intakes on a daily basis of the studied population (mother and infant) is shown in Figure 6.2. In this survey, the daily dietary intake of As through drinking water and milk was calculated using the respective volume consumed by the infants (aged: 7 months–4 years old) as 0.25–1.5 l and 0.15–0.40 l, respectively with average body weight of 4.5–13 kg (Kazi et al., 2016). The intake of cooked rice, commercial baby food (Cerelac), and homemade food mixture on a daily basis by the infants was calculated considering the respective amount consumed as 20–99 g. Singh and Ghosh (2012) considered intake of cooked rice for children aged between 5 and 10 years as 99–105 g. In a similar way, the daily dietary intake of As through drinking water and cooked rice by the mother was calculated using the daily consumption of 4 l and 750 g, respectively (Roychowdhury, 2010) with an average body weight of 55 kg (Joseph et al., 2015).

The daily dietary intake rates of As for the mothers through drinking water and cooked rice are 0.29 and 0.65 µg/kg bw/day, respectively. Likewise, for the infants the daily dietary intake rates through drinking water, cooked rice, breast milk, cow's milk, commercial food (Cerelac), and homemade food mixtures are 0.37, 0.32, 0.14, 0.49, 0.54, and 1.73 µg/kg bw/day, respectively. As a result, the survey specifies that the daily dietary intake rates of the studied mother and infant population from the exposed area are lower compared to the WHO-recommended value, i.e., 3.0 µg/kg bw/day (WHO, 2011). Hence, the studied population is presently not exposed to the toxic effect of As.

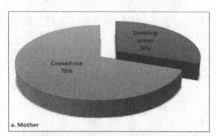 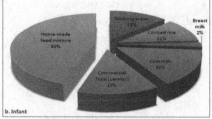

FIGURE 6.2 Arsenic content (µg) distribution as a percentage in the daily dietary intakes of the studied (a) mother and (b) infant population.

6.3.3 EFFECT OF ARSENIC TOXICITY ON THE UNEXPOSED POPULATION

6.3.3.1 Acute Exposure Level of Arsenic Toxicity

As exposure through urine is measured as the primary biomarker as it signifies the acute level of toxicity in a human body system (Vahter, 1994; Goswami et al., 2020). The half-time of As species (inorganic) is about 4 days in a human body system as it is less dependent on keratin body tissues (Goswami et al., 2020).

As concentrations in urine for the studied population of mother and infant are shown in Table 6.2. Urine samples collected from the studied population of mothers ($n = 10$) and infants ($n = 11$) showed a mean As concentration of 3.10 and 3 µg/l, respectively. Variations in urine As concentrations of the studied population (mother and infant) with their respective water As concentrations are shown in Figure 6.3. The urine As concentrations of the studied populations do not exceed the recommended value of As in urine, i.e., 3–26 µg/l (Farmer and Johnson, 1990). Regression analysis between water As and urine As of the studied mothers and infants is shown in Figure 6.4a and 6.4b, respectively. A strong significant correlation has been observed ($R^2 = 0.8992$ and 0.9084) for the mother and infant population, respectively, from the studied area. The correlation value signifies the role of consuming As-free drinking water. As a result, the valuation of urine As reveals that the studied mothers and infants are presently exposed to ingestion of As-free drinking water.

TABLE 6.2
Distribution of arsenic concentrations in biomarkers (urine, hair, and nail) of mothers and infants from the exposed area

		Biomarkers of arsenic		
Groups		Urine (µg/l)	Hair* (µg/kg)	Nail† (µg/kg)
Mother	No. of samples (n)	10	10	10
	Mean	3.10	3321	5829
	SD	0.26	2509	3184
	Range	3–3.84	1370–8300	2580–12,100
Infant	No. of samples (n)	11	8	8
	Mean	3	1655	4148
	SD	0	900	2104
	Range	3	80–2910	1810–8160

*Normal range of hair arsenic content is 80–250 µg/kg, and >1000 µg/kg in hair suggests toxic behavior (Arnold et al., 1990).
†Normal range of nail arsenic content is 430–1,080 µg/kg (Ioanid et al., 1961).

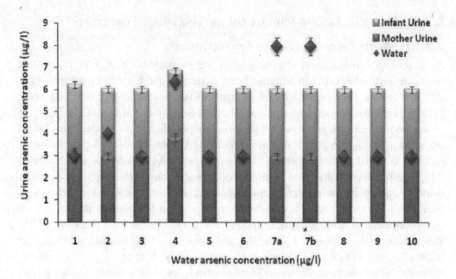

FIGURE 6.3 Variations in urine arsenic concentration of the studied population (mother and infant) with their respective water arsenic concentrations.

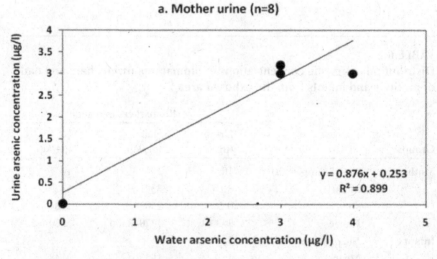

FIGURE 6.4a Regression analysis showing the relation between water and urine arsenic of the studied mother population.

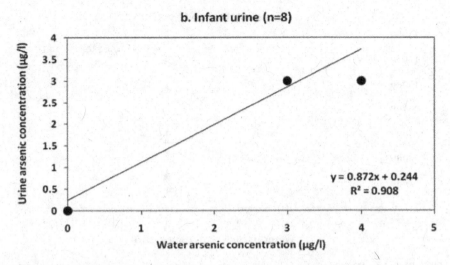

FIGURE 6.4b Regression analysis showing the relation between water and urine arsenic of the studied infant population.

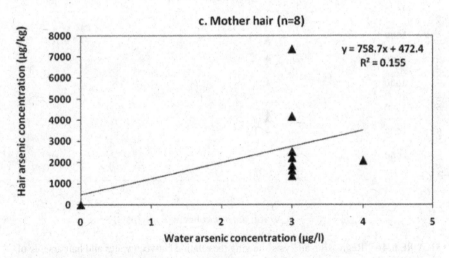

FIGURE 6.4c Regression analysis showing the relation between water and hair arsenic of the studied mother population.

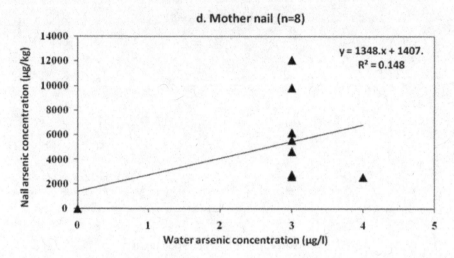

FIGURE 6.4d   Regression analysis showing the relation between water and nail arsenic of the studied mother population.

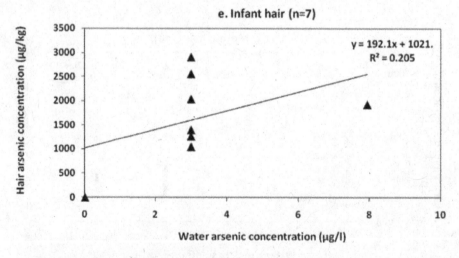

FIGURE 6.4e   Regression analysis showing the relation between water and hair arsenic of the studied infant population.

6.3.3.2   Chronic Exposure Level of Arsenic Toxicity

The chronic level of toxicity in the human body system is determined by monitoring the biomarkers (hair and nail) of As (Povorinskaya and Karpenko, 2009; Goswami et al., 2020). The deposition rate of As is fast as well as high in nails compared to hair (NRC, 1999), due to the presence of keratin protein in hair and nail body

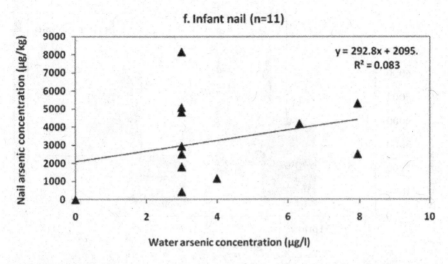

FIGURE 6.4f Regression analysis showing the relation between water and nail arsenic of the studied infant population.

tissues (Shapiro, 1967). In this study, total As in scalp hair and nails of the mother and infant was analyzed to measure the body burden depending on the rate of As exposure.

In this survey, high accumulation of As has been observed in hair and nail samples collected from the studied population (mother and infant). In our study, the hair samples collected from the mothers ($n = 10$) showed a mean As concentration of 3321 ± 2509 µg/kg, ranging from 1370 to 8300 µg/kg. Similarly, nail samples collected from the mothers ($n = 10$) showed a mean As concentration of 5829 ± 3184 µg/kg, ranging from 2580 to 12100 µg/kg. Likewise, infants from the studied area showed a mean As concentration of 1655 ± 900 µg/kg, ranging from 80 to 2910 µg/kg for hair ($n = 11$) samples. In a similar way, the nail ($n = 11$) samples collected from the infants showed a mean As concentration of 4148 ± 2104 µg/kg, ranging from 1810 to 8160 µg/kg. As distribution in hair and nail of the mother and infant individuals from the studied area is shown in Figure 6.5.

As the studied population is presently exposed to As-free drinking water, it is essential to understand the significant relation between their drinking water and chronic biological markers. No significant correlation has been observed between water As concentration and hair ($R^2 = 0.1557$) and nail As concentration ($R^2 = 0.1489$) for the mothers, respectively (Figure 6.4c and 6.4d). In the case of infant populations, no significant correlation was detected statistically between As concentration in drinking water and that of hair ($R^2 = 0.2054$) and nail ($R^2 = 0.0835$), respectively (Figure 6.4e and 6.4f). Joardar et al. (2021) reported a significant deposition of As in hair and nail samples for school children exposed to As-contaminated groundwater from an As-exposed area of West Bengal.

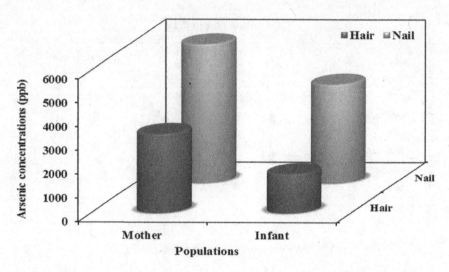

FIGURE 6.5 Arsenic distribution in hair and nail of mothers and infants from the studied area.

Children are more susceptible to adverse health effects caused by toxic elements. Borgono et al. (1977) reported that children under and over 6 years of age demonstrated a substantial amount of As deposition in hair and nail. The studied population showed no arsenical skin manifestations in this survey, but still they have a high arsenical body burden in chronic biomarkers (Table 6.2). As a result, the individuals of the studied area are considered to be sub-clinically affected due to As toxicity. In rural populations, malnutrition is held responsible for acute and chronic As toxicity. Good socio-economic status and nutritional balance result in lower arsenical health risk in the human body system (Sampson et al., 2008). The presence of vital micronutrients, i.e., zinc and selenium, in the daily dietary intake plays a dynamic role against the toxic effect of As (Roychowdhury et al., 2002). Roychowdhury (2010) highlighted that the rural Bengal population survives in conditions of poor nutrition, but as a result they suffer more from As toxicity. In our study, the populations are suffering from chronic toxicity as they lack proper nutrition in their diet on a daily basis.

6.3.4 RELATION BETWEEN DIETARY ARSENIC INTAKE AND EXCRETION

A statistical analysis named "two-tailed paired t-test" at 95% confidence level was used to evaluate the inter-relation between As dietary intake and excretion among the studied population. For the mother population, the analysis was performed to evaluate the inter-dependence between the intake of As (independent variables) through drinking water and cooked rice and excretion (biomarkers). In a similar way, for the infant population the inter-relation was evaluated between the dietary intakes of As (drinking water, cooked rice, breast milk, cow's milk, commercial baby food (Cerelac) and homemade food mixture) and excretion (dependent variable). Two hypotheses have been assumed for the statistical interpretation: the null hypothesis (H_0) signifies 'no significant dependence between As intake and excretion' whereas the alternate hypothesis (H_1) denotes 'significant dependence between As intake and excretion'. The respective t_{stat} has been evaluated against the $t_{critical}$ along with the 'degrees of freedom' (df) for the studied populations (Table 6.3).

In view of the mother population studied, no significant dependence has been observed between As intake and excretion (urine). In contrast, significant dependence was observed in the case of hair and nail (excretion) with As intake as their t_{stat} values are greater than $t_{critical}$ values. Hence, the alternate hypothesis (H_1) is accepted.

Likewise, for the infant population, no significant dependence has been observed between As intake (drinking water and cooked rice) and excretion (urine). In contrast, in the case of hair and nail (excretion) a significant dependence has been observed with As intake (drinking water and cooked rice). In a similar way, no significant dependence has been observed within the As intake (breast milk, cow's milk, commercial food (Cerelac), and homemade food mixture) and excretion (urine, hair, and nail) as their t_{stat} values are lower than $t_{critical}$ values. Hence, the null hypothesis (H_1) is accepted.

As a result, the survey specifies that food chain contamination is majorly responsible for exposure to chronic As toxicity. Hence, it can be stated that the rate of As exposure in the human body system is solely dependent on the As intake on a daily basis. Therefore, the consumption of As through daily dietary intake paves a way to be exposed to As toxicity.

6.3.5 HEALTH RISK ASSESSMENT ANALYSIS ON THE MOTHER AND INFANT POPULATION THROUGH CONSUMPTION OF DIETARY INTAKES

The potential health risk (carcinogenic and non-carcinogenic) for the studied population from their respective dietary sources is shown in Table 6.4. The mean carcinogenic risk from drinking water and cooked rice in the mother population has been observed as $1.79*10^{-4}$ and $4.04*10^{-4}$, respectively. For the infant population, the mean carcinogenic risk from drinking water, cooked rice, breast milk, cow's milk, commercial food (Cerelac), and homemade food mixture was $2.63*10^{-5}$, $2.11*10^{-5}$, $2.11*10^{-6}$, $2.85*10^{-5}$, $1.79*10^{-5}$, and $6.15*10^{-5}$, respectively. The standard range for carcinogenic risk for lifetime ranged from 10^{-6} to 10^{-4} (USEPA, 2011; Kazi et al., 2016). This study reveals that carcinogenic risk persists for a lifetime among the studied (mother and infant) population through the intake of their respective dietary sources. The potential health risk to infants through consumption of breast milk is lower compared to their other daily dietary intakes. Cancer risk assessment through ingestion of daily dietary intakes of the studied populations is shown in Figure 6.6.

TABLE 6.3
Two-tailed paired t-test showing the relation between arsenic intake and excretion among the studied groups

Group	Arsenic intakes	Arsenic excretion			Degrees of freedom (df)*	Remarks
		Urine	Hair	Nail		
Mother	Drinking water	$t_{stat}(-0.11) < t_{crit}(2.26)$	$t_{stat}(4.18) > t_{crit}(2.26)$	$t_{stat}(5.78) > t_{crit}(2.26)$	9	Null hypothesis: accepted in the case of urine.
	Cooked rice	$t_{stat}(-5.85) < t_{crit}(2.26)$	$t_{stat}(4.11) > t_{crit}(2.26)$	$t_{stat}(5.73) > t_{crit}(2.26)$	9	Alternate hypothesis: accepted for hair and nail
Infant	Drinking water	$t_{stat}(-1.53) < t_{crit}(2.36)$	$t_{stat}(6.61) > t_{crit}(2.36)$	$t_{stat}(5.57) > t_{crit}(2.36)$	7	Null hypothesis: accepted in the case of urine.
	Cooked rice	$t_{stat}(-5.01) < t_{crit}(2.36)$	$t_{stat}(6.61) > t_{crit}(2.36)$	$t_{stat}(5.49) > t_{crit}(2.36)$	7	Alternate hypothesis: accepted for hair and nail
	Breast milk	$t_{stat}(-0.93) < t_{crit}(12.7)$	$t_{stat}(3.6) < t_{crit}(12.7)$	$t_{stat}(3.17) < t_{crit}(12.7)$	1	Null hypothesis: accepted in each case
	Cow's milk	$t_{stat}(-2.89) < t_{crit}(4.30)$	$t_{stat}(2.92) < t_{crit}(4.30)$	$t_{stat}(2.06) < t_{crit}(4.30)$	2	
	Commercial food (Cerelac)	$t_{stat}(-7.97) < t_{crit}(4.30)$	$t_{stat}(3.21) < t_{crit}(4.30)$	$t_{stat}(2.24) < t_{crit}(4.30)$	2	
	Homemade food mixture	$t_{stat}(-2.55) < t_{crit}(12.7)$	$t_{stat}(2.36) < t_{crit}(12.7)$	$t_{stat}(8.62) < t_{crit}(12.7)$	1	

*Significant at α = 0.05.

TABLE 6.4
Cancer and non-cancer risk of arsenic among the studied mother and infant populations from the exposed area

Groups	Samples	No. of samples (n)	Non-cancer risk (range)	Cancer risk (range)
Mother	Drinking water	10	0.27–0.77	$1.25*10^{-4}$–$3.47*10^{-4}$
	Cooked rice	10	0.21–1.70	$9.88*10^{-5}$–$7.65*10^{-4}$
Infant	Drinking water	11	0.005–0.20	$2.41*10^{-6}$–$9.17*10^{-5}$
	Cooked rice	11	0.01–0.15	$2.56*10^{-6}$–$6.75*10^{-5}$
	Breast milk	2	0.002–0.007	$1.03*10^{-6}$–$3.19*10^{-6}$
	Cow's milk	3	0.01–0.09	$4.38*10^{-6}$–$4.34*10^{-5}$
	Commercial food (Cerelac)	3	0.01–0.08	$5.83*10^{-6}$–$3.43*10^{-5}$
	Homemade food mixture	3	0.06–0.24	$2.75*10^{-5}$–$1.09*10^{-4}$

Likewise, for the non-carcinogenic risk (HQ value) the mean value in drinking water and cooked rice observed for the mother population is 0.39 and 0.89 respectively. Similarly, in infant populations, the mean HQ values observed are 0.06, 0.05, 0.005, 0.06, 0.04, and 0.14 for drinking water, cooked rice, breast milk, cow's milk, commercial food (Cerelac), and homemade food mixture respectively. The accepted level of non-carcinogenic risk is unity (USEPA, 2005). A study has reported that when HQ values are less than 1, this signifies that the reference dose is greater than DIA and it does not carry a harmful impact for human health (Kazi et al., 2016). In our survey, as the HQ values are less than 1, so the impact of non-carcinogenic risk does not persist among the studied population. As a result, there is less chance of non-cancerous health hazards among the populations.

6.4   CONCLUSION

The present study mainly focuses on the rate of health exposure due to As toxicity on an unexposed (mother and infant) population from an As-exposed area. The studied population is presently exposed to As-free drinking water. As accumulation in cooked rice is lower compared to raw rice grain, as the cooked rice preparation was performed with As-free drinking water. Urine As concentration reflected that the studied population is exposed to a lower level of acute toxicity. The rate of As accumulation in scalp hair and nail signified the level of chronic exposure among the studied populations. The high As deposition in biological tissues (scalp hair and nail) reveals that the studied mother population had been exposed to As toxicity for a long period of time.

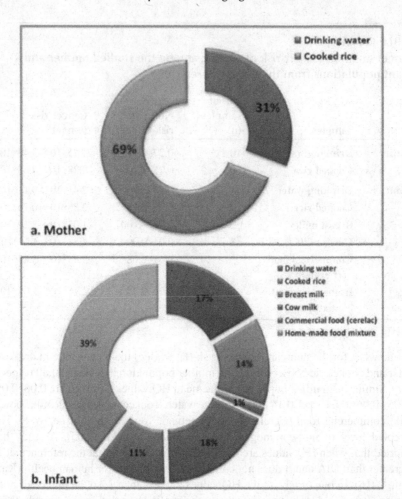

FIGURE 6.6 Cancer risk assessment through ingestion of daily dietary intakes of arsenic for (a) mother and (b) infant population.

During statistical interpretation, it was observed that ingestion of As through dietary intakes (drinking water and cooked rice) on a daily basis is a considerable exposure pathway to chronic As toxicity for the studied population. For the infant population, the high accumulation of As in the biological tissues (scalp hair and nail) indicates that they are sub-clinically affected by As toxicity. The potential carcinogenic risk persists for a lifetime among the studied (mother and infant) population through their respective dietary sources. The potential health risk to infants through ingestion of breast milk is least compared to their other daily dietary intakes. Similarly, the non-carcinogenic risk (HQ) showed values less than 1, which signifies that the studied populations are not prone to severe non-cancerous health hazards. The studied populations do not show arsenical skin lesions, as they are sub-clinically affected by As toxicity. The survey emphasized the fact that consumption of As-free drinking water is strongly to be recommended for As-exposed rural populations to struggle against the severe calamity of As pollution.

REFERENCES

Arnold, H. L., Odam, R. B., & James, W. D. (1990). Disease of the skin. In: *Clinical Dermatology,* Philadelphia: W. B. Saunders, 121–122.

ATSDR. (2007). Toxicological Profile for Arsenic. Agency for Toxic Substances and Disease Registry, Division of Toxicology, Atlanta, GA.

Biswas, A., Swain, S., Chowdhury, N. R., Joardar, M., Das, A., Mukherjee, M., & Roychowdhury, T. (2019). Arsenic contamination in Kolkata metropolitan city: perspective of transportation of agricultural products from arsenic-endemic areas. *Environmental Science and Pollution Research,* 26, 22929–22944.

Borgono, J. M., Vicent, P., Venturino, H., & Infante, A. (1977). Arsenic in the drinking water of the city of Antofagasta: epidemiological and clinical study before and after the installation of a treatment plant. *Environmental Health Perspectives,* 19, 103–105.

Carignan, C. C., Cottingham, K. L., Jackson, B. P., Farzan, S. F., Gandolfi, A. J., Punshon, T., Folt, C. L., & Karagas, M. R. (2015). Estimated exposure to arsenic in breastfed and formula-fed infants in a United States cohort. *Environmental Health Perspectives,* 123(5), 500–506.

Carlin, D. J., Naujokas, M. F., Bradham, K. D., Cowden, J., Heacock, M., Henry, H. F., Lee, J. S., Thomas, D. J., Thompson, C., Tokar, E. J., Waalkes, M. P., Birnbaum, L. S., & Suk, W. A. (2016). Arsenic and environmental health: state of the science and future research opportunities. *Environmental Health Perspectives,* 124(7), 890–899.

Chakraborti, D., Das, B., Rahman, M. M., Chowdhury, U. K., Biswas, B. K., Goswami, A. B., Nayak, B., Pal, A., Sengupta, M. K., Ahamed, S., Hossain, A., Basu, G. K., Roychowdhury, T., & Das, D. (2009). Status of groundwater arsenic contamination in the state of West Bengal, India: a 20-year study report. *Molecular Nutrition and Food Research,* 53, 542–551.

Chakraborti, D., Rahman, M. M., Das, B., Nayak, B., Pal, A., Sengupta, M. K., Hossain, M. A., Ahamed, S., Sahu, M., Saha, K.C., & Mukherjee, S.C. (2013). Groundwater arsenic contamination in Ganga–Meghna–Brahmaputra plain, its health effects and an approach for mitigation. *Environmental Earth Science,* 70(5), 1993–2008.

Chao, H. H., Guo, C. H., Huang, C. B., Chen, P. C., Li, H. C., Hsiung, D. Y., & Chou, Y. K. (2014). Arsenic, cadmium, lead, and aluminium concentrations in human milk at early stages of lactation. *Pediatrics & Neonatology,* 55(2), 127–134.

Chatterjee, D., Halder, D., Majumder, S., Biswas, A., Nath, B., Bhattacharya, P., Bhowmick, S., Mukherjee-Goswami, A., Saha, D., Hazra, R., & Maity, P. B. (2010). Assessment of arsenic exposure from groundwater and rice in Bengal Delta Region, West Bengal, India. *Water Research,* 44(19), 5803–5812.

Chattopadhyay, A., Singh, A. P., Singh, S. K., Barman, A., Patra, A., Mondal, B. P., & Banerjee, K. (2020). Spatial variability of arsenic in Indo-Gangetic basin of Varanasi and its cancer risk assessment. *Chemosphere,* 238, 124623.

Chowdhury, N. R., Das, R., Joardar, M., Ghosh, S., Bhowmick, S., & Roychowdhury, T. (2018a). Arsenic accumulation in paddy plants at different phases of pre-monsoon cultivation. *Chemosphere,* 210, 987–997.

Chowdhury, N. R., Ghosh, S., Joardar, M., Kar, D., & Roychowdhury, T. (2018b). Impact of arsenic contaminated groundwater used during domestic scale post harvesting of paddy crop in West Bengal: arsenic partitioning in raw and parboiled whole grain. *Chemosphere,* 211, 173–184.

Chowdhury, N. R., Das, A., Joardar, M., De, A., Mridha, D., Das, R., Rahman, M. M., & Roychowdhury, T. (2020a). Flow of arsenic between rice grain and water: its inter-action, accumulation and distribution in different fractions of cooked rice. *Science of the Total Environment,* 731, 138937. https://doi.org/10.1016/j.scitotenv.2020.138937.

Chowdhury, N. R., Das, A., Mukherjee, M., Swain, S., Joardar, M., De, A., Mridha, D., & Roychowdhury, T. (2020b). Monsoonal paddy cultivation with phase-wise arsenic distribution in exposed and control sites of West Bengal, alongside its assimilation in rice grain. *Journal of Hazardous Materials,* 400, 123206. https://doi.org/10.1016/j.jhazmat.2020.123206.

Das, A., Das, S. S., Chowdhury, N. R., Joardar, M., Ghosh, B., & Roychowdhury, T. (2020). Quality and health risk evaluation for groundwater in Nadia district, West Bengal: an approach on its suitability for drinking and domestic purpose. *Groundwater Sustainable Development,* 10, 100351. https://doi.org/10.1016/j.gsd.2020.100351.

European Commission. (2015). Commission Regulation 2015/1006 of 25 June 2015 amending Regulation (EC) No 1881/2006 as regards maximum levels of inorganic arsenic in foodstuffs.

EFSA. (2009). Scientific opinion on arsenic in food – panel on Contaminants in the Food Chain (CONTAM). European Food Safety Authority. EFSA Journal, 7(10), 1351.

Ettinger, A. S., Roy, A., Amarairiwardena, C. J., Smith, D. R., Lupoli, N., MercadoGarcia, A., Lamadrid-Figueroa, H., Tellez-Rojo, M. M., Hu, H., & Hernandez A. M. (2014). Maternal blood, plasma and breast milk lead: lactation, transfer and contribution to infant exposure. Environmental Health Perspectives, 22(1), 87–92.

Farmer, J. G., & Johnson, L. R. (1990). Assessment of occupational exposure to inorganic arsenic based on urinary concentrations and speciation of arsenic. *British Journal of Industrial Medicine,* 47, 342–348.

Goswami, R., Kumar, M., Biyani, N., & Shea, P.J. (2020). Arsenic exposure and percep-tion of health risk due to groundwater contamination in Majuli (river island), Assam, India. *Environmental Geochemistry and Health,* 42(2), 443–460.

Gürbay, A., Charehsaz, M., Eken, A., Sayal, A., Girgin, G., Yurdakak, M., Yigit, S., Erol, D., Sahin, G., & Aydin, A. (2012). Toxic metals in breast milk samples from Ankara Turkey: assessment of lead, cadmium, nickel and arsenic levels. *Biological Trace Elements Research,* 149, 117–122.

Halder, D., Bhowmick, S., Biswas, A., Mandal, U., Nriagu, J., GuhaMazumdar, D. N., Chatterjee, D., & Bhattacharya, P. (2012). Consumption of brown rice: a potential pathway for arsenic exposure in rural Bengal. *Environmental Science and Technology,* 46(7), 4142–4148.

Halder, D., Biswas, A., Slejkovec, Z., Chatterjee, D., Nriagu, J., Jacks, G., & Bhattacharya, P. (2014). Arsenic species in raw and cooked rice: implications for human health in rural Bengal. *Science of the Total Environment,* 497, 200–208.

International Agency for Research on Cancer (IARC). (2012). Arsenic, Metals, Fibres, and Dusts, Volume 100C.A Review of Human Carcinogens. http://monographs.iarc.fr/ENG/Monographs/vol100C/mono100C.pdf.

Ioanid, N., Bors, G., & Popa, I. (1961). Beiträge zur Kenntnis des normalen Arsengehaltesron Nägeln und des Gehaltes in den Fällen von Arsenpolyneuritis. *International Journal of Legal Medicine,* 52(1), 90–94.

Joardar, M., Das, A., Mridha, D., De, A., Chowdhury, N. R., & Roychowdhury, T. (2021). Evaluation of acute and chronic arsenic exposure on school children from exposed and apparently control areas of West Bengal, India. *Exposure and Health*, 13, 33–50.

Joseph, T., Dubey, B., & McBean, E. A. (2015). Human health risk assessment from arsenic exposures in Bangladesh. Science of the Total Environment, 527, 552–560. https:// doi.org/10.1016/j.scitotenv.2015.05.053.

Kazi, T. G., Brahman, K. D., Afridi, H. I., Arain, M. B., Talpur, F. N., & Akhtar, A. (2016). The effects of arsenic contaminated drinking water of livestock on its total levels in milk samples of different cattle: risk assessment in children. *Chemosphere*, 165, 427–433.

Kumarathilaka, P., Seneweera, S., Ok, Y. S., Meharg, A., & Bundschuha, J. (2019). Arsenic in cooked rice foods: assessing health risks and mitigation options. *Environmental International*, 127, 584–591.

Mondal, D., Banerjee, M., Kundu, M., Banerjee, N., Bhattacharya, U., Giri, A. K., Ganguli, B., Roy, S. S., & Polya, D. A. (2010). Comparison of drinking water, raw rice and cooking of rice as arsenic exposure routes in three contrasting areas of West Bengal, India. *Environmental Geochemistry and Health*, 32(6), 463–477.

NRC. (1999). Arsenic in Drinking Water. National Academy Press, Washington, D C.

Pal, A., Chowdhury, U. K., Mondal, D., Das, B., Nayak, B., Ghosh, A., Maity, S., & Chakraborti, D. (2009). Arsenic burden from cooked rice in the populations of arsenic affected and non-affected areas and Kolkata City in West-Bengal, India. *Environmental Science and Technology*, 43(9), 3349–3355.

Povorinskaya, O. A., & Karpenko, O. M. (2009). Macro and trace element status of patients of the elder age groups. *Bulletin of Experimental Biology and Medicine*, 147, 473–475.

Rahman, M. A., Hasegawa, H., Rahman, M. M., Miah, M. A., & Tasmin, A. (2008). Arsenic accumulation in rice (*Oryzasativa* L.): human exposure through food chain. *Ecotoxicology and Environmental Safety*, 69, 317–324.

Rebelo, F. M., & Caldas, E. D. (2016). Arsenic, lead, mercury and cadmium: toxicity, levels in breast milk and the risks for breastfed infants. *Environmental Research*, 151, 671–688.

Roychowdhury, T. (2010). Groundwater arsenic contamination in one of the 107 arsenic-affected blocks in West Bengal, India: status, distribution, health effects and factors responsible for arsenic poisoning. *International Journal of Hygiene and Environmental Health*, 213(6), 414–427.

Roychowdhury, T., Uchino, T., Tokunaga, H., & Ando, M. (2002). Survey of arsenic in food composites from an arsenic-affected area of West Bengal, India. *Food and Chemical Toxicology*, 40, 1611–1621.

Sampson, M. L., Bostick, B., Chiew, H., Hangan, J. M., & Shantz, A. (2008). Arsenicosis in Cambodia: case studies and policy response. *Applied Geochemistry*, 23, 2976–2985.

Shapiro, H. A. (1967). Arsenic content of human hair and nails: its interpretation. *Journal of Forensic Medicine*, 14(2), 65–71.

Singh, S. K., & Ghosh, A. K. (2012). Health risk assessment due to groundwater arsenic contamination: children are at high risk. Human and Ecological Risk Assessment: An International Journal, 18(4), 751–766.

Sun, G. X., Williams, P. N., Zhu, Y. G., Deacon, C., Carey, A. M., Raab, A., Feldmann, J., & Meharg, A. A. (2009). Survey of arsenic and its speciation in rice products such as breakfast cereals, rice crackers and Japanese rice condiments. *Environmental International*, 35(3), 473–475.

USEPA. (2001). Baseline human health risk assessment Vasquez Boulevard and I-70 superfund site, Denver CO. www.epa.gov/region8/superfund/sites/VB-170-Risk.pdf. Accessed 01/20/2011.

USEPA. (2005). Guidelines for Carcinogen Risk Assessment. Risk Assessment Forum. United States Environmental Protection Agency, Washington, DC. EPA/630/P-03/001F

USEPA. (2011). Screening Level (RSL) for Chemical Contaminant at Superfound Sites. Washington, DC: U.S. Environmental Protection Agency.

Vahter, M. E. (1994). Species differences in the metabolism of arsenic. *Environmental Geochemistry and Health*, 16, 171–179.

Vahter, M. E. (2009). Effects of arsenic on maternal and fetal health. *Annual Review on Nutrition,* 29, 381–399.

WHO. (2011). Evaluation of certain contaminants in food. Seventy second report of the Joint FOA/WHO expert committee on food additives, WHO technical report series No. 959. World Health Organization (WHO), Geneva.

Zhao, F. J., Stroud, J. L., Eagling, T., Dunham, S. J., McGrath, S. P., & Shewry, P. R. (2010). Accumulation, distribution, and speciation of As in wheat grain. *Environmental Science and Technology*, 44, 5464–5468. https://doi.org/10.1021/es100765g.

Unit III

Climate Change and Human Health

A Perspective

7 Climate Insecurity, Health and Well-Being Among Ganga–Meghna–Brahmaputra Delta Communities

Debojyoti Das and Upasona Ghosh*

CONTENTS

7.1   INTRODUCTION: CLIMATE AND HEALTH INTER-LINKAGES

Life in the Ganga–Meghna–Brahmaputra (GMB) delta is like the edge of a knife. This is an environmentally vulnerable, densely populated area which has recently become the ground zero of climate change. During the 19th century the deltas was reclaimed from the sea and resettled by colonial revenue officials to shore up the fiscal coffers of the Bengal Presidency. Such land policy exposed

* Corresponding author: Debojyoti Das. ukdebodas@gmail.com

DOI: 10.1201/9781003095422-7

peasants and sharecroppers to tropical cyclones. Two significant political events of the 20th century, the partition of India in 1947 and the 1971 Bangladesh liberation war auxiliary, imposed pressure on the region's limited land resource and ecology from East Bengal migrant refugees. Ever since, the marginalized littoral communities of the Bengal delta, mostly composed of Dalits and other outcaste communities, are facing triple betrayals from geography, politics, and social marginality. In recent years, the impact of tropical cyclones such as Sider (2007), Nargis (2008), Aila (2009), Mahasen (2013), Amphan (2020) and Yash (2021) enforced worrying concerns among delta community members, policy makers, civil society actors and medical professionals working on the fragile delta ecosystem.

Worldwide states are calling for transformational approaches to deal with challenges posed by climate change. Among the countless impacts, community health is one crucial sphere where climatic changes are already having a detrimental impact. Changes in extreme weather events, under-nutrition, and increasingly climate-sensitive diseases are projected to intensify morbidity and mortality by 2030 (WHO 2010). The Lancet Commission in their 2009 report stated that climate change would be "the biggest global health threat of the 21st century" (The Lancet 2009). The Commission urged that all countries should strengthen their health systems to expand their reach in order to achieve United Nations Sustainable Development Goal 3 (healthy lives and wellbeing) and universal health coverage. However, policy response in this regard is crucial, especially in developing and under-developed countries as access to resources here is sensitive to societal intersections. Vulnerability towards climate change impacts varies according to social vulnerabilities which can be determined by several factors, such as livelihood, class, caste, ethnicity, geographic location, gender, and socio-economic status. The intensity of these determinants of vulnerabilities is not uniformly distributed; rather it varies according to contextual structure. Therefore, efforts to respond to, mitigate, or adapt to health impacts of climate change will need to address issues of equity and social justice posing challenges for policy making.

Before moving on to the next section we would like to present an ethnographic vignette in order to contextualize the health care challenges faced by delta dwellers in their everyday life. These chronicles were recorded firsthand from interlocutors and hosts during our fieldwork sojourn in the Sundarbans. During 2012–13 and 2017 fieldwork in Sundurbans Dayapur village we were supported by my host late *dalit* intellectual, poet and intellectual Mukunda Gayne. He migrated from East Pakistan, present-day Bangladesh, in 1946 just before the eve of partition. His family exchanged land with another Muslim household in this part of the Sundarbans. We stayed in his mud hut to conduct our eight-month-long fieldwork in Dayapur and the surrounding villages of the Gosaba block.

After returning from the field the lead author made another field trip in 2017 when Mukunda's son Prodosh shared a disturbing story of the death of his infant daughter a few days after delivery. She died of a rare medical condition, meconium aspiration syndrome. Meconium is the first feces, or stool, of the newborn. Meconium aspiration syndrome occurs when a newborn breathes a mixture of meconium and amniotic fluid into the lungs around the time of delivery. Meconium aspiration syndrome, a leading cause of severe illness and death in the newborn, occurs in about 5 -10% of births. It typically occurs when the fetus is stressed during labor, especially when the infant is past its due date. The parents cited medical neglect and lack of care in the village delivery center as the main cause of their child's death. When they complained their concern was silenced by officials who claimed that they were ignorant villagers and had no knowledge of science and medicine. The doctors declined to interact with us and as usual blamed the villagers for their ignorance, belief in superstition, and lack of education and hygiene that transmits to such accidents. The experience left the couple and my host heartbroken. Such traumatic pregnancy and complicated delivery are common in Sundarbans where health care centers are far apart, and women often cannot make it to the delivery center or hospital on time in complicated cases where constant monitoring and care is needed.

Mukunda's son was not the only person who had experienced such a fate; there were others in the village who regularly faced such problems. His testimony made me realize the precarious health care facilities in the delta. If we look back, the islands in Gosaba were reclaimed from the mangrove forest by a Scottish Zamindar Sir Daniel Mackinnon Hamilton, who was the head of P&O cruise operations in Bombay and had bought three islands from the British Indian government to develop settlements through free land grants to landless peasants who came from central India and the Medinipur district of West Bengal during 1910 to 1920. Besides establishing schools and agricultural institutions, Hamilton also established health clinics in the settled villages. After India's independence the Zamindari was run by upper-caste landlords like Sudanshu Bushan Mazundar, who became the defecto trustee and owner of the estate. During the 1970s Gopinath Burman, locally known as daktar babu, became the trustee of the Hamilton estate in Gosaba. He revolutionized the maternal health care system in the island by introducing the red data book. During our visit to the Hamilton archives, we discovered many files that contained patients' details and meticulous notes on the development of the pregnancy until birth. Such record keeping helped clinicians in his hospital monitor meticulously maternal health and reduced the number of pre- and post-natal deaths in Gosaba and its neighboring villages. Gopinath Burman introduced the book on the advice of his daughter who was at that time graduating as a pediatrician from the USA. We also saw newspaper clippings in the record room showcasing how he treated people who were attacked by tigers in the Sundarbans and he soon became a household name, a hero and savior doctor. His achievements were covered by the local newspaper, and he soon became a very popular physician in Gosaba. Soon after his death these established practices were no longer followed by other government doctors who rarely come to attend the clinic. These days there is a general dispiritedness among doctors not to become a resident doctor in the islands because of poor pay and opportunities in Sundarbans village.

In the past decade non-government organizations (NGOs) and community-based organizations have filled the gap by organizing health camps and building hospitals in the region. Many of these organizations have dalit entrepreneurs who are planning to create local health care facilities. During our field study we observed health camps set up to treat cataract patients and blood donation camps that were aimed to help village people in need. As we toured the villages in and around Gasabo we realized that the health care facility in the region was dismal with limited trained medical staff. The NGO Tagore Society for Rural Development (TSRD) had a medical clinic in Rangabelia while the BM Foundation was planning another one in the region. The concrete structure of the hospital building was half complete and dilapidated as the organization had run out of money and was in the process of raising funds from the Bengali diaspora. Faith based NGOs and religious missionaries also volunteer to provide first aid and humanitarian assistance to villagers after a disaster strikes and often fill the vacuum left by the scanty presence of state functionaries. Given this backdrop we will discuss the health care system in the Indian part of the Sundarbans delta that is susceptible to climate change and the grand challenges posed to health and wellbeing in the region. For this we will first examine the social determinants of health (SDH).

7.2 SOCIAL DETERMINANTS OF HEALTH

At the core of these complexities, some striking social factors run through different layers of society (Marmot 2005), especially in low- and middle-income countries. Hence, in the last 35 years, the SDH approach describing non-medical factors like socio-economic status, race and ethnicity, gender, cultural beliefs, education and information, climate and environment has emerged as an approach to explain health as a social problem and persisting health inequalities at individual and community level. International organizations, namely United Nations, European Union, and World Health Organization (WHO), are committed to bring about health equity by acting on SDH.

The WHO Commission on Social Determinants of Health (CSDH) (CSDH 2008) defines SDH as "the conditions in which people are born, grow, live, work and age, including the health system." The CSDH (2008) divides social determinants into two broad areas: structural determinants and intermediate determinants. Structural determinants refer to the socio-economic and political factors where inequalities regulate the access and distribution of resources as per social status and dynamics of power. The major structural determinants pointed out by CSDH are livelihood, education, economic status, gender, ethnicity, and cultural practices. Structural determinants are mediated by a series of factors which are termed as intermediary social determinants by CSDH. Structural determinants are causally antecedent to these intermediary determinants, which are linked to a set of individual-level influences, including social ties, health behaviors, physiological factors, access to information, and climate (WHO 2010).

According to the WHO (WHO 2010), SDHs include social gradients, stress, early childhood development, social exclusion, unemployment, social networks, addiction, availability of quality food, and healthy transportation. Later in 2010, WHO addressed two broad areas of SDH in the CSDH report. First was living conditions, including healthy physical environment, quality employment and decent work, social protection throughout life, and health care access. The other area was decentralization of power, money, and resources, including equity in health programs, public financing, gender equity, political empowerment, and a balanced prosperity of nations. Again, the US Centers for Disease Control and Prevention (2009) define SDH as "life-enhancing resources, such as food supply, housing, economic and social relationships, transportation, education, and health care, whose distribution across populations effectively determines length and quality of life" (Centers for Disease Control and Prevention 2009).

In 1948 the WHO acknowledged the significance of social and economic factors in human health and urged for the collaboration between allied sectors like livelihood, shelter, and welfare protection. However, during the 1950s and 1960s WHO and other global health leaders were not that concerned about the social context while implementing various health interventions. The concept again came to light in 1978 after the Alma Ata Declaration and Health for All movement to reassess the social factors to achieve health equity and social justice (WHO-UNICEF, Alma-Ata, Geneva: WHO 1978). Many countries welcomed this approach under the Health for All program; however, countries with neo-liberal market models of the 1980s posed challenges to incorporating vulnerable marginalized sub-groups in mainstream heath sectors. Around this time prominent literature by scholars such as McKeown (1976), Illich (1976), the Black report (Department of Health and Social Security 1980), and Marmot et al. (1978) marked considerable understanding of the importance of social factors in existing health inequalities in Britain. For the next two decades, the understanding became strongly established in other European countries through significant work (Whitehead 1990; Marmot et al. 1991) which finally began to address SDH around the 1990s. Within decades, the concept had traveled beyond European boundaries and spread across other developed European countries and under-developed countries from Africa and Central and South-East Asia to take a policy stand on reducing health inequalities (Tajer 2003).

In 2004 WHO in the World Health Assembly positioned the CSDH as a key mechanism to reduce health inequalities, especially in countries from the Global South. In 2008, the CSDH produced their report on health inequalities which was welcomed by countries across the world to formulate their health policies as per guidelines suggested in the report.

Environment and climate play a decisive role in accessing health care but often overlooked are their cascading impacts which mediate other social factors and affect human health. In conventional literature, geographical factors are often identifiable and viewed as major intervening aspects for access to medical care and resultant health outcomes, specifically for the disadvantaged population from both low and middle-income countries (Peters et al. 2008). Regional variations in access to health care due to distance and travel time, linked to uptake of services and sometimes health outcome or even rate of mortality, have been widely documented in the existing literature (Wong et al. 1987; Wilson and Rosenberg 2002; Soeung et al. 2012). Climate can affect the geographic distribution of vector-borne diseases (Anderson and Main 2006) such as malaria, dengue, and schistosomiasis. For these evident health outcomes, children were more vulnerable than their adult counterparts. Scholars like Neira et al. (2008) stated that children are one of the groups that are most susceptible to adverse environment-related health outcomes. Shea in 2003 pointed out the reason behind children's vulnerability. According to this scholar, while growing up physically and cognitively, children are more vulnerably exposed to biological, chemical, and physical environments (Shea 2003).

However, an alternate school of thought suggests that the role of geographical accessibility in hindering health care access differs as per perceived health needs of the community. Therefore, a higher perceived need often seems to overcome the influence of geographic inaccessibility (Arcury et al. 2005). Evidence from India and other developing nations indicates that for childbirth and maternal health needs in particular, customs related to care seeking often overpower geographic accessibility of services (Basu 2000; Furuta and Salway 2006).

The aforementioned factors facilitate or hinder the access and utilization of health services, and influence people to behave differently in terms of their health. Voluminous evidence reflects the crucial impacts of community factors on health, though the definitive knowledge of impact pathways is partial. The knowledge gap also exists on which factors influence others in a given context.

7.3 THEORETICAL UNDERPINNING OF HOW CLIMATE AS A SOCIAL DETERMINANT EMERGED TO LIMIT CAPABILITY OF A PERSON TO ACCESS HEALTH CARE

The philosophical discourses around SDH have mainly built upon John Rawls' "theory of justice" (Rawls 1971) and Amartya Sen's "capability perspective" (Sen 1985). In his theory of justice, Rawls stated that justice necessitates a fair and equal supply of principal goods, among which health is one of the crucial goods. His concept stated that people of a lower social stratum are often in a "veil of ignorance" about their position, hence unknowingly tend to choose the minimum facilities. Rawls term this behavioral pattern as the "social lottery of life" (Rawls 1971). While applying Rawls' theory in SDH, Daniels and his colleagues (Daniels et al. 2000; Daniels 2002) argued that "justice can only be achieved if the circulation of primary goods like health can be implemented through a wider approach across the socio-economic strata assuring far more than a decent minimum" (Daniels et al. 2000). They argued further that social determinants, for example, socio-economic status, should be equally distributed firsthand as health inequalities are the byproducts of this determinants (Daniels 2002). Hence, according to them, the aim should be equal distribution of basic services like education, housing, and employment and poverty eradication (Daniels et al. 2000).

Critics of Rawlsian analysis of SDH have pointed out that reducing health inequality only through the improvement of socio-economic conditions is not that linear; rather it needs greater political and policy reforms to reduce systematic health inequalities (Angell 2000; Emanuel 2000; Kamm 2001). Similarly, critics like Anand and Peter (2000) and Gakidou et al. (2000) stated that, to address health inequality, reform should incorporate justice across and within different social intersections – race, ethnicity, and gender – and not just across socio-economic groups (Brock 2000). Brock in 2000 provided a much clearer critique in this regard by saying that justice on health inequality as a philosophical framework requires inclusion of tradeoffs between different inequalities instead of being built around only socio-economic inequalities (Brock 2000). A more fundamental critique of the Rawlsian approach has been provided by Amartya Sen in 1985 and by Michael Marmot in 2008. Both these scholars argued that resources and the means to achieve those resources have no innate value; hence, access to health care as a primary good depends upon one's individual characteristics (Sen 1985). Sen further argued that:

> account would have to be taken not only of the primary goods the persons respectively hold, but also of the relevant personal characteristics that govern the conversion of primary goods into the person's ability to promote her ends. For example, a person who is disabled may have a larger basket of primary goods and yet have less chance to lead a normal life (or to pursue her objectives) than an able-bodied person with a smaller basket of primary goods.
>
> **(Sen 1999)**

Sen continued that identifying health as a byproduct of justice (Rawls 1971) is over-simplifying the actual demands of health equity, which in turn limits widespread desire for social justice (Sen 1999). Amartya Sen through his seminal works developed the capability approach applied to SDH, rooted in Aristotle's political theory (Sen 1985). This concept is, according to various SDH scholars, more nuanced, practical, and people-centered (Ruger 1998, 2006). This approach expands the fundamental values of health by not looking at it as essential goods like employment or health care, but by incorporating individuals' capabilities like education, political freedom, or participation in trade or production (Ruger 1998, 2006).

Marmot and colleagues also supported the concept of SDH by adding that the aforementioned capabilities may be associated with individuals but often have great importance, either jointly or individually, on the health of that particular individual (Marmot et al. 1991; Marmot and Wilkinson 2001). Sen's view on "Development of Freedom" (Sen 1999) thus incorporates complete freedom of individuals as a social being to perform their own choices to live a life they value. Sen stated that freedom in one sphere of life can enhance other spheres; at the same time disadvantages in one sphere may lead to a decline in freedom in other spheres of life (Sen 1999). Hence, Sen's capability approach implies the agency-oriented view to take action individually or collectively to exercise complete freedom (Sen 1999).

Reducing social inequalities cannot be the stand-alone process for reducing health inequalities. It requires a much broader approach for transforming the overall situation of people to perform choices about a healthier life for themselves and for the future generation (Sen 1999; Marmot 2008; Ruger 2006). This is the exact converse of the view that treated individuals as passive recipients of health care facilities and other policy implementations (Rawls 1971).

As the concept of SDH progresses, it has incorporated the different capabilities of individuals within its domains. WHO's CSDH framework thus incorporates a life course approach. The approach traced upon a strong foundation to start the life of every child, including pregnant mothers, prenatal childcare, early-life care and education, and an overall childcare system (WHO 2010). The approach also emphasizes the later stages of life by incorporating individual and collective empowerment, employment, reducing stress in the workplace, and social isolation.

The new SDH framework (WHO 2010) incorporates the wider society for collective action on health by improving local-level social solidity and resilience. The framework emphasizes inter-generational equity, especially for determinants like environment. Effective convergence between stakeholders inter- and intra-country should be the key to governance of a health care delivery system, as suggested by the framework (Alliance for Health Policy and Systems Research 2004). Theoretical discourses of the SDH concept have a strong focus on policy implications from the very beginning. The discourses suggest greater actions to improve people's health by engaging in reduction of inequalities in socio-economic status and also taking a widespread approach towards improvement in every sphere of life of an individual which, according to Sen, is capabilities of freedom (Sen 1999).

7.4 CASES OF INDIAN SUNDARBANS

7.4.1 BACKGROUND

The literature has suggested strong evidence of climate change impacts on children's health. Hoddinott and Kinsey (2001) found that the 1994–95 droughts in Zimbabwe significantly lowered annual growth rates for children, and the effects lasted for four years after the drought. Similarly, Story et al. (2020) found that during the drought in Ethiopia from 1996 to 1997, the prevalence of child stunting increased. Heltberg and Lund (2009) in their study in Pakistan found that, out of various shocks faced by the study household, health shocks dominated in frequency, costliness, and severity of outcome. Alderman et al. (2006) established a causal relationship between a child's height and adult height and schooling by manipulating external events like civil war and droughts in Zimbabwe. Datar et al. (2013) examined the impact of natural disasters on children's health in rural India at a household level through a time series analytical approach which identified three-way impacts of natural disasters on children: (1) direct impact such as various morbidity patterns and fatality; (2) sub-optimal delivery of health care; and (3) a negative correlation between demand for health care and decreasing socio-economic status. These factors are highly dependent on both individual and household characteristics. The study found factors such as a child's gender and age, mother's education, and household ethnic status differ significantly between northern and southern Indian states.

The climate and environmental threats are gaining strong footholds, especially on the health of children from the Global South, as we are still unable to manage climate change. Hence, as regards the health of children, which significantly depends on social determinants such as impoverishment, safe drinking water, unhygienic sanitation, and inadequate healthcare systems, the outcome became worse (McMichael et al. 2007). As changes in the climate seems to be continuing into the foreseeable future, impacts on children's health in terms of physical and mental trauma, communicable water-borne and vector-borne diseases, under-nutrition, and stunting are expected to increase (Sheffield and Landrigan et al. 2011; Smith et al. 2014).

Exposure of a significant number of households to major climatic shocks is an integral part of any discourse on the Sundarbans. Nature often takes its toll in terms of cyclonic storms and floods that breach the banks, inundate localities, render people homeless, and make agricultural lands completely unusable for the next few years. However, these manifestations of climate changes are not linearly placed. Several crucial pathways have been found to hinder child health outcomes and overall development of the children of the Sundarbans. The climatic changes which are stereotypically intermediate determinants of child health turn to be the most crucial structural one by mediating other determinants such as parents' livelihood and health-seeking behavior.

7.4.2 CLIMATE IMPACTS ON CHILD HEALTH IN INDIAN SUNDARBANS

The Indian Sundarbans is one of many unique empirical grounds to understand how climatic changes are actually heightening existing structural inequalities to make children vulnerable to long- and short-term impacts. Climate change in Sundarbans produces two magnitudes of impact on child health. First is the immediate impact; for example, a sudden rise in the prevalence of water-borne and vector-borne diseases; the health care infrastructure makes the already weak system more inaccessible, and deprives affected children of timely or quality-assured medical attention (Kanjilal et al. 2013). This also erodes the livelihood opportunities of the affected parents and sucks the poor households deeper into a vicious poverty cycle and resulting food and nutrition insecurity (Kanjilal et al. 2013). The second is a more long-term impact originating from the immediate impacts. These immediate impacts, in combination, trigger child under-nutrition and strengthen the vicious cycle between recurrent morbidity and under-nutrition. We argue that children in the climatically vulnerable pockets of Indian Sundarbans have to face recurrent health shocks due to frequent climatic events like cyclones, floods, and daily tidal inundation more than their mainland counterparts. They also have to face shortages of required food intake to maintain a balanced nutritional status due to the loss of their parents' livelihood options as a result of the changing climate. Male out-migration and other local-level adjustments are being undertaken by the parents to deal with socio-economic changes. More so, parents have fewer choices about service delivery options in terms of both formal and informal health providers impacting their care-seeking behavior.

The health care delivery system, on the other hand, is equally being hampered by frequent climatic events in terms of losing infrastructure and human resources and becomes less prepared to cope with further impacts. Central to the aforementioned conceptualization of climate impact on child health in Sundarbans, we argue about two types of vulnerabilities: (1) clinical vulnerability that makes children susceptible to various diseases; and (2) social vulnerability which holds back children from getting over their illness with desirable treatment choices.

7.4.3 THE CLIMATIC CONTEXT OF THE SUNDARBANS: A DETERMINANT IN ITSELF

The legacy of colonial oppression and neglect is still continuing in post-colonial rules and political regime shift in the Sundarbans. The changes are taking place in an always dynamic political environment. The Sundarbans are part of the North 24 Parganas and South 24 Parganas districts of West Bengal – districts with the dubious distinction of having arguably witnessed large numbers of deaths due to political clashes. This political tussle on the issue of compensation of land and areas to be earmarked for embankments is being carried out by the islanders themselves following the wishes of their state political heads in Kolkata. The islanders believe nature makes their life uncertain but, paradoxically, also adds an element of certainty to their livelihood. Cumulative imposition of restrictions by policy makers on fishing, prawn catching, etc. on the entreaty of preserving biodiversity has only served to intensify the climate-induced uncertainty afflicting the lives of these people.

The idea of climate change, which has become a scientific discourse among scientists, is a mixture of extremes. One group of academicians based their postulates on three cornerstones which have been affected by global warming: rising sea surface temperature, rate of sea level rise, and net erosion and accretion rates. In contrast, the other group points out that the change is minimal and that it is mostly human-made factors that have done most damage to the islands. These two conflicting views among academicians have in turn divided policy makers and policy implementers down to sub-divisional level. The believers in climate change have actually used the evidence to justify inertia of inaction to help islanders cope with limate shock following the theory that this is common for a coastal belt and that human settlements bordering the embankments should be forthrightly evacuated.

The debate among civil society, particularly international agencies, is also pronounced and is increasingly being drawn along the lines of pro- and anti-conservationists. A section of civil society, mostly belonging to the tiger conservation lobby, has forecast that a planned resettlement plan for one-third of the islands is urgently needed. One of the reasons cited is that the Sundarbans delta is riverine ecology and only suitable for the flora and fauna that are the true inhabitants of the islands and are resilient to their climate and riverine topography. However, the islanders view what they term as "weather change" through the lens of their daily chores and what affects their livelihood. Fishers would cite turbulent weather at unlikely times in the year, farmers cite uncertain rainfall periodicity and frequencies, and women are concerned about rises in water levels during high tides inundating their homestead ponds with saltwater. The debate on climate has been high on the agenda ever since cyclone Aila and the resultant attention of outsiders which even women in the remotest islands are aware of. Recently, after cyclone Amphan happened in May 2020, the common people gained more significant experiential knowledge about the impacts of large environmental events.

The livelihood of the islanders has perhaps been the worst hit by climate change. There is perhaps not a single house in the deltaic parts of the Sundarbans that remained unscathed by cyclone Aila and cyclone Amphan within a decade. During Aila, in some of the worst-hit remote islands where the saline water sweeps into homes at high tide, most male members between the ages of 18 and 50 have migrated outside, leaving behind women to fend for the family. For these women – the most vulnerable and disadvantaged of the islanders – depleting livelihood options and daily threats to shelter seem to be not of as much concern as the mustering of the few necessities that would keep them going each day. To an outsider like the researcher, they may complain about their precarious existence and uncertain future, but what really matters to them is the present and the myriad struggles involved in keeping it alive. In this situation, proper care of children is – needless to say – the toughest problem.

After Amphan, the situation became even more complicated as just before the cyclone there was an influx of reverse migration due to COVID-19 lockdown measures which limited the option of out-migration as a livelihood alternative. Evidence on the gradual and long-term impacts of Amphan are yet to be generated; in time this may provide a future lead on climate change impacts on health and development of the people of Sundarbans.

In the Sundarbans the debate on the different discourses regarding socio-economic development amidst climate change is not unlike the mud layers that make up the fragile embankments. The complexity of the situation is heightened by the fact that there is scarcely any homogeneity even within the present situation: not in the distribution of vulnerabilities, nor in the perceptions of the islanders and policy makers. This discrepancy in understanding leads to unplanned actions like male migration or making the scattered earthen embankments. Children of the Sundarbans suffer all these uncertainties from the very beginning of their life and do not get enough requisite societal safeties required to sustain a healthy life under such uncertainties.

7.4.4 Climate Change Moderating Other Determinants of Health

Climate change and its impacts on the life of the Sundarbans people have now become overarching phenomena. In a nutshell, in the case of Sundarbans, climatic changes are producing two types of impact on child health. It is controlling everything: sometimes individually; sometimes in combination with other determinants. First is the immediate impact, for example, a rise in the incidence of flood-related diseases (e.g., diarrhea and respiratory infections). The second is a long-run extension of the immediate effect. The coastal regions of Sundarbans are facing food resource crunches by losing agricultural and fishing products due to frequent salinity ingression and rapid land erosion, breaking the economic backbone of households by altering traditional livelihoods and increasing social vulnerability which in turn increases the burden of under-nutrition.

However, the risk is still not well reflected in the malnutrition status of the children due to the range of short-term coping strategies taken by the parents. Findings revealed a direct link between malnutrition status of the children in the studied regions along with the household food security which in turn correlated with climatic vulnerability (Ghosh et al. 2018). These effects, in combination, trigger child under-nutrition and strengthen the vicious cycle between recurrent morbidity and under-nutrition.

7.4.5 Health Care Delivery System: Sub-Optimal to Cater Generally as Well as Climate-Sensitive Health Care Services

The current health care delivery system notion of categorizing child health with general reproductive health care is a well-tested one. However, in the present context of geographical inaccessibility, existing structural inequality, and climate change, child health issues are often diluted due to extra emphasis on birth delivery care (pre- and peri-natal care of mothers). This is especially true for the general services provided to people of all ages (for example, outpatient care in the block health facility), where the lack of focus manifests in different ways, such as inadequacy of pediatric beds, absence of child-related critical equipment at the primary health centers, untrained (in critical child care) staff, and so on. The deficiency in supply structure, as this research has already highlighted, is particularly visible in neonatal care for home-born babies. Similarly, for nutritional services, a large number of children in the critical age group (0–2 years) remain virtually unreached by the Integrated Child Development Services (ICDS) service centers. As presented in the research done by Ghosh et al. in 2018, the focus on child health is equally tilted, if not more so, in the services provided by voluntary agencies and other private providers which are unable to meet the needs of geographically inaccessible areas.

On the other hand, what the health care delivery system of Sundarbans fails to understand is that, though climate change is a physical phenomenon, it is mediated through socio-cultural and economic systems in a given context. Within the contextual vulnerabilities, there are layers of structural vulnerabilities which may change the experience of climatic adversities and consequences it has created on different determinants of health. In most cases, as in Sundarbans, the health care delivery system has failed to understand these factors and has processed a more generalized implementation plan. Though climatic changes have become more visible in the last two decades in the Sundarbans, the health care system lacks the knowledge required to link the changes with the sufferings of the children and the different layers of social vulnerabilities within it. The top layers of the delivery system are uncertain, both about the local effects of the global climate change in coastal vulnerable pockets, as well as lacking a nuanced understanding of the dynamic coping strategies of the islanders. The lack of convergence between the different health care delivery actors like civil societies and informal care providers has resulted in a lack of structural and sustained dialogue with the local-level implementing institutions. The growing dichotomy between the perceptions of the policy makers and the grassroots institutions have prevented a re-evaluation of the threat and risk perceptions due to the ever-changing nature of uncertainties that is manifested in new challenges in the domain of health and its social determinants amidst climate change in the Indian Sundarbans.

7.4.6 CONCLUSION

Climate change-related impacts and uncertainties are increasing with time through the perception of people and through secondary analysis of scientific articles. For local people in the Sundarbans, uncertainty is not a new phenomenon in itself. It is part of life and has been so for many generations. Still climate change and other anthropogenic interventions (e.g., infrastructure development like roads, commercial overfishing, and top-down bureaucratic interventions) are increasing the vulnerabilities of local people. While marginalized people are constantly coping with variability and present ecological realities, they also have to live with uncertainties arising due to changes in their livelihoods and restrictions imposed on access to commons.

Supposedly our study is also a critique of the Rawlsian approach (Rawls, 1971), which argued that SDH are the byproduct of socio-economic inequalities and can be improved through enhancement of socio-economic conditions (Daniels et al. 2000). The study argues that addressing SDH requires incorporating tradeoffs (Brock 2000) of inequalities like climatic vulnerability, social cohesion, and responses of health care delivery system, rather than a merely linear understanding of socio-economic deprivation.

Reflecting on Sen (1985) and Marmot (2008) – these authors proposed that the "individual characteristics" of a person determine his/her health. In children, not only their own characteristics but some of their parents' characteristics also acted as the determinants of their health. In the Sundarbans, a child is born with his/her individual characteristics, like caste or religion, and even the economic condition of the household, just as is every other child beyond the region. However, the biggest characteristic they have which will influence whether they achieve good health or not is that they are the children of the Indian Sundarbans. Their health is governed by a number of structural as well as context-specific factors which make them unique and difference from their state-level counterparts, more or less in the way Marmot and colleagues proposed in 2000.

If we wish to see how much the health of the Sundarbans children is closer to the "life course approach' proposed by WHO (2010) under the CSDH framework, we can see complete failure in this regard. The approach emphasizes a healthy start in life for every child, including pregnant mothers. It also emphasizes pre-natal child care and early-life care. The approach is based on proper education and easy availability of all child care systems (WHO 2010). It also incorporates wellbeing during the later stages of life to maintain good health, such as individual and collective empowerment, employment, and reducing stress at work and social isolation. This unique framework is well suited to Sen's approach of "development as freedom" (Sen 1999). A typical child is born in Sundarbans in a geographically hostile resource-scarce setting which is now facing uncertainties in almost every sphere. Structural characteristics like cultural beliefs, economic conditions, and availability of quality care services determine whether he/she is going to be born into safe hands or not. His/her healthy birth also depends upon the health and nutritional status of the mother, which is again determined by structural forces like gender and cultural beliefs. After birth, his/her neonatal, prenatal, and nutritional care initiation is determined by cultural practices and penetration of formal health care in terms of availability and acceptability. During the initial years of life, soon after the weaning period contextual factors like repeated climatic shocks, livelihood depletion of household, and household-level food insecurities start to determine the child's health and general wellbeing. These contextual forces, though significantly strong and in places like climatically vulnerable pockets, supersede individual characteristics like caste, religion, and economic condition. One can view a crucial tussle between structural determinants and contextual determinants in this regard. In some cases the contextual forces win, such as when the general caste households of remote islands cannot secure enough food for their children. In other cases the structural forces have swept over contextual ones, such as the Muslim households which have failed to achieve a secure shelter in their neighboring Hindu hamlet during climatic emergencies.

The battle between structural forces and contextual forces is ever increasing with growing uncertainties due to climate impacts and failure in policy and planning to handle these impacts. These in turn determine the later stages of the life of the Sundarbans' children, manifested in dropping out from school, early marriage (for girls), out-migration at a very young age (for boys) without any proper skilled employment, and sustaining stressful livelihood flexibily within the island. Under these circumstances, the mothers of the Sundarbans, especially the young-generation mothers, have shown promising increments in their negotiations with various social ties for accessing available resources. The mothers, mainly whose husbands have out-migrated, now became de facto household heads. Even in cases where the husband is present, more and more women are joining the workforce to restore their livelihoods. The women are feeling economically empowered and socially more active as they step beyond the household boundaries by breaking strict gender norms of this traditionally patriarchal society. This is indeed a positive drive towards increments of mothers' bargaining powers and seems to have a positive impact on child health outcome, which is a fact already established by scholars.

The chapter re-established the argument proposed by Subramanian and colleagues (2008) that, in a South Asian context, SDH should not be taken as the byproduct of socio-economic stratification. The present chapter is also commensurate with Subramanian and colleagues' findings that caste and gender are slowly determining their controlling power as per child health as a concern. And we arguably add climate change as a newly emerged social determinant. However, the study added that gender is still prevailing as a determinant in later stages of life, though probe the requirements of more in-depth research. Subramanian and colleagues identified two important focuses for the SDH approach in the Indian context: the life course of a particular community and contextual determinants of the life course. Hence, we have added further knowledge in this regard by presenting the case of Sundarbans on how contextual determinants individually as well as jointly with structural forces determine the health of the children. We argue that Indian health policy making needs to come out from the traditional poverty reduction path and should provide traces of a more nuanced micro-level planning. If incremental changes are needed for most of the country, transformational changes require dealing with especially vulnerable regions like Indian Sundarbans.

The authors hope that this analysis will inform scientists, researchers, and policy makers to design and implement appropriate and socially just welfare measures / interventions in the Sundarbans. The authors strongly feel that empowering communities, especially women, with information, technological skills, education, and employment is the best way to address reduction of social vulnerability to cope with present-day uncertainties which will ultimately lead towards better child health outcomes. The authors believe that the local observations described above will provide a clear direction for future research, development planning, and adaptation programs that consider the interests and priorities of the children of the vulnerable islanders as the starting point. It is important that multiple knowledge framings and approaches are considered to address crucial determinants of child health in the Sundarbans to promote equity and socially just initiatives towards contextual diversities amidst climate change.

REFERENCES

Alderman H, Hoddinott J, Kinsey B. Long term consequences of early childhood malnutrition, Oxford Economic Papers 2006; 58, 450–474.

Alliance for Health Policy and Systems Research. Strengthening health systems: the role and promise of policy and systems research. Geneva, Switzerland, 2004.

Anand S, Peter F. Equal opportunity. Boston Review 2000; 25 Available from: http://bostonreview.net/BR25.1/anand.html.

Anderson JF, Main AJ. Importance of vertical and horizontal transmission of West Nile virus by *Culex pipiens* in the northeastern United States. Journal of Infectious Diseases 2006; 194, 1577–1579.

Angell M. Pockets of poverty. Boston Review 2000; 25 Available from: http://bostonreview.net/ BR25.1/angell.html.

Arcury TA, Gesler WM, Preisser JS, Sherman J, Spencer J, Perin J. The effects of geography and spatial behavior on health care utilization among the residents of a rural region. Health Service Research 2005; 40, 135–155.

Basu S. Dimensions of tribal health in India. Health and Population – Perspectives and Issues 2000; 23(2), 61–70.

Brock D. Broadening the bioethics agenda. Kennedy Institute of Ethics Journal 2000; 10, 21–38.

Centers for Disease Control and Prevention. Addressing Social Determinants of Health: Accelerating the Prevention and Control of HIV/AIDS, Viral Hepatitis, STD and TB. External Consultation Meeting Report. Atlanta, Georgia: Centers for Disease Control and Prevention; April, 2009.

CSDH. Closing the gap in a generation: health equity through action on the social determinants of health. Final Report of the Commission on Social Determinants of Health. Geneva: World Health Organization, 2008.

Daniels N. Justice, health, and health care. In: Rhodes R, Battin MP, Silvers A, ed. Medicine and Social Justice: Essays on the Distribution of Health Care. New York: Oxford University Press; 2002, pp. 6–23.

Daniels N, Kennedy B, Kawachi I. Justice is good for our health: how greater economic equality would promote public health. Boston Review 2000; 25. Available from: http://bostonreview.net/ BR25.1/daniels.html.

Datar A, Liu J, Linnemayr S, Stecher C. The impact of natural disasters on child health and investments in rural India. Social Science and Medicine 2013; 76(1), 83–91.

Department of Health and Social Security. Inequalities in Health: Report of a Research Working Group. London: Department of Health and Social Security, 1980 (Black report).

Emanuel EJ. Political problems. Boston Review 2000; 25. Available from: http://bostonreview.net/ BR25.1/emanuel.html.

Furuta M, Salway S. Women's position within the household as a determinant of maternal health care use in Nepal. International Family Planning Perspectives 2006; 32(1), 17–27. doi: 10.1363/3201706. PMID: 16723298.

Gakidou E, Frenk J, Murray C. A health agenda. Boston Review 2000; 25. Available from: http://bostonreview.net/BR25.1/frenk.html.

Ghosh U, Vadrevu L, Mondol A. Children of Uncertain Climate, FHS-IIHMR, 2018. https://opendocs.ids.ac.uk/opendocs/bitstream/handle/20.500.12413/14327/CCH%20Report_Final%20version_UG%20revisions.pdf?sequence=3&isAllowed=y.

Heltberg R, Lund N. (2009). Shocks, coping, and outcomes for Pakistan's poor: health risks predominate. Journal of Development Studies 45(6), 889–910.

Hoddinott J, Kinsey B. Child growth in the time of drought. *Oxford Bulletin of Economics and* Statistics 2001; 63(4), 409–436.

Illich I. Medical Nemesis: The Expropriation of Health. New York: Pantheon, 1976.

Kamm FM. Health and equality of opportunity. American Journal of Bioethics 2001; 1, 17–19.

Kanjilal B, Bose S, Patra N, Barman D, Ghosh U, Vadrevu L, Mandal A, Sengupta P. How healthy are the children of Indian Sundarbans? Institute of Health Management Research (IIHMR) 2013; 79.

Marmot M. Social determinants of health inequalities. Lancet Public Health 2005; 365, 1099–1104.

Marmot M. Achieving health equity: from root causes to fair outcomes. Lancet 2008; 370(9593), 1153–1163.

Marmot M, Wilkinson RG. Psychosocial and material pathways in the relation between income and health: a response to Lynch et al. British Medical Journal 2001; 322(7296), 1233–1236.

Marmot M et al. Employment grade and coronary heart disease in British civil servants. Journal of Epidemiology and Community Health 1978; 32, 244–249.

Marmot M et al. Health inequalities among British civil servants: the Whitehall II study. Lancet 1991; 337, 1387–1393.

McKeown T. The Modern Rise of Population. New York: Academic Press, 1976.

McMichael AJ, Powles JW, Butler CD, Uauy R. Food, livestock production, energy, climate change, and health. Lancet 2007; 370(9594), 1253–1263. doi: 10.1016/S0140-6736(07)61256-2. PMID: 17868818.

Neira M, Bertollini R, Campbell-Lendrum D, Heymann DL. *The year 2008. A breakthrough year for health protection from climate change?* American Journal of Preventive Medicine 2008; 35, 424–425.

Peters DH, Garg A, Bloom G et al. Poverty and access to health care in developing countries. Annals of the New York Academy of Sciences 2008; 1136, 161–171.

Rawls J. A Theory of Justice. Cambridge, MA: Harvard University Press; 1971.

Ruger JP. Aristotelian justice and health policy: capability and incompletely theorized agreements. PhD thesis. Cambridge, MA: Harvard University; 1998.

Ruger JP. Health, capability, and justice: toward a new paradigm of health ethics, policy and law. Cornell Journal of Law and Public Policy 2006; 15(2), 403–482.

Sen AK. Commodities and Capabilities. Amsterdam: North-Holland; 1985.

Sen AK. Development as Freedom. Oxford: Oxford University Press; 1999.

Shea E. Living with a Climate in Transition: Pacific Communities Plan for Today and Tomorrow. Honolulu: East-West Center; 2003.

Sheffield PE, Landrigan PJ. Global climate change and children's health: threats and strategies for prevention. Environmental Health Perspectives 2011; 119, 291–298, doi:10.1289/ehp.1002233

Smith KR, Woodward A, Campbell-Lendrum D, Chadee D, Honda Y, Liu Q, Olwoch J, Revich B, Sauerborn R. Human health: impacts, adaptation and co-benefits. In Field CB, Barros V, Dokken D, Mach KJ, Mastrandrea MD, Bilir TE, Chatterjee M, Ebi KL, Estrada YO, Genova RC et al., eds. Climate Change 2014: Impacts, Adaptation, and Vulnerability. Volume I: Global and Sectoral Aspects. Contribution of Working Group II to the Fifth Assessment Report of the Intergovernmental Panel on Climate Change, Cambridge, UK: Cambridge University Press, 2014; Chapter 11.

Soeung SC, Grundy J, Sokhom H, Chang Blanc D, Thor R. The social determinants of health and health service access: an in depth study in four poor communities in Phnom Penh Cambodia. International Journal of Equity and Health 2012; 11, 1–10.

Story WT, Tura H, Rubin J, Engidawork B, Ahmed A, Jundi F, Iddosa T, Abrha TH. Social capital and disaster preparedness in Oromia, Ethiopia: an evaluation of the "Women Empowered" approach. Social Science & Medicine 2020; 257. 111907, ISSN 0277-9536. https://doi.org/10.1016/j.socscimed.2018.08.027.

Subramanian SV, Ackersonet L, Subramanyam M, Sivaramakrishnan K. Health inequalities in India: the axes of stratification. Brown Journal of World Affairs 2008; xiv(2).

Tajer D. Latin American social medicine: roots, development during the 1990s, and current challenges. American Journal of Public Health 2003; 93(12), 1989–1991

The Lancet. A commission on climate change. The Lancet 2009; 373(9676), 1659. DOI: https://doi.org/10.1016/S0140-6736(09)60922-3.

Whitehead M. The concepts and principles of equality and health. Copenhagen: WHO Regional Office for Europe (EUR/ICP/RPD 414), 1990.

WHO. WHO called to return to the Declaration of Alma-Ata, 1978. www.who.int/teams/social-determinants-of-health/declaration-of-alma-ata.

Wilson K, Rosenberg MW. Exploring the determinants of health for First Nations peoples in Canada: can existing frameworks accommodate traditional activities? Social Science & Medicine 2002; 55(11), 2017–2031.

Wong EL, Popkin BM, Gullkey DK, Akin JS. Accessibility, quality of care and prenatal care use in the Philippines. Social Science and Medicine 1987; 24, 927–944.

Unit IV

Industrial Safety and Occupational Health Issues

8 Occupational Hazards in Alternative Medicinal Industry
An Exploratory Study

*Abha Arya**

CONTENTS

8.1 INTRODUCTION

Global environmental changes have an impact on different medicinal systems and the health-seeking behaviour of the population. Gradually, global demand for alternative medicinal products has risen. The increasing side effects of allopathic medicine have also made a significant contribution to this shift. Production of the alternative medicinal industry has risen, but guidelines for manufacturing units are still evolving. The industrialization of the medicinal industry of Ayurveda, Siddha, and Unani started in the pre-independence period and the guidelines for manufacturing have developed over a period of time. Regulation and legislation have not been adequately discussed. The chapter discusses occupational health and industrial safety in factory and non-factory spaces for production of herbomineral–metallic formulations. This subject has not been explored previously, especially in the context of the alternative medicinal system. The topic is important to discuss in

* Corresponding author: Abha Arya. abha@sihspune.org

DOI: 10.1201/9781003095422-8

today's scenario when multiple industrial chemicals pollute the human body and the ecosystem, impacting environmental health.

The debate on usage of heavy metals, minerals, and chemical components, and their impact on human bodies and the environment is not only restricted to manufacturing units and pharmacies, but extends to the laboratories of academia. The chapter captures institutional normative behaviour and discusses the role of multi-stakeholders in making a policy related to occupational health for the working class. The context of health and its intersections with the ecosystem has long been debated in the field of the pharmaceutical industry and drug development; however, those people working in close proximity with these compounds and their state of functioning have not been contemplated appropriately.

The following sections will explore the alternative medicinal industry in India and occupational health for the working class. The literature available on the subject and data collected in the field have been analysed to explore the intersections in the fields of alternative medicinal industry and occupational health, as well as different methods which have been used in the industry to prevent occupational hazards.

8.2 AYUSH INDUSTRY: OVERVIEW ON OCCUPATIONAL HEALTH

AYUSH stands for Ayurveda, yoga and naturopathy, Unani, Siddha and homeopathy medicinal systems. The emergence of the industry in India can be traced back to the pre-independence period, when several practitioners of Ayurveda started their own factory which not only offered diagnosis and treatment but also manufactured Ayurvedic medicines and prescribed the same to patients. For instance, Shri Dhootapapeshwar Limited was established in 1872 (Shree Dhootpapeshwar Limited, n.d.), Dabur India Limited was set up in 1884 (Dabur Limited, n.d.) and Arya Vaidya Sala was founded in 1902 (Arya Vaidya Sala, n.d.). These knowledge systems are derived from ancient Ayurvedic books like *Bhaishajya Ratnavali, Bhava Prakasha, Rasaratna Samuchaya*, and so forth. These factories and/or pharmacies were established at a modest level and few have now started manufacturing drugs on a large scale. The revenues of some of these firms have also increased tremendously. The Government of India's policies have supported their industrialization. In 1969, Chapter IV A of the Drugs and Cosmetics Act 1940 (DCA) was introduced as a separate chapter for the Ayurveda, Siddha, and Unani (ASU) medicinal system (Ministry of Health and Family Welfare, 2005). In the same year, they came up with the First Schedule in Drugs and Cosmetics Act (1940) which consists of the name of the authoritative books belonging to Ayurveda, Siddha, and Unani systems. In the Ayurveda section, the government recognized 54 ancient textbooks. This recognition facilitated manufacturers to prepare formulations which are mentioned in this schedule and that are categorized as classical medicines. Moreover, recommendations from the Bhore Committee (Bhore, 1946) and Udupa Committee (Udupa, 1958) emphasize the importance of traditional medicines to cater to the demands of such a large population. Traditional medicines are not only used in the healthcare system and home remedies but also for scientific breakthroughs in discovering new formulations and drugs.

The traditional medicinal industry depends on authoritative textbooks and the traditional methods of manufacturing medicines; however, with time and the development of new equipment, manufacturing methods have changed. Similarly, the practices of maintaining the premises have also changed. Schedule T of the Drugs and Cosmetic Rules (1945) mentions manufacturing practices and infrastructure of the manufacturing unit. Schedule T has sections on the usage of equipment and machinery for manufacturing medicine. Similarly, it has the provision for manufacturing premises needed for production. With recent debates on permissible limits of alcohol and heavy metals, the schedule has sections on supplementary guidelines for manufacturing of herbomineral-metallic compounds. These compounds consist of metals and/or minerals mixed with herbal concoctions. The supplementary guidelines are for herbomineral-metallic compounds like *bhasma, sindura, kupipakwa*, etc. These are different formulations and dosage forms. The discourse on heavy metals has been raised because of the ingredients used in its making. Such formulations have raised concerns about the content of heavy metals like mercury, arsenic, etc. For example, two important ingredients of *sindur* are mercury and sulphur.

A few were moved by Saper et al.'s work of 2008 and Sébastia's work of 2015, whereas another group opined that it was a sensationalist approach (Saper et al., 2008; Sébastia, 2015). Thereby, manufacturing of a few kinds of complicated medicines came into focus and recently standard operating procedures have been published by the government. Some debates attracted attention to the effectivity of Ayurvedic medicines, thought to be due to bad manufacturing practices, taking into consideration that ancient textbooks mentioned each and every step precisely and carefully. There were also debates on the presence of heavy metals, alcoholic compounds, less scientific data for proving efficacy, and so on. This became the reason for clinical evaluation of the most used products like *chyawanprash* (Clinical Trials Registry, India, 2020).

The occupational health institution in India, National Institute of Occupational Health, was established in 1970 as a collaborative effort with the World Health Organization (Saha, 2018). Moreover, National Policy on Safety, Health and Environment at Work Places (2009) provided guidelines for maintaining safety culture in the workplace for all types of stakeholder. Good manufacturing practices (GMPs) for Ayurveda, Siddha, and Unani medicines production discuss the safety of factory workers and also make provision to ensure better health for employees working inside the firm. The guidelines for proper disposal of bio-waste showcase their willingness towards improving public health. The schedule has safety measures for workers in factories manufacturing Ayurveda, Siddha, and Unani medicines and it also has a separate provision for the *bhasma*-manufacturing unit. Further, medical services provisions are specified in the guidelines; they stipulate that workers must have a periodical check-up and the firm should maintain records (Central Council for Research in Ayurvedic Sciences (CCRAS), 2018).

However, the implementation of these guidelines has not been discussed in depth in the research domain. As discussed earlier, occupational health in the pharmaceutical industry has not been adequately explored. Similarly, the AYUSH industry and associated occupational health have not been discussed in detail. Moreover, drug-manufacturing units have guidelines written for workers in close proximity with machineries, assembly lines, and chemicals. These guidelines are debated and formulated in the World Health Organization and Indian organizations like the Indian Association of Occupational Health.

Furthermore, constitutional provisions for the safety and health of workers are enshrined in the form of Directive Principles of State Policy (DPSP) articles 42 and 43. It is mentioned that the aim is "endeavouring to secure for workers a living wage, humane conditions of work, maternity relief, a decent standard of life and full enjoyment of leisure and social and cultural opportunities" (Kashyap, 2001). DPSP is significant in understanding the efforts of the Indian state to improve the quality of life and health of a worker since the establishment of the Indian Constitution. However, the guidelines for ASU workers materialized at a later stage, when the industry emerged in the pre-independence era. This delay is due to the attitude associated with the AYUSH medicinal system which talks about minimal side effects. Moreover, the upheaval caused by the work of a few authors like Robert Saper has raised arguments about the presence of heavy metals in *bhasma* formulations. Debate about its safety led the state to formulate provisions to standardize and regulate *bhasma* productions (Saper et al., 2008).

8.2.1 INTERSECTION WITH ONE HEALTH

One Health approach is an interdisciplinary concept which came into existence due to increasing global health emergencies. This approach focuses on human–animal relationships and their role in the environment. With the emergence of new infectious diseases and chronic diseases as well as the threat of environmental pollution, the significance of protecting the interface of human–animal ecosystem relations is immense. One Health approach is crucial to understanding non-communicable chronic diseases, as it captures certain factors responsible for their occurrence, such as lifestyle, environmental pollution, stress, etc. This holistic approach is necessary because of the increase in human population: "industrialization, and geopolitical problems that accelerate global changes causing significant damage to biodiversity, extensive deterioration of ecosystems, and considerable migratory movement of both mankind and species in general" (Destoumieux-Garzón et al., 2018). This approach also recognizes that it is difficult to maintain public health and wellbeing on a "polluted planet-suffering from social or political instability and ever-diminishing resources" (*ibid*). Moreover, the emphasis should be to safeguard the ecosystem and environment of the world as well as to ensure prevention of environmental hazards; and to include preventive and promotive measures in all policies.

This reminds us of the approach of Health in All policies to include health-related decision making at all national and supra-national levels for all kinds of policies (WHO, n.d.). In low- and middle-income countries, it has been observed that pesticides and fertilizers have been abused in agricultural practices as a manifestation of the industrialization of agriculture. The present chapter takes inspiration from the One Health concept to attain public health and wellbeing by making policies for better environmental health. Environmental degradation and pollution are the result of human intervention in the forest for industrialization and to generate profits. In order to balance development with sustainable living with the ecosystem, different stakeholders must come together to resolve this issue.

The ASU medicinal industry, which includes large manufacturing units as well as small pharmacies, comes under the radar of regulatory bodies which work to prevent environmental pollution. States have taken steps to relocate factories to industrial estates like State Infrastructure and Industrial Development Corporation Uttarakhand Ltd. (SIIDCUL, n.d.). Moreover, the steps which the state has taken regarding occupational health and the impact on workers in ASU-manufacturing units are discussed in this chapter.

Against this backdrop, we are trying to explore: (1) the method to prevent issues of occupational health in alternative medicinal industry manufacturing metal-based formulations, both formally and informally, through existing regulations and health-seeking behaviour of workers and experts; and (2) intersections between the norms in the alternative medicine industry and occupational health.

8.3 METHOD

For the purpose of studying these research questions, a qualitative research method was adopted to explore these questions, represented in Figure 8.1. In-depth interviews were used to collect data, and papers and government guidelines were studied to comprehend the state of workers in the ASU industry. Ten respondents were interviewed in three cities: Jaipur, Delhi, and Varanasi. These respondents belonged to different categories, such as academic scientists and firm owners. The firm owners fell into the categories of micro, small, and medium enterprises (MSMEs). The categories of ASU firms on the basis of small annual turnover ranged from Rs 1 to 5 cr revenue, whereas medium-sized enterprises had revenue falling in the range of Rs 5–50 cr (Goraya and Ved, 2017). Moreover, questions were mostly limited to the conditions of workers in close proximity to the herbomineral-metallic formulation-manufacturing units.

8.4 CURRENT SCENARIO ON OCCUPATIONAL HEALTH IN THE AYUSH INDUSTRY

The literature available on the topic has been reviewed and analysed, and it has been realized that not many scholarly papers have been published on the topic. Thus, government documents were utilized for the purpose of this study. Further, the data were collected through in-depth interviews and inductive approach in qualitative analysis was used.

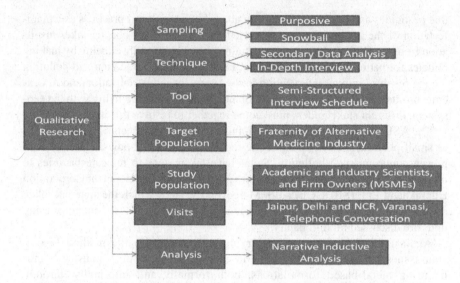

FIGURE 8.1 Research methodology. MSMEs, micro, small and medium enterprises; NCR, National Capital Region.

8.4.1 LITERATURE AVAILABLE ON OCCUPATIONAL HEALTH

In the 1960s, Ayurvedic medicines came under the DCA of 1940 and introduced sections 3a and 3h. Section 3a is defined as the classical preparations of ASU, which are mentioned in the extant ancient textbooks recognized by the Government of India in First Schedule of Drugs and Cosmetics Act 1940, where 3h defines patents and proprietary medicines. Gradually, the government came up with various guidelines appropriate for the larger fabric of the regulatory framework. This includes establishment of the Ayurvedic Pharmacopoeia Committee in 1962, emergence of modern codification in the form of Ayurveda Pharmacopoeia of India and Ayurveda Formulary of India, and various guidelines for Ayurveda medicinal system. The liberalization of trade gave the Indian AYUSH industry the opportunity to expand their sales in the global market. To make it a regularized industry, GMP guidelines were laid down in the form of Schedule T in Drugs and Cosmetics Rules (1945). Section (v) of Schedule T provides an exemption where *vaidyas*, *siddhas*, and *hakeems* "who prepare medicines on their own to dispense to their patients and are not selling such drugs in the market are exempted from the purview of G.M.P" (CDSCO, 2016).

Further, in the section called "Health Clothing, Sanitation and Hygiene of Workers" in Schedule T, it is mentioned that all workers employed in the factory shall remain free from infectious diseases. The workers shall be provided with clean and suitable uniform for the kind of work and the environment. This should include a covering for head, hands, and feet whenever and wherever needed. Facilities for personal cleaning shall be adequately given. Schedule T Part II.D.5 includes

"Medical Examination of the Employees", which suggests that medical examination at least once a year is necessary for employees who manufacture metal and mineral compounds. During the GMP inspection, the report should be made available to the statutory inspectors.

There is nothing more on workers' code of conduct. However, the above-mentioned excerpts of Schedule T and guidelines on GMP lead us to two parts of the story. One is the factory setup and the other is non-factory setup (and they are exempted from the purview of GMP).

8.4.2 IMPLEMENTATION IN A FACTORY

The implementation of Schedule T of the Drugs and Cosmetics Rules of 1945 has been discussed in this section. Besides coming under the purview of Schedule T, these factories also come under the ambit of the Factories Act of 1948. Section 41B is on the "Compulsory disclosure of information by the occupier", which suggests that the occupier of every factory should disclose all the information regarding dangers of hazardous processes, including health hazards. This is followed by another point that, at the time of registering the factory, the owner should lay down the policy in front of the Chief Inspector and local authority for the health and safety of workers. The popular practice of industry is laid down as follows:

1. Soft jobs like packing and filling, and so forth, are done by women. Jobs done in the close proximity of machines are done by men. Not many female *vaidya* could be seen in the industry.
2. One of the major characteristics of the industry is the number of manufacturing units. There is no unanimity in the number of manufacturing units in existence. Moreover, 8610 was the approximate number of manufacturing units based on the consumption of herbal raw materials (Goraya and Ved, 2017: 12). Several of them do not exceed the number of labourers to avoid the Factory Act of 1948. It has been observed that most of the firms stay less than 10. This avoids the schedules which relate to occupations and processes prohibited in the Factories Act 1948. For instance, Part B of industrial activity mentions manufacturing processes using toxic metals and substances like lead, mercury, asbestos, etc.
3. The fraternity of the Ayurveda industry should define hazardous processes or risks in handling of materials like metals (mercury, arsenic, iron, etc.) and minerals (mica), which are dangerous in the longer run for labourers.

8.4.3 PRACTITIONERS EXEMPTED FROM GMP

As enshrined in Schedule T, practitioners who manufacture for inpatients are exempted from the guidelines of GMP for ASU medicines. Most of them prepare classical drugs or 3a drugs. Moreover, such practitioners and their establishments do not come under the Factories Act of 1948. However, the number of patients who visit these establishments may vary according to the influence and popularity of the *vaidya*. The lack of a regulatory framework for these firms is evident. In manufacturing units which are exempted from GMP, the production of various dosage forms including herbomineral-metallic compounds can be seen.

8.4.4 OBSERVATIONS FROM THE FIELD

The data were collected from firms that had a varied understanding of the subject. Most individuals said that there is no impact on them, despite working in close proximity with heavy metals and handling compounds without any protective gear. Moreover, this narrative was published by one of our respondents, who observed that his father was a *vaidya* and that tradition was carried forward by him. He had seen mercurial formulations and also helped his father in making them. However, he had never suffered from any issues with health as a result. "Making mercurial preparations was a routine in my family; all of us were used to living with these ongoing activities of ayurvedic practice" (Prakash, 2013).

Moreover, I interviewed students of the National Institute of Ayurveda, Jaipur and saw them handling the equipment in the laboratory area with ease and casually handling these heavy metals with bare hands. They believe exposure to the chemical agents will not make any change to their health. Similar observations were made in the Banaras Hindu University, where students were comfortable in handling heavy metals with precision, and they believed that exposure to these metals had never impacted their health in a negative manner.

A common subject discussed in the interview was the role of commercialization and how it could impact on production processes, as commercialization also includes profit and gains associated with the marketing of the drugs. An interview with an industrial scientist from a big firm recalled that his firm had maintained a proper diet for the workers (including bananas and milk), who manufacture herbomineral-metallic compounds. Further, in a traditional setup where *bhasma* formulations are prepared continuously in small amounts, the worker or *vaidya* takes precautions with a diet which consists of milk and bananas. They believe that the elements present in this diet detoxify the metals in the body and can ensure good health. Also, they regularly change the worker's shift in the production unit every 15 days. However, this was not discussed in any other firm. With the measures provided to them in Schedule T, every firm has to maintain records for an annual inspection. It has also been observed that factories have recruited workers who have worked in the same production unit for 15–20 years because of the perfection of the preparations.

It has been seen that inpatient manufacturing units do not come under the guidelines of Schedule T of Drugs and Cosmetics Rules (1945), and they also do not come under the ambit of the Factories Act of 1948 as the number of workers is mostly fewer than ten. They keep the number of workers limited. A field narrative on the subject was shared by an academician, who noted that his relative could not get proper treatment for pancreatitis from allopathic institutes so they adopted

Ayurvedic means. Someone had mentioned that a *vaidya* treats patients with pancreatitis but unfortunately the treatment didn't work. The important point here is that a larger section of people of poorer economic status visit the *vaidya* for an assured cheap treatment. Moreover, as the practitioner does not come under any regulatory guidelines, he used to sell medicines without disclosing their name and ingredients. These places are not covered by any regulatory mechanisms like that of manufacturing and consultancy. In the same vein, some of the proprietary medicines with proper clinical evaluation reports sell their drugs in such establishments which are run by godmen. (By godmen is meant those charismatic faith gurus and leaders like demigods who have a cult following.) This method of selling is adopted by some *vaidyas* to get wider sales.

Moreover, the normative behaviour of the *vaidyas*, whether in academia, as consultants, or as clinicians attached with inpatient facilities, is that they believe that handling mercury or other metals is not poisonous. There are several secondary literatures on the experiences of *vaidyas* who claim that they have been handling such poisonous metals since their childhood (as their families carried expertise in *ras-shastra* [the knowledge of herbo-mineral and metallic drugs]). Only a few in the fraternity believe that it is harmful and workers' health should be taken in priority.

8.5 CONCLUSION

This chapter discusses the state of workers in production units of the ASU medicinal industry. We have discussed the regulations available on guidelines for GMP and Schedule T of Drugs and Cosmetics Rules, 1945. It has been observed that the occupational health of workers has not been discussed explicitly. However, there is other legislation in place to look after occupational health and safety of workers, including Factories Act of 1948. The chapter analyses the present state of workers in two ways. It comprehends the legislation and regulations associated with the ASU medicinal industry. Industries that deal with heavy metals and hazardous chemicals have to take certain precautions. However, when we talk about this industry, the same safety and precautions are seldom taken literally. Therefore, legislature is required for both factory and non-factory setup for proper handling of mineral and metal-based formulations. Though guidelines on medical checkups are available for workers on an annual basis, it is for those manufacturing units which come under the purview of Schedule T. However, if a pharmacy prepares medicines for their inpatients, *vaidyas* are exempted from Schedule T. Thus, uniformity in the regulatory framework is also required. Based on the responses and some papers it can be said that change in diet and rotational shifts can be useful in preventing any occupational health hazard.

Nevertheless, all those practitioners who prepare drugs at home may have conflicting viewpoints regarding metal poisoning. But how will one measure metal poisoning when it is not in free form but in a compound state? The effect will be pharmacologically different. For larger-batch preparation, these practitioners hire labourers to work. It is written in several ancient textbooks and also mentioned by P. C. Ray (1982 [1918]) that *vaidyas* are needed for supervision. In any manufacturing unit, the *vaidyas* supervise and the workers get involved in the medicine production. Whether a factory follows GMP or a pharmacy is exempted from such rules, the owner should take care of health and safety measures for workers. The normative behaviour of the fraternity of ASU is that metal handling is neither poisonous nor hazardous to the health of workers. This is problematic due to the reasons mentioned above. It is important to explore this area and make appropriate guidelines for labourers working in a factory as well as spaces which are exempted from GMP preparing the herbomineral-metallic compounds.

Through these arguments we can understand the intersectional point in both disciplines. The occupational health issues related to heavy metals have long been under debate, especially mercurial compounds. The shift in medicinal system will not change the science behind the chemical reaction of heavy metal to the human body. Similarly, workers who are constantly exposed to these chemical compounds, in any form, cannot be taken for granted. The lack of evidence and research shows the unwillingness of the state regulatory bodies on the subject. Normative behaviour is not always supported by scientific data and that is the reason for occupational health in ASU medicines becoming an important topic worthy of discussion.

The occupational health of workers in the ASU medicinal industry cannot be improved if we look from the regulator's point of view only. A strict and uniform regulation is helpful in building a better system for manufacturing and working conditions for labourers. Moreover, a multi-stakeholder approach is required to develop an inclusive system and workers are among the important stakeholders in the production of herbomineral-metallic compounds. Moreover, to make guidelines inclusive and provide a bottom-to-top approach, it is necessary to take workers' viewpoints into consideration. Further, exposure to different chemical compounds is not merely dangerous for workers but may also pollute the environment as a result of large-scale production of *bhasma* to cater for the demands of domestic and global markets.

Also, the management of bio-waste in ASU medicinal industry has not been discussed in depth. The impact of heavy metals in workers' life has increased due to industrialization and globalization of the market and the holistic approach of One Health is crucial to understand the balance between human activities and the ecosystem, and to attain better occupational health and wellbeing of workers.

REFERENCES

Arya Vaidya Sala, Kotakkal. (n.d.). About Us. Retrieved December 03, 2020, from www. aryavaidyasala.com/about-us.php.

Bhore, J. W. (1946). Bhore Committee, 1946: National Health Portal of India. India: *Ministry of Health and Family Welfare*.

CDSCO. (2016). The Drugs and Cosmetics Act, 1940 and Rules, 1945. Retrieved September 20, 2020, from https://cdsco.gov.in/opencms/export/sites/CDSCO_WEB/Pdf-documents/acts_rules/2016DrugsandCosmeticsAct1940Rules1945.pdf.

Central Council for Research in Ayurvedic Sciences (CCRAS) (2018). Guidelines Series I. General Guidelines for Drug Development of Ayurvedic Formulations Ministry of AYUSH. New Delhi: Government of India.

Clinical Trials Registry, India. (2020). Clinical Trials Registry, India, ICMR- National Institute of Medical Statistics. Retrieved December 3, 2020, from http://ctri.nic.in/ Clinicaltrials/pdf_generate.php?trialid=11066&EncHid=&modid=&compid=%27, %2711066det%27.

Dabur Limited. (n.d.). Our Founder. Retrieved October 2, 2020, from www.dabur.com/in/ en-us/about/leadership/our-founder.

Destoumieux-Garzón, D., Mavingui, P., Boetsch, G., Boissier, J., Darriet, F., Duboz, P., ... Voituron, Y. (2018, February 12). The one health concept: 10 years old and a long road ahead. *Frontiers in Veterinary Science*. https://doi.org/10.3389/fvets.2018.00014.

Factories Act. (1948). New Delhi: The Ministry of Labour and Employment, Government of India.

Goraya, G. S., & Ved, D. K. (2017). *Medicinal Plants in India: An Assessment of their Demand and Supply*. Dehradun: National Medicinal Plants Board, Ministry of AYUSH, Government of India, New Delhi and Indian Council of Forestry Research and Education.

Kashyap, Subhash C. (2001). *Our Constitution: An Introduction to India's Constitution and Constitutional Law*. India: National Book Trust.

Ministry of Health and Family Welfare. (2005). Government of India Ministry of Health and Family (Department of Health). *The Drugs and Cosmetics Act and Rules*. Cosmetics, 1940.

National Policy on Safety, Health and Environment at Work Place. (2009). India: Ministry of Labour and Employment, Government of India.

Prakash, V. B. (2013, September 7). Growing up with mercury in an ayurvedic family tradition in Northern India. *Asian Medicine*. Brill Academic Publishers. https://doi.org/ 10.1163/15734218-12341275.

Ray, P. C. [1982 (1918)]. Chemistry in Ancient India, In *Studies in the History of Science in India*, edited by Debiprasad Chattopadhyaya. Volume I, pp. 344–355. New Delhi: Editorial Enterprises.

Saha, R. K. (2018). Occupational health in India. *Annals of Global Health*. Levy Library Press. https://doi.org/10.29024/aogh.2302.

Saper, R. B., Phillips, R. S., Sehgal, A., Khouri, N., Davis, R. B., Paquin, J., ... Kales, S. N. (2008). Lead, mercury, and arsenic in US- and Indian-manufactured Ayurvedic medicines sold via the internet. *JAMA – Journal of the American Medical Association*, 300(8), 915–923. https://doi.org/10.1001/jama.300.8.915.

Sébastia, B. (2015). Preserving identity or promoting safety? The issue of mercury in Siddha medicine: A brake on the crossing of frontiers. *Asiatische Studien – Études Asiatiques*, 69(4), 933–969. https://doi.org/10.1515/asia-2015-1043.

Shree Dhootpapeshwar Limited. (n.d.). *SDL Corporate Movie*. Retrieved on December 3, 2020, from www.youtube.com/channel/UCkYxpuwKiVI0A8Jdx8f9nvg.

SIIDCUL. (n.d.). About Us. Retrieved October 1, 2020, from www.siidcul.com/.

Udupa KN. (1958). *Udupa Committee Report on Indigenous Systems of Medicine*, New Delhi: Ministry of Health Government of India.

WHO. (n.d.). Health Promotion: Health in All Policies. Retrieved October 1, 2020, from www.who.int/healthpromotion/frameworkforcountryaction/en/.

9 Silicosis
An Occupational Health Crisis Among Stone Grinders

Chetan Kumar Joshi*, Madhur Mohan Ranga
and Surbhi Ranga

CONTENTS

9.1 INTRODUCTION

Industrial development is the index of the physical development of a nation; in this development the contribution of the workforce is present in organized and unorganized sectors. There are poor workplace conditions among unorganized workers in various industries in all dimensions such as space, ventilation, illumination, temperature, humidity, hygiene and cleanliness, as well as safety against accidents as compared to the organized sector (National Commission for Enterprises in the Unorganized Sector (NCEUS), 2008). The situation is more severe in micro, small and medium enterprises (MSMEs), especially those dealing with hazardous substances and which have an unsuitable workplace environment. One such industrial field is stone crushing, in which crushed and powdered stone is produced to

* Corresponding author: Chetan Kumar Joshi. cjoshisk@gmail.com

DOI: 10.1201/9781003095422-9

act as the raw material for various construction and manufacturing activities (Patil, 2001). Small-scale enterprises produce fine powders of various grades from a variety of minerals such as quartz, feldspar, mica, and clay which are utilized or transported to other industrial units as raw material for manufacturing products such as ceramics, chemicals, glass and refractory materials etc. (Mamoria and Mishra, 2007). These units generate mineral dust during the production, storing and packaging of mineral powder. The workers are exposed to this workplace environment and inhale air along with dust particles. We inhale 5 liters of air per minute and since 40 square meters of alveolar space are constantly being exposed to the air pollutants that we breathe, there is involuntary entry of pollutants into the human body.

Particulate air pollutants are responsible for different forms of occupational disease. The aerodynamic size of dust particles and convective flow are the main determinants of where in the respiratory passage the particle will come to settle, when inhaled. Due to the smaller diameter of dust particles, they can penetrate deeper into the lung alveolar surface. Dust particles deposit within the respiratory tract by five mechanisms: inertial impaction, sedimentation, diffusion, electrostatic precipitation and interception (Mohanraj and Azeez, 2004). Particulate matter of aerodynamic size less than 10 nm (PM_{10}) suspended in the air atmosphere is subjected to Brownian action due to bombardment by gas molecules. A large percentage of PM_{10} is deposited in bronchi and lungs and can cause lung disease.

Particles smaller than 2.5 µm ($PM_{2.5}$) can penetrate deeper into the gas exchange region of lungs. Particles inserted into the respiratory tract up to the bronchioles are captured in the mucous membranes and taken to the mucociliary ladder to be expelled in a cough. Small particles that are immersed deep in the non-ciliated air path are engulfed by lung macrophages and removed slowly, as the macrophages move the particles to the mucociliary ladder or to the lymphatic system.

In humans, inhaled dust particles are stored between the lungs. There is a correlation between the amount of air polluted or particle matter and the type and level of reaction produced in the lung tissue. When a fraction of particles inserted into a sensitive area within the lungs exceeds the tolerance limit, it causes lung disease (Mohanraj and Azeez, 2004). Semple et al. (2008) investigated crystalline silica respirators and dozens of other metrics at work and in rural areas. This situation is critical in view of the health risks of workers exposed to stone dust, which can lead to various diseases. It is therefore necessary to assess and evaluate the impact of grinding and packaging on employee health.

One of the major health problems that developing and underdeveloped nations worldwide are facing is occupational health injuries. The problem is much more severe in developing countries. Bernadino Ramazzini, an Italian scientist, first identified silicosis in 1705. He is known as the founder of occupational medicine. The full name of silicosis is "pneumonoultramicroscopicsilicovolcanokoniosis," the longest word in the English language. Silicosis is a lung infection caused by inhaling very small pieces of ash or dust. It is often misdiagnosed as Tuberculosis. The name of the disease changes depending on the type of dust the person is exposed to. Crystalline silica causes fibrogenic effects in the lungs. Other materials such as asbestos, soft coal, jute or hemp dust, iron dust, animal or vegetable origin dust and other materials have also been reported to have the same effect but these conditions are given different names. For example, iron dust causes siderosis; Coal dust leads to pneumoconiosis and organic dust such as cotton, jute, flax or hemp dust causes byssinosis. Dust from animals or vegetables, such as animal hair, flour, fungus, pollen, feathers, and mold causes bronchial asthma or aleveolitis. These are all lung diseases.

Silicosis is one of the oldest known occupational diseases. Silica is a product of flint, sandstone, slate and many common building materials such as mud, clay bricks and concrete. Silicon dioxide (SiO_2) or crystalline silica is the basis of granite, sand, quartz and rock. The three most common types of crystalline silica observed in the industry are cristobalite, quartz and tridymite. Silica causes diseases when workers inhale small particles floating in the air of dust produced by cutting, grinding, drilling or blasting rocks. Workers may also be exposed to silica dust while working on highway construction, dumping and dragging or crushing stones, demolition or concrete or stone structures, loading, grinding or cutting stone. Working in mines, ceramics, foundries, quarries and construction sites, glassmaking, hard powders and masonry workshops is especially dangerous. Silica particles are very small and can only be seen with a microscope, and because of their light weight they can stay in the air for a long time. Silica can therefore travel long distances through the air and pose a risk to people who exposed.

It has long been expected that this chronic lung disease caused by inhaling dust from the air containing free crystalline silica is irreversible and that the disease will continue even if exposure stops. Silicosis continues to be a real danger to people constantly and still kills thousands of workers around the world every year. But it can be prevented.

9.2   SOURCES OF SILICA

Silica is often found in nature as sand, generally in the form of quartz. It is a natural compound and has crystalline characteristics and can be found in beach sand. The quartzite is a metamorphic rock of sedimentary origin and is essentially composed of quartz grains. Crystalline silica is found in stone soil and sand. For mineral extraction industrial units use different stones for different commercial purposes. The two important mineral classes are silicate and carbonate; the former includes quartz, feldspar (sodium and potassium), talc, mica, amphibole, olivine and pyroxenes. The other subclass of silicates includes nesosilicates, sorosilicates, inosilicates, cyclosilicates, phylosilicate and tectosilicate. The carbonate class of minerals includes dolomite, calcite, nahcolite, aragonite, magnesite and rhodo-chrosite. In the silicate class of minerals especially quartz, feldspar and talc have more silica compared to others. In the carbonate class of minerals dolomite and calcite also have silica content.

In the workplace environment, workers have personal exposure to dust, since they are involved in various operations including dressing (crushing of stones to pebble size), feeding (manual feeding of stone in stone-feeding soot), collection and bagging. Since the workers are directly exposed to mineral dust the quantity of total suspended particle and respirable suspended particulate matter is important. It can be estimated by gravimetric analysis.

Out of many chemical components present in various rocks, silica (SiO_2) is the common form which occurs in amorphous or in crystalline form. Crystalline silica occurs in many polymorphs, among which quartz (CAS No. 14808 – 60-7) is most common (World Health Organization (WHO), 2000). Geologically, quartz is the commonest mineral of the Earth's crust after feldspar. It is present in igneous and sedimentary rocks.

9.3 PROPERTIES OF SILICA

Silica is clearly visible in gray and odorless dust, which is most commonly found on the surface of the Earth. Oxygen and silicon are two of the commonest elements on the Earth's surface. In total they weigh 74.32% and 83.77% of the crustal rocks. When the eyes and skin are exposed to silica, it causes irritation. Breathing causes irritation to the lungs. It is especially dangerous when exposed to the elements. This airborne silica poses serious health risks and has been known for over a century. Throughout the history of occupational diseases crystalline silica is the most widely studied chemical substance. It is a mineral that forms rocks and is found in abundance in nature in a variety of ways. Free silica, also called quartz, is found in India in large quantities.

9.4 SILICA GENERATION BY HAZARDOUS INDUSTRIES

Release of respirable crystalline silica with diameter <10 μm is a part of many occupational settings. Numerous reports have been published by the United States National Institute for Occupational Safety and Health (Shamim et al., 2017), details of which are summarized in Table 9.1. People working in masonry mines directly inhale the dust of silica (Figure 9.1). The grinding of stones results in the release of large dust clouds containing fine silica particles in plenty.

9.5 THE HARMFUL EFFECTS OF SILICA DUST

In 1997, crystalline silica dust was classified by the International Agency for Research on Cancer (IARC, 1997) as a Group 1 human lung carcinogen. In most cases a common form of silicosis develops after long exposure to relatively low concentrations. Once the person has been exposed to silica dust and the disease has started, it will continue to growth even if the worker is isolated from further exposure. Initial contact with silica particles causes irritation of the eyes, throat and nose, as with most other dusts. However, if extensive amounts of particles of silica with dust come in close contact with the lungs over a period of time, this can result in damage to the lung and its tissue. In mild cases the disease can remain

TABLE 9.1
Hazardous industries and activities that generate silica dust and their sources

Serial no.	Activity/sector	Specific activity/task	Source
1	Agriculture	Ploughing, harvesting, use of machinery	Soil
2	Mining and related milling operations	Most occupations (underground, surface, mill) and mines (metal and non-metal, coal)	Ores and associated rock
3	Quarrying and related milling operations	Crushing stone, sand and gravel processing, monumental stone cutting and abrasive blasting, slate work, diatomite calcination	Sandstone, granite, flint, sand, gravel, slate, diatomaceous earth
4	Construction	Abrasive blasting of structures, buildings	Sand, concrete
		Highway and tunnel construction	Rock
		Excavation and earth moving	Soil and rock
		Masonry, concrete work, demolition	Concrete, mortar, plaster
5	Glass, including fiberglass	Raw material processing	Sand, crushed quartz
		Refractory installation and repair	Refractory materials
		Raw material processing	
6	Cement	Raw material processing	Clay, sand, limestone, diatomaceous earth
7	Abrasives	Silicon carbide production	Sand
		Abrasive product fabrication	Tripoli, sandstone
8	Ceramics, including bricks, tiles, sanitary ware, porcelain, pottery, refractories, vitreous enamels	Mixing, molding, glaze or enamel spraying, finishing	Clay, shale, flint, sand, quartzite, diatomaceous earth
9	Iron and steel mills	Refractory preparation and furnace Repair	Refractory material

(continued)

TABLE 9.1 Continued
Hazardous industries and activities that generate silica dust and their sources

Serial no.	Activity/sector	Specific activity/task	Source
10	Silicon and ferro-silicon	Raw material handling	Sand
	Foundries (ferrous and non-ferrous)	Casting, shaking out	Sand
		Abrasive blasting, fettling	Sand
		Furnace installation and repair	Refractory material
11	Metal products including structural metal, machinery, transportation equipment	Abrasive blasting	Sand
12	Shipbuilding and repair	Abrasive blasting	Sand
13	Rubber and plastics	Raw material handling	Fillers (Tripoli, diatomaceous earth)
14	Paint	Raw material handling	Fillers (Tripoli, diatomaceous earth, silica flour)
15	Soaps and cosmetics	Abrasive soaps, scouring powders	Silica flour
16	Asphalt and roofing felt	Filling and granule application	Sand and aggregate, diatomaceous earth
17	Agricultural chemicals	Raw material crushing, handling	Phosphate ores and rock
18	Jewelry	Cutting, grinding, polishing, buffing	Semi-precious gems or stones, abrasives
19	Dental material	Sand blasting, polishing	Sand, abrasives
20	Automobile repair	Abrasive blasting	Sand
21	Boiler scaling	Coal-fired boilers	Ash and concretions

Source: International Agency for Research on Cancer (IARC), 1997: 63.

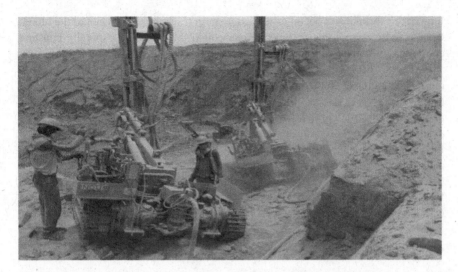

FIGURE 9.1 Laborers working in masonry mines (Prajapati et al., 2020).

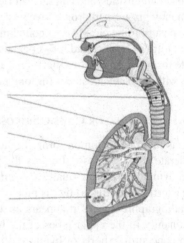

Rhinitis and laryngitis

Tracheitis, bronchitis and Bronchiolitis

Asthma and COPD

Cancer

Interstitial Disease

FIGURE 9.2 The affected parts of the respiratory system as a result of silica particle exposure. COPD, chronic obstructive pulmonary disease (Shamim et al., 2017).

symptom-free for 10–20 years after exposure; only breathlessness during exercise is observed. People with the disease are also at higher risk of developing lung cancer. The size of the silica dust particles is significant in causing the disease. Larger particles are generally prevented from reaching the lung's small air sacs. The smaller particles (less than five-thousandths of a millimeter) are the most risky.

The dust of silica causes inflammation in the lungs and prevents gas exchange by damaging the lung sacs, which affects normal breathing (Figure 9.2). The damaged lung tissue shrinks and becomes less efficient in transporting oxygen to the blood. Characteristic symptoms include serious cough, blood-stained sputum, constant chest pain and rapid weight loss, leading to untimely death later.

Workers who are in contact with silica dust have respiratory ailments, especially chronic coughing and phlegm, chest congestion, irritation of the throat and dyspnea (Wagh et al., 2006). Other clinically proven diseases are silicosis, silico-tuberculosis and chronic obstructive pulmonary disease (COPD) (Preller et al., 2010). Clinical examination of workers indicates that silicosis disease is evidenced as bilateral upper-lobe disease, with excessive calcification (Chopra et al., 2012), basal hyperlucency and miliary nodules. Similar investigations are also seen in silico-tuberculosis, with the exception of basal hyperlucency, but the entire lung remains filled with nodules. Hyperlucency is also reported throughout the lung in COPD. Cowie and Mabena (1991) reported obstructive changes in lung with silica exposure.

9.6 SILICOSIS TYPES

Silicosis is categorized into three common forms: chronic, accelerated and acute. These are the clinical and pathologic expressions of silicosis which reflect differing exposure intensities, and natural histories and latency periods. The chronic or classic form may progress to progressive massive fibrosis, caused by one or more decades of exposure to respirable dust containing quartz. The second type, the accelerated form, follows heavier and shorter exposures and progresses more speedily. The last acute form may arise after short-term, intense exposure to high levels of respirable dust with high silica content for long periods like months rather than years.

9.6.1 CHRONIC OR CLASSIC SILICOSIS

This is the most common form of silicosis. It may show up decades after low to moderate silica exposure. Initially the person may be asymptomatic or may show mild symptoms that gradually worsen. Common symptoms are cough (progressive exertional dyspnea) that is mostly mistakenly attributed to the aging process. In radiographic images it appears as small round opacities (<10 mm), more predominantly in the upper lobes of the lungs. In chronic silicosis, silicotic nodules with concentric whorls of hyalinized collagen fibers with a cell-free central part are the pathologic hallmark. Such nodules are surrounded by connective tissues and reticulin fibers. Chronic silicosis sometimes progresses to progressive massive fibrosis, also termed complicated silicosis, decades after termination of silica particle exposure.

9.6.2 ACCELERATED SILICOSIS

This is an aggressive, debilitating and potentially lethal variety of the disease. It occurs due to intense exposure to or inhalation of large quantities of very fine respirable silica particles. This condition develops even after a short exposure duration of 5–10 years. Symptoms including physiological expression and radiological findings are similar to those of chronic silicosis. This form of silicosis is characterized by rapid lung deterioration, further accompanied by mycobacterial infection in many patients. Accelerated silicosis is often associated with auto-immune conditions like scleroderma or systemic sclerosis.

9.6.3 Acute Silicosis

This condition may result from short-term exposure of high levels of silica. It may develop from silica inhalation of a few months to 5 years. Individuals working in mining, tunneling, quarrying, stone cutting, foundry work and ceramics are more prone to develop this condition. Symptoms of acute silicosis include weakness, dramatic dyspnea and weight loss. Clinically it is associated with rapid progression to severe hypoxemic ventilatory failure causing death. In radiological examination diffuse alveolar filling is seen that differs from chronic forms of silicosis. Histologically, pulmonary alveolar proteinosis and extrapulmonary abnormalities are often reported.

9.7 INDIAN SCENARIO OF SILICOSIS

In Kolar gold mines the first case of silicosis was reported in 1934 by C. Krishnaswami Rao (Antony, 1942). Dr. Anthony Caplan detected silicosis during 1940–1946 among 3472 out of 7643 workers. Epidemiological surveys are usually conducted to get correct information which has revealed that the trouble is more serious in unorganized areas of the country. Great fluctuations were observed in frequency of disease spread after the survey. These fluctuations result from the type of job, exposure timing and density of silica dust around or in working area. Brief study and prevalence of disease silicosis in India can be summarized in Table 9.2.

9.8 WORLD SCENARIO OF SILICOSIS

China recorded more than 5 million cases of silicosis from 1991 to 1995 (WHO, 2018). During this period more than 6000 cases were observed every year and around 24,000 deaths occurred every year, especially among older workers. Thus lung diseases are one of the most frequent occupational diseases in China. In the state of Minas Gerais in Brazil, more than 4500 workers have been detected with silicosis. In the state of Rio de Janeiro when a quarter of shipyard workers were reported with silicosis, sandblasting was banned. A total of 37% of miners in Latin America were found to be affected by this disease (Srivastava and Fareed, 2009). The National Institute of Occupational Safety and Health (NIOSH) estimates that in the USA around 1.7 million persons are exposed on a daily basis to free crystalline silica at their workplace; 1 million of these are sandblasters. The estimated data from the US Department of Labor is that 300 people die each year from silicosis and related disease, and the true number is still in question (Occupational Safety and Health, 2017).

TABLE 9.2
List of industries reporting cases of silicosis in India

Serial no.	Type of industrial sector	References
1	Gold mines	Caplan and Burden, 1947
2	Manganese mines	Ministry of Labor (GoI), 1960
3	Lead and zinc mines in Rajasthan	Government of India, Ministry of Labour and Employment, Office of the Chief Advisor (Factories), India 1961
4	Stone cutters, Jammu and Kashmir	Saini et al., 1984
5	Stone cutters	Sethi and Kapoor, 1982
6	Stone cutters	Gupta et al., 1972
7	Ordnance factory	Viswanathan et al., 1972
8	Agate workers in Khambat	Patel and Robbins, 2011
9	Glass bangle factories	Srivastava et al., 1988
10	Slate pencil workers	Saiyed et al., 1985
11	Mica mines and mica processing	Gangopadhyay et al., 1994
12	Quartz crushing	NIOH, 1986
13	Stone quarry	NIOH, 1986
14	Ceramics and potteries	Saiyed et al., 1995

Source: ICMR Bulletin (1999), Shamim et al. (2017).

9.9 MITIGATION MEASUREMENTS FOR PREVENTION OF SILICA DUST EXPOSURE

In order to overcome direct exposure of workers to silica-rich mineral dust in the workplace environment it is essential to formulate and implement both short-term and long-term planning. It is essential to find suitable substitutions for stone powder, especially in ceramics. The suggestions are:

- Machine manufacturers must ensure proper design and manufacturing of machines to control dust completely during operations.
- Engineering controls such as industrial ventilation or water should be used to mitigate exposure levels.
- Workers access to high-exposure areas should be limited.
- Workers should be provided with respirators if silica exposure mitigation controls are not sufficient.
- The density of quartz-grinding units in a specific area should also be prescribed.

- Special conditions for ventilation and height of shades should also be decided according to the rules.
- Installation of machinery layout as well as minimum areas of quartz-grinding unit and standardization thereof should be specified. The concentration of silica dust will be less when the area of these factories is greater.
- The filter system should be efficient, its efficiency should be specified and it should be examined repeatedly by a competent person.
- Maximum vibrations of equipment used in quartz-grinding factories should be prescribed because an important cause of airborne silica is machine vibration. Skilled persons may also be appointed to submit vibration reports on these machines to the area inspector regularly.
- The name, age and address of workers with their photograph, signature and occupier's signature should be regularly submitted to an area inspector within a month of employment of such workers in quartz-grinding units.
- It is equally important that the occupier should maintain a register regarding this along with a health record for such worker.

REFERENCES

Antony, C. (1942). A Critical Analysis of Collapse in Underground Workers on the KGF. Kolar Gold Field Mining and Metallurgical Society, Bulletin No. 54, Vol. 1.

Caplan, A., Burden, D.J. (1947). Proceedings of Conference on Silicosis, Pneumoconiosis and Dust Separation. London: Institute of Mine Engineering and Institute of Mineral Metallurgy, p. 5.

Chopra, K., Prakash, P., Bhansali, S., Mathur, A., Gupta, P.K. (2012). Incidence and prevalence of silicotuberculosis in western Rajasthan: a retrospective study of three years. National Journal of Community Medicine 3(1): 161–163.

Cowie, R.L., Mabena, S.K. (1991). Silicosis, chronic airflow limitation, and chronic bronchitis in South African gold miners. American Review of Respiratory Disease, 143(1): 80–84. doi: 10.1164/ajrccm/143.1.80. PMID: 1986688.

Gangopadhyay, P.K., Majumdar, P.K., Bhattacharya, S.K., Ahmad, S., Chatterjee, M.K. (1994). Highly dusty mica processing and occupational health problems. Indian Journal of Industrial Medicine, 40(4): 124–134.

Government of India, Ministry of Labour and Employment, Office of the Chief Advisor (Factories), India. (1961). Report No. 21. Silicosis hazard in a lead and zinc mine in Rajasthan. Annals of Occupational Hygiene, 6(3): 147–148.

Graham, R.E., Rowley, L.S. (2017). Occupational Safety and Health. Orland Park, Chicago, IL: American Technical Publishers.

Gupta, S.P., Bajaj, A., Jain, A.L., Vasudeva, Y.L. (1972). Clinical and radiological studies in silicosis: based on a study of the disease amongst stonecutters. Indian Journal of Medical Research, 60(9): 1309–1315.

ICMR Bulletin. (1999). Silicosis – An Uncommonly Diagnosed Common Occupational Disease. Retrieved April 1, 2017, from http://icmr.nic.in/busep99.htm.

International Agency for Research on Cancer (IARC). (1997). IARC Monographs on the Evaluation of Carcinogenic Risks to Humans, Silica, Some Silicates, Coal Dust and Para-Aramide Fibrils, p. 63: 1–475. PMID:9303953. France: IARC.

Mamoria, C.B., Mishra, J.P. (2007). Advance Geography of India, 14th edition. Agra: Sahitya Bhawan, p. 762. ISBN: 81-8298-X.

Mohanraj, R., Azeez, P.A. (2004). Health effects of airborne particulate matter and the Indian scenario. Current Science, 87(6), 25 September.

National Commission for Enterprises in the Unorganized Sector (NCEUS). (2008). Report on Conditions of Work and Promotion of Livelihoods in Unorganized Sector. Academic Foundation; p. 390. India: Government of India.

NIOH. (1986). Annual Report, India, 1986–87. Cincinnati: NIOSH.

Patel, J., Robbins, M. (2011). The agate industry and silicosis in Khambhat, India. New Solutions, 21(1): 117–139. doi: 10.2190/NS.21.1.l. PMID: 21411429.

Patil, M.A. (2001). Environmental management scenario in stone crusher industry sector and cleaner production possibilities. TERI Information Monitoring Environmental Science (TIMES), 6 (2): 83–92.

Prajapati, S.S., Nandi, S.S., Deshmukh, A., Dhatrak, S.V. (2020). Exposure profile of respirable crystalline silica in stone mines in India. Journal of Occupational and Environmental Hygiene, 17:11–12, 531–537. doi: 10.1080/15459624.2020.1798011.

Preller, L., van den Bosch, L.M.C., van den Brandt, P.A., Kauppinen, T., Goldbohm, R.A.S. (2010). Occupational exposure to silica and lung cancer risk in the Netherlands. Occupational and Environmental Medicine, 67(10): 657–663. https://doi.org/10.1136/oem.2009.046326.

Saini, R.K., Yousuf, M., Allagaband, G.Q., Kaul, S.N. (1984). Silicosis in stone cutters in Kashmir. Journal of the Indian Medical Association, 82(6): 198–201.

Saiyed, H.N., Parikh, D.J., Ghodasara, N.B., Sharma, Y.K., Patel, G.C., Chatterjee, S.K., et al. (1985). Silicosis in slate pencil workers: an environmental and medical study. American Journal of Industrial Medicine, 8(2): 127–133.

Saiyed, H.N., Ghodasara, N.B., Sathwara, N.G., Patel, G.C., Parikh, D.J., Kashyap, S.K. (1995). Dustiness, silicosis and tuberculosis in small scale pottery. Journal of Medical Research, 102: 138–142.

Semple, S., Green, D.A., Mc Alpine, G., Cowie, H., Seaton, A. (2008). Exposure to particulate matter on and Indian stone crushing site. Occupational Environmental Medicine, 65: 300–305.

Sethi, N.K., Kapoor, S.K. (1982). Mass miniature radiographs vs. standard sized chest films for the detection of silicosis. Indian Journal of Industrial Medicine, 29(1): 69.

Shamim, M., Alharbi, W., Tariq, P. Nour, M. (2017). Silicosis, a monumental occupational health crisis in Rajasthan – an epidemiological survey. International Journal of Research – Granthaalayah, 5: 554–583. 10.5281/zenodo.841120.

Srivastava, A.K., Fareed, M. (2009). A perspective on silicosis in Indian construction industry. Construction Journal of India, March.

Srivastava, Z.I., Mathur, N., Rastogi, S.K. (1988). Case control study of chronic bronchitis in glass bangle workers. Journal Society of Occupational Medicine, 38(4): 134–136. doi: 10.1093/occmed/38.4.134.

Viswanathan, R., Boparai, M.S., Jain, S.K., Dash, M.S. (1972). Pneumoconiosis survey of workers in India: ordnance factory in India. Archives of Environmental Health, 25(3): 198–204.

Wagh, N.D., Pachpande, B.G., Patel, V.S., et al. (2006). The influence of workplace environment on lung function of flour mill workers in Jalgaon urban center. Journal of Occupational Health, 48: 396–401.

WHO. (2018). Hazard Prevention and Control in the Work Environment: Airborne Dust. Retrieved August 8, 2018, from www.who.int/occupational_health/publications/airdust/en/.

World Health Organization (WHO). (2000). Crystalline Silica, Quartz. Concise International Chemical Assessment Document 24. www.who.int/ipcs/publications/cicad/en/cicad24.pdf.

Unit V

Food Safety and Impacts on Health and Environment

10 Impact of Climate Change on Food Safety
A Review

Rinku Moni Devi*

CONTENTS

10.1 INTRODUCTION

Climate change is a global concern impacting all natural ecosystems and human-kind and it has implications for global development. Climate change effects can be seen, such as changes in rainfall, elevated temperature and increasing extreme events. According to Mbow et al. (2019), the temperature increased by 0.85°C between 1880 and 2012 and rainfall has reduced over the years globally. Additionally, projections for the 21st century have shown a rise in average global temperature by 1.8–4°C and this has adverse impacts on agricultural production and destroy food systems due to changes in climate variables. Furthermore, vulnerable poor people risk their lives due to insufficient food availability and malnutrition as a result of climate change (FAO, 2008).

The change in climatic variables will upset the occurrence, pattern and persistence of viruses, bacteria, fungi, harmful algae, parasites and vectors, leading to foodborne diseases and toxic contamination. Changes in climate variables have an effect on the ecology of microbes, the growth, redistribution and intensification of pest infestations, and host susceptibility results in food-related diseases and

* Corresponding author: Rinku Moni Devi. rinku.devi.fri@gmail.com

zoonosis (FAO, 2008; Tirado et al., 2010). The impacts vary widely by pathogen and differ geographically. Additionally, diverse crop varieties, methods of cultivation, soils, redistribution of sediments, heavy metals, persistent organic pollutants and long-range atmospheric transport increase the risk of food contamination. It impacts agriculture, health of crops and plants, animal health, animal production, aquaculture, fisheries, food manufacturing, trade and processing. Hence, implications are both direct and indirect for food production, food safety, food security and different stages of the food chain, placing public health at risk.

The climate change risks are inequitably distributed and mostly originate as a result of human behavior, mostly from developed countries. However, developing and poor countries have to bear the brunt of the public health burden and pay the cost (Campbell-Lendrum et al., 2007). Moreover, developing countries are more vulnerable due to low adaptation measures, lack of financial resources and technological constraints. Thus, these impacts in turn create major distress in public health, and in economic, social and environment sectors. Hence, a clear understanding of all related changes regarding climate change along with its variability is the most vital step safeguarding preparedness for emerging food risks.

Thus, this paper reviews the potential impact of different climate factors on various sectors, food contamination, foodborne diseases, and related food safety risks at different stages in the food chain and recommends food safety strategies regarding climate change.

10.2   IMPACTS OF CLIMATE CHANGE ON IMPORTANT SECTORS

10.2.1   AGRICULTURE AND LIVESTOCK

Alteration in climate factors can have both direct and indirect effects on agriculture and livestock. Around 80% of the world's crops depend on rain, so farmers depend on weather for agriculture. Further, any change in climate variables, such as an increase or fall in temperature, rainfall, flood, drought and extreme events, may cause crop damage and reduce yield. In many regions in the world inhabitants are suffering from high rates of hunger and food insecurity. However, the greatest decline in food production is observed in sub-Saharan Africa and South Asia (Schmidhuber and Tubiello, 2007; Nelson et al., 2009; Gornall et al., 2010).

Climate change affects ecosystems and their services; for example, in agriculture, pollination and natural predators control pests. Also, there is a threat of extinction of numerous wild plant species used in domestic plant breeding (Jarvis et al., 2008). Heat stress intensifies diseases, reduces fertility and decreases milk production. Pastures, feed supplies and quality of forage are impacted due to drought conditions affecting livestock and production. Furthermore, plant growth is stimulated by rising CO_2, which alters the nutritional value of food crops and the concentrations of essential minerals and proteins. The latest IPCC climate change and land use report (Mbow et al., 2019) states that 25–30% of global food produce is wasted, not all of it for the same reasons, resulting in gas emissions.

In developed countries, food is discarded if it is "excess" or "surplus". However, developing countries lack proper refrigeration, resulting in wastage. Additionally, various pests, weeds and fungi flourish in warmer temperatures and CO_2 levels increases in wetter climates; thus, the ranges and distribution increase with climate change. Climate change affects zoonoses in diverse ways, such as increasing the transmission cycle of many vectors as well as the range and prevalence of vectors and animal reservoirs (FAO, 2008). Moreover, it may result in the establishment of new diseases in some regions, while changes in feeding practices alter the ecological situation, leading to changes in nutritional benefits.

10.2.2 CROP PRODUCTION

The microbial population of the macro-environment is impacted by change in climate. Important factors like soil, air, water and pest population or other vectors are affected by climate change which creates an upsurge in biotic diseases. Additionally, the health of crops and their nutritional value are affected due to abiotic factors like air pollutants and temperature/moisture extremes. Furthermore, the food chain is ultimately impacted by chemical residues and contaminants.

Thus, crop production is extremely vulnerable to climate change and food crop safety and production are affected. The IPCC (Mbow et al., 2019) estimated a likely reduction in yields and damage to crops in the 21st century because of climate change. However, the impacts will be differ globally and regionally.

10.2.3 FISHERIES

An increase in temperature and changes in levels of CO_2, ocean currents and nutrient value have resulted in fish migrating in search of appropriate conditions and altering the spatial distribution of fish stocks. The productivity of aquaculture systems is affected and thus, cultured fish have become more susceptible to diseases which ultimately reduce the returns to farmers. Climate change intensifies eutrophication, causing phytoplankton growth and an upsurge in toxic species of algal blooms. These toxins, accumulated by filter feeders followed by consumption of these products by humans, cause serious health issues. Furthermore, rising water temperature encourages the growth of organisms such as *Salmonella*, *Vibrio vulnificus* and *Campylobacter* and increases the risk from handling or consuming fish grown in these waters (Paz et al., 2007; FAO, 2008).

10.3 FOOD HANDLING, PROCESSING AND TRADING

Climate change directly affects primary production, food manufacturing and trade. Due to variability in climatic factors like temperature and moisture, the hygiene risks linked with distribution of food commodities and storage also increase. Although there are audits to test the validity of hygiene programs and guidelines, challenges arise in adaptation strategies and risk management measures which make developing countries more vulnerable.

10.4   MICROBIOLOGICAL FOOD CONTAMINATION AND ASSOCIATED FOODBORNE DISEASES

There are numerous uncertainties regarding the relations between climate variability, food safety, food contamination and foodborne diseases as the association is very complex. Thus, this section reviews the impacts of climate change on microbiological and chemical food contamination and related foodborne diseases. Climate change impacts the sources, growth, modes of transmission, survival and the food matrix (FAO, 2008).

- **Salmonella** – *Salmonella* causes salmonellosis, which is a type of bacterial infection associated with common diarrhea. It can spread easily by consuming raw and undercooked items like contaminated raw fruit, vegetables, eggs, meat, raw milk and other dairy products that are made with unpasteurized milk. Furthermore, *Salmonella* bacteria spreads easily if appropriate hygiene and cooking methods are not maintained. The bacteria exists in the intestinal tract of humans and other animals and prevails easily.
- **Clostridium perfringens** – *Clostridium perfringens*, common in our environment, grows very fast under appropriate conditions. Older adults, infants and young children are at high risk. It causes diarrhea and abdominal cramping when contaminated foods are consumed. *C. perfringens* is also called a "buffet germ" as it has the fastest ability to grow in large portions of food, such as casseroles, stews and gravies which have been kept at room temperature for a long time. Proper refrigeration and cooking at the right temperature are important.
- **Campylobacter** – *Campylobacter* causes common diarrhea which is related to eating raw, untreated water or contaminated produce, unpasteurized dairy products, undercooked meat or cross-contamination of other foods by these items. The number of *Campylobacter* bacteria on raw meat may be reduced by freezing, but complete killing is done only by proper heating of foods. Campylobacteriosis mostly occurs in the summer and most common in infants and young children. Cooking food properly and washing raw fruit and vegetables is necessary.
- **Staphylococcus aureus** – *Staphylococcus aureus* bacteria is found on the throat, skin, and nostrils of healthy people and animals. It causes illness by multiplying and producing harmful toxins on transmission to food products. Stomach cramps, nausea, vomiting and diarrhea are major symptoms. The bacteria can be destroyed by cooking, but their toxins are heat-resistant. Individuals with chronic conditions such as lung disease, diabetes, vascular disease, cancer and eczema are at greater risk.
- **Escherichia coli** – *Escherichia coli* or *E. coli* is a large group of bacteria mostly associated with food-poisoning outbreaks due to drinking contaminated water, eating raw or undercooked beef or drinking unpasteurized beverages or dairy products. Most strains of *E. coli* are harmless, but

some are responsible for sickness, e.g. the effects of *E. coli* O157:H7 are extremely severe.

- ***Listeria monocytogenes*** – *Listeria monocytogenes* bacteria causes listeriosis, associated with a high risk of food poisoning caused by eating contaminated food. *Listeria* has the capability to grow at low temperatures where most other bacteria cannot grow, i.e. refrigerator temperatures. The bacteria is found in refrigerated, ready-to-eat food like meat, hot dogs, raw sprouts, dairy products, unpasteurized milk and raw/undercooked seafood and poultry.
- **Norovirus** – Norovirus results in food poisoning and is associated with symptoms similar to stomach flu. Major symptoms include stomach cramping, vomiting, nausea and diarrhea. Important sources are fresh produce, ice, shellfish, fruit and ready-to-eat foods, especially sandwiches, salads and cookies. The virus spreads easily in crowded areas if an individual comes into contact with a norovirus-infected person. Good kitchen hygiene, properly cooked food and washing vegetables and fruit are necessary to avoid transmission.
- ***Toxoplasma gondii*** – Toxoplasmosis is caused by the *Toxoplasma* parasite that results in serious health problems with food poisoning. Infants, pregnant women, older adults and individuals with a reduced immune system are at higher risk. Symptoms are similar to flu, and include swollen lymph glands, muscle aches, pains for a long period and impacts on the eyes, including reduced or blurred vision or pain, redness or tearing. Sources include eating undercooked food, drinking contaminated water, eating contaminated meat or using utensils or cutting boards that have been in contact with raw meat and coming into contact with feces from an infected cat. A mother can infect her infant if she becomes infected before becoming pregnant or during the pregnancy. The risk can be minimized by cooking food, washing fruit and vegetables, freezing meat at the correct temperature, avoiding unpasteurized dairy products, maintaining good hygiene and consulting a physician in relation to health issues.
- **Prions** – Prions are proteins containing infectious agents associated with neurodegenerative disease. "Mad cow disease" in cattle is caused by bovine spongiform encephalopathy, and variant Creutzfeldt–Jakob disease (vCJD) is the major cause in humans. Prion agents are transmitted to humans by consumption of bovine products such as brain tissue.
- **Chemicals** – Chemicals include toxins which occur naturally and pollutants in the environment causing health concerns in humans.
- **Naturally occurring toxins** – These include marine biotoxins, cyanogenic glycosides, mycotoxins and toxins present in mushrooms. Mycotoxins, ochratoxin and aflatoxin are found in staple foods like cereals and corn. The mold produced on grain affects normal development and the immune system, causing cancer.

- **Persistent organic pollutants** – These are highly toxic compounds found worldwide which persist in the body of humans and in the environment. Polychlorinated biphenyls and dioxins are highly toxic by-products of industrial processes and waste incineration. They are present in our environment and accumulate in animal food chains. They cause cancer, hormonal issues and reproductive and developmental problems and damage the immune system.
- **Heavy metals** – Air, soil, and water pollution is associated with heavy-metal contamination in food. Lead, cadmium and mercury are major heavy metals which cause neurological and kidney damage.

10.5　FOODBORNE DISEASES, HEALTH AND SAFETY MEASURES

The economies of developing and developed countries mostly underestimate or under report issues related to foodborne disease which have become a serious health concern in this era. WHO (2015) reported the disease burden estimates due to 31 foodborne agents (viruses, bacteria, parasites, chemicals and toxins) globally and regionally. Another report by the World Bank (Jaffee et al., 2018) on the economic burden of foodborne disease stated that low- and middle-income countries face total productivity loss due to foodborne disease. It has been observed that urbanization, changing consumer habits, travel and changes in lifestyle have encouraged people to procure and eat unhealthy foods and prefer to eat food in public places. Additionally, consumer demand for diverse varieties of foods has grown due to globalization, leading to longer and complex global food chains. Increasing population, industrialization and strengthening of agriculture meet the growing demands for food, creating both challenges and opportunities for food safety. These challenges put more responsibility on handlers and food producers to safeguard food safety. International emergencies quickly evolve from local incidents because of the speed and range of product distribution. Similarly, globalized trade in many continents has amplified outbreaks of foodborne disease, converting them to serious outbreaks. There is a global health threat from unsafe food which causes danger for every individual, particularly pregnant women, infants, elderly people and young children, who are more vulnerable. Safe food supplies sustain trade, national economies and tourism, contribute to food and nutrition security and strengthen sustainable development.

The IPCC report cited different mitigation and adaptation measures to reduce the adverse impacts of food and dietary preferences on climate change (Mbow et al., 2019). There is a need for sustainable food production, no-tillage farming practices, reduction in food waste, forest management and carbon sequestration in agriculture. International conferences and forums have discussed the significance of food safety in achieving the United Nations Sustainable Development Goals and prioritizing government policies and regulatory frameworks for effective response and planning. Furthermore, policy makers maintain and build adequate food safety systems, risk management and infrastructure in order to manage the entire food chain, including during emergencies. Although there are uncertainties and challenges in understanding and addressing food safety implications linked with climate change and its variability, many countries are proactively active in promoting and strengthening the present food safety management programs. Thus, such efforts will offer a base for action to address the emerging risks. Different initiatives, like inter-sectoral coordination, monitoring, surveillance, predictive modeling, risk assessment, good hygiene practices, risk management agriculture practices and emergency preparedness, were used to avoid the risks.

10.6 CONCLUSION AND RECOMMENDATIONS

Thus, from the above discussion and review it is clear that the challenge of climate change is a global threat. Alteration in climate parameters like temperature, rainfall, humidity and CO_2 level has increased the risk and impacted different sectors such as agriculture, livestock, crop production and fisheries. The effect on food management and safety is of prime concern as human beings and animals depend directly on food for their survival on this planet. Climate change distresses zoonoses in various ways, such as in the emergence of new diseases, upsurge in the cycle of transmission of various vectors, range, occurrence of vectors and animal reservoirs. Thus, variations in climatic factors impact various sectors, such as food contamination and disease occurrence, and associated food safety risks at different stages of the food chain are affected by variability in climate. Hence, there is a risk to human health and survival.

Many international organizations play an important part in safeguarding synchronized approaches regarding all aspects of food safety in developed and developing countries. Priority has been given to strengthening existing food management programs, maintenance of strategic food stocks, storage management and food quality. Smart sustainable agriculture, animal husbandry, use of organic food and efficient veterinary practices safeguard the quality of products and safety. More focus should be given to research, the application of predictive modeling, innovations in scientific technology, awareness and exchange of data at both international and national level to develop a greater level of understanding of food safety and management issues. Improved early-warning systems, monitoring and risk management are crucial to minimize the risk due to climate change.

REFERENCES

Campbell-Lendrum, D., Corvalan, C., & Neira, M. (2007). Global climate change: implications for international public health policy. Bulletin of the World Health Organization 85, 235–237.

FAO. (2008). Bioenergy, Food Security and Sustainability – Towards an International Framework. Paper prepared for the High-Level Conference on World Food Security: The Challenges of Climate Change and Bioenergy, 3–5 June 2008.

Available from: www.fao.org/fileadmin/user_upload/foodclimate/HLCdocs/HLC08-inf-3-E.pdf.

Gornall, J., Betts, R., Burke, E., Clark, R., Camp, J., Willett, K., & Wiltshire, A. (2010). Implications of climate change for agricultural productivity in the early twenty-first century. *Philosophical Transactions of the Royal Society B: Biological Sciences*, *365*(1554), 2973–2989.

Jaffee, S., Henson, S., Unnevehr, L., Grace, D., & Cassou, E. (2018). *The safe food imperative: Accelerating progress in low- and middle-income countries*. Washington, DC: The World Bank.

Jarvis, A., Upadhyaya, H. D., Gowda, C. L. L., Agrawal, P. K., Fujisaka, S., & Anderson, B. (2008). *Climate change and its effect on conservation and use of plant genetic resources for food and agriculture and associated biodiversity for food security*, pp. 1–26. Monograph. Food and Agriculture Organization of the United Nations, UK. Available from: http://oar.icrisat.org/id/eprint/5810.

Mbow, C., Rosenzweig, C., Barioni, L. G., Benton, T. G., Herrero, M., Krishnapillai, M., & Tubiello, F. N. (2019). Food security. In *Climate change and land: An IPCC special report on climate change, desertification, land degradation, sustainable land management, food security and greenhouse gas fluxes in terrestrial ecosystems*. IPCC. Working Group III Technical Support Unit, UK. Available from: www.ipcc.ch/site/assets/uploads/2018/07/sr2_background_report_final.pdf.

Nelson, G. C., Rosegrant, M. W., Koo, J., Robertson, R., Sulser, T., Zhu, T., & Magalhaes, M. (2009). *Climate change: Impact on agriculture and costs of adaptation* (Vol. 21). Washington, DC: International Food Policy Research Institute.

Paz, S., Bisharat, N., Paz, E., Kidar, O., & Cohen, D. (2007). Climate change and the emergence of *Vibrio vulnificus* disease in Israel. *Environmental Research*, *103*(3), 390–396.

Schmidhuber, J., & Tubiello, F. N. (2007). Global food security under climate change. *Proceedings of the National Academy of Sciences*, *104*(50), 19703–19708.

Tirado, M. C., Clarke, R., Jaykus, L. A., McQuatters-Gollop, A., & Frank, J. M. (2010). Climate change and food safety: A review. *Food Research International*, *43*(7), 1745–1765.

WHO (2015). World Health Day 2015: Food Safety; 2015. Available from: who.int/foodsafety/en/#story02.

World Health Organization. (2008). *Viruses in food: Scientific advice to support risk management activities: Meeting report*. Geneva: World Health Organization. Available from: www.who.int/foodsafety.

11 Flourishing Amidst Ecological Pressures

Insights from the Experience of the Solegas of Karnataka, India

Shreelata Rao Seshadri*, Dhanya B.,
Sheetal Patil and Raghvendra S. Vanjari

CONTENTS

* Corresponding author: Shreelata Rao Seshadri. shreelata.seshadri@azimpremjifoundation.org

DOI: 10.1201/9781003095422-11

11.1 INTRODUCTION

Traditional food systems, which were the basis for food and nutritional security of communities for millennia, have undergone tremendous transformation over time. Various structural and policy initiatives have transformed the agroecology and the conditions under which food is sourced and produced. This, combined with larger socio-cultural trends, has impacted the diets and taste preferences of society, as well as the way in which food is accessed, exchanged and consumed. While the impetus for change varies from region to region, its effects on societies have been fairly uniform changes in the local agroecology have transformed traditional food systems and shaped dietary preferences. In turn, this has impacted the diversity and adequacy of dietary inputs and, consequently, nutritional and health outcomes.

Referring specifically to the interlinkages between agroecology and food systems of indigenous people of North America, Kuhnlein and Receveur (1996) create three categories of drivers: (1) food availability, which refers to ways in which food is produced or accessed, including crop/wildlife potential, types and quantity of food species in existence, food-cropping/harvesting practices and methods of food distribution; (2) food selection, which refers to the cultural beliefs, tastes and preferences around types of food that are deemed acceptable for consumption, and the affordability of such foods; and (3) the biological need for certain types of food, depending on age, health status and nutritional sufficiency. These challenges create the overarching discourse in the arena of food and nutrition, which privileges conversations around "food security" to the exclusion of a culturally appropriate, locally accessible and nutritionally satisfying diet that is central to traditional food systems. It is now widely accepted that the imbalances and inequities in health and nutritional outcomes are the result of the manner in which the producer–consumer relationship has changed in response to the emphasis on macro-scale planning and policy in agriculture and food security with little respect for ecological and social realities and household-level changes in tastes and preferences, and influenced heavily by multinational economic interests (Kuhnlein et al., 2009). Food and nutritional security, therefore, have broader implications that are environmental, social, cultural, physical, cognitive, psychosocial and economic and encompass state–society interactions at both local and global level (FAO, IFAD and WFP, 2014).

The global discourse around food sovereignty best captures this broader view (Pimbert, 2019) and exhorts communities to assert their right to more just and sustainable access to a diverse and culturally appropriate diet. La Via Campesina, the global movement campaigning for food sovereignty, states the following:

Long-term food security depends on those who produce food and care for the natural environment. As the stewards of food producing resources, we hold the following principles as the necessary foundation for achieving food security. Food is a basic human right. This right can only be realized in a system where food sovereignty is guaranteed. Food sovereignty is the right of each nation to maintain and develop its own capacity to produce its basic foods respecting cultural and productive diversity. We have the right to produce our own food in our own territory. Food sovereignty is a precondition to genuine food security.

(Via Campesina, 1996, quoted in Patel, 2009, p. 665)

Using the experience of the Solegas[1] of the Biligirirangana hills (BR hills) of Karnataka (South India), this chapter traces their journey with regard to transformations of their food systems. The Solega lifestyle and socio-cultural practices have been in a state of constant flux, despite the community's continuing struggle for rights to land and forest produce and to manage the forests in accordance with traditional practices. Recognizing the transitions in food systems as symptomatic of the interplay between multiple underlying drivers, this chapter: (1) lays out the current understanding of how and why the food systems of Solegas have changed, based on an exhaustive review of literature; (2) generates a conceptual framework that ties the different threads of the literature together and identifies areas of divergence and synergy; and (3) identifies the possibilities of meaningful interventions to ensure food and nutritional security, sovereignty and justice among Solegas.

11.2 METHODOLOGY

Acknowledging the wealth of extant scientific literature on Solegas, we conducted a systematic literature review to consolidate the available knowledge pertinent to forests, agroecology and food systems and to identify knowledge gaps in these domains. The software package Publish or Perish (PoP)[2] was used to search for publications, considering its easy-access features and smart interface to work with (Harzing, 2010). Keywords applied for the search in Google Scholar database included "Solega", "Sholega", "Sholaga", "Soliga", "Soligaru", "BRT", "BRTWS", "Biligiri Rangaswamy Temple (BRT) Wildlife Sanctuary", "traditional food system" and "Indigenous people in Karnataka". Literature from sources including peer-reviewed academic journals, books (in both English and Kannada languages), reports and the popular press that were published in the timeline 1970–2020 were explored. The publication list was downloaded from PoP to Bibtex format and extracted into the Zotero program[3] to create a bibliography.

Appropriate materials were selected for review after screening for the following criteria related to research questions: (1) the item must relate to Solegas in BR hills specifically, not elsewhere; and (2) it must deal with aspects such as forests and biodiversity, agriculture, health and nutritional wellbeing and socio-cultural practices that are related to food systems. Among a total of 281 hits, 217 research articles and a report that were found to be irrelevant were thus excluded. A total of

69 items across books (11), papers (45), the popular press including magazines (3), reports (6) and theses (4) were reviewed.

11.3 FOREST, FARMING AND FOOD SYSTEMS OF SOLEGAS: TEASING OUT THE INTERLINKAGES

The Biligiri Rangaswamy Temple (BRT) Wildlife Sanctuary (notified as a Tiger Reserve in 2011) is located in Chamarajanagar district of Karnataka state (refer to location map in Figure 11.1). The sanctuary spans an area of 540 km^2 with elevations ranging from 600 to 1800 meters above sea level. BRT is a unique bio-geographical entity straddling the Western and Eastern Ghats and is part of the Nilgiri Biosphere Reserve (Madegowda & Rao, 2017). The landscape is home to 16,487 Solegas living in 62 *podus* (settlements) within and on the periphery of BRT (Madegowda, 2009). Historically, Solegas practiced shifting cultivation, gathered honey and berries from forest and hunted occasionally (Buchanan, 1807). Following the declaration of a wildlife sanctuary in BR hills, shifting cultivation was banned in 1974 and with the support of conservation non-government organizations (NGOs) and other organizations, the tribe was settled in villages where they started practicing settled agriculture. Solegas have a rich repository of traditional knowledge about agriculture and sustainable harvest of forest produce, biodiversity conservation and traditional health care (Jadegowda & Ramesh, 2008).

The literature review yielded interesting perspectives on the Solegas' interactions with the forests and agroecology at BR hills. The review is presented here under three main heads – forests, farming and food systems.

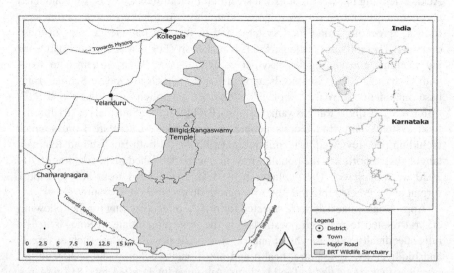

FIGURE 11.1   Location map for Biligiri Rangaswamy Temple (BRT) Wildlife Sanctuary.

11.3.1 FORESTS OF BR HILLS: LIFELINE OF SOLEGA SUSTENANCE

'"The forest is our home', is a statement that all Solega will, no doubt, agree on."

(Si, 2015, p. 28)

Perhaps the best fleshed-out aspect about the Solegas is their intricate cultural and livelihood linkages with the forest. The BR hills landscape is a place of deep cultural, social and economic meaning for the Solegas (Rai & Madegowda, 2018). The socio-cultural, ecological and livelihood roles of forests in BR hills and the trajectory, drivers and outcomes of changes in the Solegas' interactions with forest ecosystems are summarized under the following headings.

11.3.1.1 Ecological and Cultural Diversity of BR Hills Landscape

Extensive records exist of the ecological resources of BR hills, including wild food and medicinal resources and culturally important species. Ramesh (1989) classified the natural vegetation of BR hills into five types: dry deciduous forest, scrub, grasslands, wet evergreen and high-altitude montane forest, of which seasonally dry forests comprising the scrub savanna and deciduous forests constitute approximately 90% (Ganesan & Setty, 2004). Solega speakers distinguish between some 14 habitats (*kadu*) on the basis of plant and animal life, geological and topographic features and human use cycles (Si, 2015). The biodiversity of the area is rich, with at least 1,400 species of higher plants (Ramesh, 1989), 27 species of mammals, over 100 species of butterflies and around 250 species of birds (Si, 2015). Documentations of 108 medicinal plant species used in traditional health care – of which seven are endangered and three endemic (Nautiyal et al., 2016), 71 different crop varieties of pulses, cereals, millet and vegetable crops as part of mixed and multistoried subsistence agriculture (Jadegowda & Ramesh, 2008) and 24 different species of non-timber forest products (NTFPs) (Hegde et al., 1996) – are other notable records on the culturally salient biological wealth of BR hills. Participatory mapping of cultural diversity of the forests showed more than 500 sites of cultural significance (Mandal et al., 2010).

11.3.1.2 Extraction of Non-Timber Forest Products – Livelihood and Ecological Implications

Collection of NTFPs is a major livelihood activity of Solegas, from both subsistence and commercial angles. More than 7,500 Solega families make a living by collecting NTFPs from the sanctuary (Misra, 2006). NTFPs play a major role in traditional food systems and contribute to nearly half of the gross annual income of Solega households (Hegde et al., 1996). Honey, lichens (moss), soap nut (*Acacia sinuata*), *magaliberu* (*Decalapis hamiltonii*), *amla* (*Phyllanthus emblica* and *Phyllanthus indofischeri*), soap berry (*Sapindus trifoliatus*), *arale* (*Terminalia chebula*), tamarind (*Tamarindus indica*), broom grass (*Thysanolaena maxima*), gum (*Gum arabica, Gum karaya*) wild turmeric (*Curcuma angustifolia*), *tarekai*

(*Terminalia bellirica*), *jamun* (*Sygizium cumini*), silk cotton (*Bombax ceiba*) and wild mango (*Mangifera indica*) are some of the major NTFPs collected from the forests (Madegowda, 2009). Some of these are marketed through cooperative societies known as Large-scale Adivasi Multipurpose Societies (LAMPS) supervised by government officials, while some are marketed directly or collected for own use (Hegde et al., 1996). Solegas have traditionally followed sustainable practices of NTFP harvest; for instance, honey is extracted only by skilled collectors leaving two to five colonies unharvested for the sustenance of bee populations. Similarly, while collecting fruit, roots and tubers, small plants are left untouched, and enough of the produce is left on the ground and the trees to support regeneration of plants and wild animals that depend on these food resources (Madegowda, 2009).

Notwithstanding the prevalence of such sustainable practices among Solegas, a series of articles published during 1996–1998 in the journal *Economic Botany* drew attention to the multifarious impacts of produce extraction on the population and community structure of forests and regeneration of important NTFP species such as *amla* and fuelwood-yielding species in BR hills (Murali et al., 1996; Ganeshaiah et al., 1998; Shankar et al., 1996, 1998). Uma Shaanker et al. (2004) in a detailed analysis of the ecological consequences of forest use, at different levels from genes to ecosystem, confirm poor regeneration of NTFP species and intense landcover changes at peripheries with high human disturbance, pointing to population and ecosystem level impacts. No clear pattern of loss of genetic diversity was apparent. However, these studies did not clearly establish NTFP extraction as the sole causal factor and other drivers such as fire, grazing and competition with weeds were also proposed to be contributing to the vegetation decline (Murali et al., 1996). Between 1973 and 2014 the core area of BR hills was found to have greened due to invasion of the weed *Lantana camara* (*Lantana* henceforth), while the periphery and wildlife corridors browned, owing to factors including human habitation, historical forest management practices and policies, resource extraction, cattle grazing, drought and forest fires (Mallegowda et al., 2015).

Though none of these studies offered conclusive evidence of NTFP extraction as the sole driver of observed vegetation changes, early researchers hypothesized low incomes from NTFPs to largely drive their unsustainable extraction. NTFP extraction was not found to be a preferred vocation among Solegas as they obtained low wages for their extractive efforts and, given the lack of value addition, the price appreciation varied widely for different products (50% in *magaliberu* to as high as 255% in soap nut). NTFP extraction decreased with the percentage of educated family members and income from other vocations and increased with family size (Hegde et al., 1996). Subsequently suggestions had been put forth to involve Solegas directly in processing and marketing NTFPs through cooperatives; part of these profits could be distributed to Solegas in proportion to the quantity of produce collected and participation in the processing industry, and the rest spent for community welfare and silvicultural work for forest protection (Shankar et al.,

1998). Some of the later interventions in this regard are detailed under Section 11.5, below.

11.3.1.3   Fire and Invasive Species: Major Drivers of Forest Ecosystem Changes

Changes in the fire regime and spread of the ubiquitous invasive species *Lantana* have been areas of considerable interest for ecology research in BR hills. The annual dry-season fires were used by the Solegas to burn forests and to promote the growth of fresh fodder for grazing and to facilitate NTFP collection. Fires cleansed the forests, controlled the spread of hemi-parasites on gooseberry trees and spurred the growth of native trees and grasses by fertilizing the soil with ashes and enhanced the availability of food for local wildlife (Hiremath & Sundaram, 2005; Madegowda, 2009; Sundaram et al., 2012). The repeated burns ensured that the fires stayed close to the ground, not affecting the tree canopies (Rai & Madegowda, 2018). Following the declaration of Wildlife Sanctuary in 1973, the traditional fire practice of *taragu benki* (litter fire) was stopped. Subsequently the risk of destructive canopy fires started increasing from the high fuel load in the forests, stimulating invasion by fire-tolerant alien species (Chatterjee, 2008). *Lantana* possesses several characteristics of fire-adapted invasive species such as re-sprouting on being burnt, year-round flowering and fruiting producing copious quantities of seeds that are readily dispersed by frugivores, and efficient nutrient uptake and use (Hiremath & Sundaram, 2005). The mean density of *Lantana* increased almost fourfold from 1997 to 2008, accompanied by changes in the population structure of native tree species and visible consequences for forest structure and composition, including reduction in sapling density, alterations in species richness, diversity and evenness (Sundaram & Hiremath, 2012; Sundaram et al., 2015).

The traditional knowledge of Solegas about the *Lantana*–fire relationship is very nuanced, in contrast to scientific knowledge that considers fires as promoting *Lantana* uniformly. Solegas observe that fires suppress *Lantana* when its density is low, while dense *Lantana* fuel destructive canopy fires that further enhance its spread. Solegas believe that *Lantana* invasion in BR hills is due to the decrease in the frequency of fires that killed *Lantana* plants and seeds in soil, while leaving native species that are historically exposed to fires untouched (Sundaram et al., 2012). The prolific fruit output and seed dispersal of *Lantana*, and historical extraction of grass and bamboo, were also cited as reasons by Solegas for *Lantana*'s expansion. Several perceptions of Solegas on the repercussions of *Lantana*'s spread are confirmed by research studies, such as reduction in density and regeneration of *amla* and other NTFP species (Setty et al., 2008; Ticktin et al., 2012) and increase in crop raiding by wild herbivores due to reduction in forage availability in forests (Ticktin et al., 2012; Madegowda & Rao, 2014; Mundoli et al., 2016). *Lantana* has replaced the former grass understorey and has made it difficult to see and move around in the forest for NTFP collection (Madegowda & Rao, 2014). Thus, the fallout of *Lantana* colonization spills over the forest boundaries to adversely impact the farming practices that now have to respond to crop depredation by wildlife, and livelihoods and dietary practices that are impoverished by the decreasing abundance of important forest produces. For Solegas, *Lantana* is even a metaphor for the influx of foreign cultural influences into their world, that devoured large tracts of their forest understorey, sites of religious and utilitarian values and old forest trails, driving many culturally important species of plants and animals to local extinction (Si, 2015).

11.3.1.4 Social and Ecological Impacts of Conservation Policies

BR hills have seen a slew of policy interventions, primarily aimed at conservation of forests, in response to national-level legal mandates for protection of biodiversity and ecosystems. The outcomes of many of these policies in terms of ecological integrity of the forests and sustainability of Solega livelihoods are far from desirable. Many such interventions had often overlooked the deep embeddedness of the Solega way of life in the ecology of the forests and failed to accommodate the Solega cultural schemas and views about forests' ecological processes that are often in contradiction to the state's outlooks. For instance, for Solegas a "good" forest would be an open-canopy savanna woodland that supports a multitude of livelihood, dietary and socio-cultural requirements, whereas for the Forest Department (FD) on the other hand, a closed forest is the ideal condition, resonating with the global goals of carbon storage and biodiversity preservation (Rai & Madegowda, 2018).

A review of the various forest-related laws (Table 11.1) unequivocally reveals the piecemeal approaches of forest policies with immense socio-ecological repercussions for the forests and their people. Using a web of relationships approach, Rai et al. (2019) confirmed that the effects of restrictions on livelihood activities following establishment of a protected area have been unfavorable for people and ecosystems (as shown in Table 11.1), while the state seems to have benefitted from revenue generation through tourism. They conclude that centralized policies have affected the relationships between people, forests and the state.

11.3.2 Farming Systems of Solegas

Although NTFP collection is the major source of livelihood of Solegas in BR hills, they have been involved in subsistence agriculture since time immemorial. Shifting cultivation in the earliest times and in later settled agriculture with mixed food crops using minimum amounts of external input were the key features of the Solega farming system. This section highlights the transitions in Solega farming systems and management regimes and their links with forest ecology.

11.3.2.1 Traditional Agricultural and Animal Husbandry Practices

Traditionally known to be hunter-gatherers, the Solega community practiced subsistence farming throughout their existence in BR hills. Earliest writings about the farming practices of Solegas mention that they practiced shifting (*podu*) cultivation

TABLE 11.1
Impacts of various forest-related laws and policies on Solega livelihoods

Policies and laws	Implications
Indian Forest Act 1927	Livelihood uses of the forests were allowed, Solegas practiced shifting cultivation inside forests and collected minor forest produce
Wildlife Protection Act 1972	Biligiri Rangaswamy Temple (BRT) reserve forest was notified as BRT Wildlife Sanctuary in 1974. Traditional practices such as shifting cultivation and *taragu benki* was banned, Solegas were relocated to settlements outside the forest and a few were given houses and land without relevant records. Non-timber forest product (NTFP) collection continued, under the aegis of Large-scale Adivasi Multipurpose Society (LAMPS), set up in 1982 under an integrated tribal development program
National Forest Policy 1988	Eco-development committees were formed that carried out afforestation activities, though these were short-lived
Amendment to Wildlife Protection Act in 2003	NTFP collection for commercial purposes was banned in 2004 and strictly enforced in 2006. Livelihoods of 16,000 Solegas were affected. They resorted to migration to Kerala and Tamil Nadu to work as agricultural laborers in plantations in the absence of alternative employment. A total of 33% of families migrated, for 10–300 days a year, affecting children's education, food, health, culture, etc.
Scheduled Tribes and Other Traditional Forest Dwellers (Recognition of Forest Rights) Act (FRA), 2006	In 2008, Solegas claimed rights to NTFPs, grazing, fishing, forest management, intellectual property and worship at cultural sites and cultivated land for individual households. Almost all households that claimed received rights to cultivated land. In October 2011, in what was the country's first case of rights granted to a community in a protected area under the FRA, community forest rights were granted to 32 Solega settlements. An additional ten settlements received the rights in 2018, and 20 settlements are yet to receive community forest rights
Mahatma Gandhi National Rural Employment Scheme, 2009	Though not directly related to forest conservation, the employment of Solegas for *Lantana* removal from forests in 2009 and 2011 under this scheme helped them to tide over the lean period following the NTFP collection ban in 2006 to some extent and helped in enhancing native grass recovery
Declaration of BRT Tiger Reserve in 2011	340 square kilometers of the sanctuary's core zone were declared as critical tiger habitat. Eight settlements in the core zone faced relocation to outside the protected area

of millet and pulses, and were dependent mainly on forests for vegetables, fruit, roots and tubers, honey and meat (Morab, 1977). Their cultivation practices are believed to have benefitted the community and the forest ecology (Madegowda, 2009). Morab (1977) observed that Solegas were reluctant to share any of their knowledge with the outside world and this was experienced repeatedly by many researchers studying their traditions and culture. Bhat (1997) traced the socio-economic changes in Solega tribal settlements between 1965 and 1990 to highlight the vast difference in a short time span, chiefly owing to resettlement to forest peripheries following sanctuary declaration (Table 11.2).

Following the resettlement of Solegas to peripheries, the forest–farm production system shifted to a purely farm-based settled agriculture system with support from government and NGOs to overcome the knowledge and skill barriers. Even then Solegas continued to practice low-input organic subsistence farming in mixed and multilayered cropping systems of traditional varieties of millet, pulses, vegetables, oilseeds and tubers. Most of the Solega land holdings are small and rainfed. They hardly use chemical inputs or improved seeds. Jadegowda and Ramesh (2008) confirmed that inadvertently sustainable practices, including maintaining diverse crop varieties and using indigenous inputs and harvest methods, were integral to traditional farming practices. Solegas applied their traditional knowledge of soil fertility, water and pest management in their farming practices. The agrobiodiversity was reflected in their dietary practices as well as in cultural rituals.

Livestock herding is not common in Solega community. They occasionally domesticated a small number of goats, cattle and fowl. Goats and fowl were reared for sacrificial rituals, and cattle for agricultural activities and milk. Milk is consumed only in tea and coffee and preparation of curd and other milk products is rare in the community. Somagond et al. (2019), in a comparative study on animal husbandry in the core and buffer zones of BR hills, highlighted constraints such as lack of grazing land, restrictions on grazing in forests and non-availability of feed and veterinary services that resulted in viewing cattle and goat rearing only as safety nets during an emergency, than as permanent livelihood options.

11.3.2.2 Traditional Knowledge, Perceptions and Attitudes towards Farming

Culturally, farming activities of Solega community are strongly embedded in their festivals and rituals. Collective celebrations during clearing of land, sowing, weeding and harvesting of new crops are performed with certain rituals (Rathod et al., 2011). Different clans perform different rituals for the deity; some prepare and offer food every day while others clean the premises and draw fresh water for the deities. Solegas worship forest, waterbodies, wildlife, fire and rain and continue to celebrate festivals for seeking divine blessings for good crops, rain, forest products and safety from wildlife. *Rotti Habba*, which marks the harvest of *ragi* (finger millet) every year from February to May, is celebrated by clans over two days – *Rotti puja* and big *Rotti Habba*. *Hosa Ragi Habba* is celebrated every year

TABLE 11.2
Socio-economic changes in Solega settlements from 1965 to 2016

	1965	1990	2016
Podus	Nine *podus* inside forest	All nine resettled in core zone	61 *podus* in total in both core and buffer zones
Farming	Shifting cultivation	Plough and settled farming	Settled agriculture with more emphasis on cash crops (Mundoli et al., 2016)
Crops	Subsistence – millet and maize	Along with subsistence crops coffee plantations and sericulture	More coffee and pepper compared to subsistence food crops (Mundoli et al., 2016)
Crop loss	Insignificant (from pest attacks)	50% of produce lost to wildlife attacks	79% in millet-producing *podus*, 4% in coffee-producing *podus* and 25% in *podus* with mixed crops (Rai et al., 2019)
Animal husbandry	Not prominent	Government schemes for animal husbandry failed since Solegas are not used to keeping animals	Comparatively more in core zone than in buffer zone (Somagond et al., 2019)
Education	School started by Vivekananda Girijana Kalyana Kendra (VGKK) in 1981 focusing on alternative ways of education	Same school with more students	Anganwadis in most of the *podus*. Government primary school and VGKK high school are functional
Health	VGKK hospital with capacity to treat 20,000 people in a year	Government hospital also operates in addition to VGKK's	Government and private hospitals at taluk and district level, VGKK hospital
Community organization	Forest laborers' cooperative	Solega Abhivrudhi Sangha (SAS)	SAS, Large-scale Adivasi Multipurpose Society (LAMPS), women's self-help groups (Madegowda & Rao, 2017)
Socio-economic and cultural aspects	Solegas exploited by traders from plains. Most also worked as daily wage laborers with the Forest Department	Most transactions are in terms of money. Livelihood options have increased. Social events are losing importance. Changes in names, dress and ornaments and food. Solega no longer isolated from rest of society	Changes in lifestyle, food consumption patterns, livelihood choices and health status (Krishna Raj et al., 2017)

from the November to January after *ragi* is harvested. The produce harvested is first offered to the deities before being used at home.

Every ritual is celebrated with songs and dances that reflect the rich indigenous knowledge of flora and fauna. The songs narrate the importance of different species so that knowledge is easily transferred to the next generation. Traditional knowledge about weeds, wildlife, water management, sustainable harvest, monsoon, forest fire and sacred sites (Madegowda, 2009) has also contributed significantly in their farming activities. The custom of sharing farm produce helped Solegas in two ways – first in sustaining the rich genetic diversity of crops and second in ensuring nutritional supply.

More than 80% of the produce is stored for subsistence until the next year's harvest using ten different storage methods. Naveena et al. (2017) estimated grain loss from insect pest infestation, especially in pulses, to be 10–100% in the samples that were studied, even after careful storage. The diversity of pests increased with number of food grain types stored by each household (Naveena et al., 2015). Food grain sharing habits among Solegas and improved accessibility to markets in towns, often resulting in purchase of infested grains that facilitate the spread of storage pests, were reported to be the reasons for grain loss. The culture of sharing food grain ensured nutritional supply, but at the same time was also found to contribute to loss of grains.

A study by Ranganath (2002) revealed that the use of indigenous farming practices varied from high to low, with more or less the same proportion of farmers represented in each group. While the shift from indigenous practices was mostly due to socio-economic factors (type of family, economic motivation, value orientation towards farming, exposure to mass media, etc.), the constraints for following such practices were largely related to environment (improper water management practices, wildlife menace and small landholding size) and governance (irregular extension services).

11.3.2.3 Shift to Commercial Crops – Drivers, Status and Impacts

Solega farming systems have undergone multiple transformations, partially driven by natural phenomena such as climate variation, but more importantly by a range of social, political and governance factors. When Solegas started settled agriculture in the forest peripheries, they faced crop loss due to wildlife depredation that prompted a switch to commercial crops like coffee in wet zones and cotton in dry areas. In response to exploitation by middlemen and price fluctuations in these two commercial crops, other crops like maize and banana were adopted later. The capability of Solegas to adapt quickly to alternative options in difficult circumstances was noted by Mundoli et al. (2016). They concluded that the social resilience of community against various external stressors – political, environmental and social – was enhanced by support from NGOs for indigenous practices such as mixed cropping systems and welfare services from the state. The most recent and much celebrated intervention is the recognition of land rights through the Forest Rights Act (Table 11.1) that provided the opportunity for intensifying cultivation of commercial crops like coffee on Solega lands.

Bose (2017) narrated the story of the arrival of coffee in Solega farmlands rather dramatically. Although there were large coffee estates in the region owned by well-known business families of the country, Solegas were never inclined towards growing coffee themselves, even when they were residing in the forest core zone. Resettlement to the buffer zone and crop raids by wildlife made them try their hands at coffee growing. Unlike the large estates, Solega's first stock of coffee did not come from FD nurseries or the Coffee Board. They were just saplings collected from the edges of those large estates, most probably carried by wildlife. Even without a meticulous management plan, coffee planted by Solega thrived only with goat manure, which was commonly available. Slowly other companion plants and trees to coffee, such as pepper vine (*Piper nigrum*) and silver oak (*Grevillea robusta*), made their entry into Solega farms. Native species like *nandi* (*Spathodea campanulata*), *mathi* (*Terminalia elliptica*), *honne* (*Pterocarpus marsupium*) and *honge* (*Millettia pinnata*) were also retained in coffee plantations.

According to recent estimates there are about 540 Solega families cultivating coffee and pepper over 2,500 acres of land, producing about 40 tonnes of coffee annually (Kaggere, 2020). Each family earns anywhere between Rs 40,000 and Rs 50,000 a year by selling coffee to middlemen. Apart from the presence of ready markets, traders at the farmgate and quick cash income, the preference for coffee was driven by its low vulnerability to wildlife raids and ease of cultivation. But agrobiodiversity loss and shift from food to commercial crops have had negative implications on food sovereignty and nutritional security (Mundoli et al., 2016).

11.3.3   Food, Health and Nutrition Among Solegas

According to the National Family Health Survey (Round 4; 2015–16), 44% of tribal children <5 years old in India were stunted and 45% were underweight. The same data show that, in Karnataka, 12.2% of tribal children were wasted as compared to 10.3% of non-tribal children; 19.4% were stunted as compared to 16.3% of non-tribal children; and 14.1% were underweight as compared to 11.6% of non-tribal children. A total of 63.7% of tribal children were anemic as compared to 60.5% of non-tribal children. While information on the health and nutrition of both Solega children and adults is fairly limited, two major threads of evidence can be identified from the available literature:

* Dietary diversity and nutritional status of Solega adults and children
* Health status and access to services among the Solega community.

11.3.3.1   Dietary Diversity and Nutritional Status

An important concern is whether Solegas are able to access adequate food, given that their access to the forest has been seriously curtailed. The special Public Distribution System (PDS) rations provide *ragi*, lentils, eggs, oil/ghee and sugar. Apart from possible disruptions during the COVID-19 pandemic-induced lockdown, access to PDS has been reported to be quite satisfactory. However, the evidence shows that Solegas have been dependent on the forest as a food source, and it is a principal means of diversifying their diet. While their food habits are fairly monotonous, with consumption of *ragi* balls and *sambar* for lunch and dinner, they regularly supplement this with 8–10 varieties of green leafy vegetables, 10–12 varieties of fruit and 4–5 types of tubers, all of which have been gathered from the forest (Yankanchi & Channesh, 2017). Often this is augmented by vegetables, along with fruit like bananas, guavas and jackfruit, from a small kitchen garden.

Both adequacy and diversity of diet are of interest in as much as they are major determinants of nutritional outcomes. Perhaps as a result of the regular availability of staples through the PDS, recent findings did not show a severe deficiency in the consumption of different categories of major nutrients (Krishna Raj et al., 2017). Based on a survey of 1000 respondents, the researchers analyzed food consumption according to recommended daily allowance (RDA) and found that the mean consumption of nutrients by Solega men met the requirement for energy (105.0%), iron (128.8%), calcium (153.2%) and vitamin C (161.7%). However, consumption of protein (88.2%) and fat (84.8%) was less than RDA. With regard to Solega women, mean consumption of nutrients met the requirement of adequacy for energy (103.8%), calcium (149.0%) and vitamin C (166.5%). Here also, consumption of protein (88.2%), fat (84.8%) and iron (80.5%) was less than RDA.

However, measures such as levels of anemia and body measurement of children indicate a significant shortfall in the nutritional adequacy of the diet. A hematological and anthropometric study by Prabhakar and Gangadhar (2016) found that the overall prevalence of anemia was 91.4%: 7.2% mild, 74.3% moderate and 9.9% severe anemia. A higher proportion of girls was severely anemic in the age group of 9+ and 10+ years than boys. Unusually, about 94.3% of children with normal body mass index were anemic. The study concluded that anemia among Solega children is a cause for concern. A related issue was the impact of malnutrition on other health conditions. Although this has not been well studied among the Solegas, there is some evidence to show that there was a greater incidence of mental illness such as depression among malnourished adults (Narendran et al., 2019).

11.3.3.2 Health Status and Access to Services

A study specific to the Solegas of BR hills showed a 30% prevalence of hypertension in the sample of tribal adults surveyed as compared to 34.5% among non-tribal people (Prashanth et al., 2020). In addition, Solegas have specific health challenges such as sickle cell anemia. About 4.5% of Solegas have some form of sickle cell disease, which requires specific types of (usually) hospital-based interventions which are not available in BR hills (Madegowda & Rao, 2013).

Access to health services is a major issue for the Solegas. For example, in the case of sickle cell anemia, they have taken recourse to natural control of the disease with different types of folic acid-rich green leaves, fruit and tubers in their daily diet due to the lack of medical services (Madegowda & Rao, 2013). In fact, traditional medicine such as castor (*Ricinus communis*) oil, *manasige habbu* (*Todalia asetiea*) leaf decoction, *kakke* (*Cassia fistula*) bark, *hulisoppu* (*Oxalis corniculata*) decoction, *hurigilu beru* (*Chloroxylon swetneides*) root and many other traditional medicines have been the first line of treatment for sickle cell disease. The same was true of other common disease conditions as well, such as water-borne diseases or even animal attacks: the treatment was largely diet-based, with tubers, fruit, leaves, honey, mushrooms, bamboo shoots and seeds in their everyday diet or using medicinal plants (Madegowda & Rao, 2015). Traditional methods were also commonly used in childbirth, with cultural practices playing an important role in health-seeking behavior (Zaraska, 1997).

A common thread in several studies looking into the choice of health-seeking behavior among Solegas has stressed the transformation brought about by the Vivekananda Girijana Kalyana Kendra (VGKK) hospital set up by Dr. H. Sudarshan in 1979. A Vivekananda follower, the doctor was able to combine his spiritual commitment with very secular activities such as implementing the Health for All principle of the Alma Ata declaration and getting funding from the Government of Karnataka (and later many other governments) to run their primary health centers according to his principles. Later, VGKK was able to engage with many other aspects of Solega life, including land rights, housing, livelihoods and so on, inspiring a great deal of trust and dedication from the Solega community (Bose, 2006). Importantly, the introduction of modern medical practices through the VGKK hospital, along with the changing ecological environment as a result of changes in forest rights, shifted the Solegas' relationship with traditional medicine. Overall, however, it seems as if good health, as a desirable social outcome, is not as salient in the Solegas' daily life as issues such as forest rights and access to NTFP (Seshadri et al., 2019).

Ghosh et al. (2007) found that the overall health status of the Solegas had improved with the use of modern medicine, based on improvements in health indicators such as infant mortality rate and prevalence of sickle cell disease. They also found that there had been a shift in preference for modern medicine, largely due to its relatively easy availability and longer effect. They concluded that the reduction of reliance on traditional medicine was due to lengthy treatment protocols as well as the reduced number of practitioners, rather than a decline in the availability of medicinal plants. This is despite several efforts to revive traditional medical knowledge and preserve agroecological systems by the World Health Organization, VGKK and Ashoka Trust for Research in Ecology and the Environment (ATREE) and the production and propagation of traditional medicines by VGKK (Roy et al., 2015).

11.4   FRAMING THE RELATIONSHIP BETWEEN FORESTS, FARMING AND FOOD SYSTEMS OF SOLEGAS

This extensive review of literature leads to the realization that the relationship between the forest, farm and food systems of the Solegas is multidimensional. For instance, the cascading impacts of the ban on litter fires after the declaration of Wildlife Sanctuary in 1974 is well documented. Discontinuance of fire led to a regime shift in the forest ecosystem to a *Lantana*-dominated state. Apart from this, the proliferation of *Lantana* has affected the growth of grasses where wildlife used to shelter and the regeneration of native fruit trees, tubers and bamboos. This has substantially reduced the availability of wild foods for both humans and animals. In addition, the thick bushes impede the movement of tribal people within the forest, constraining their ability to gather whatever forest produce is still available.

Another impact of *Lantana* is that it has driven wildlife out of the forest; plus, the Wildlife Protection Act prohibits hunting or even culling of wildlife such as boar and small animals that were earlier part of the tribal diet. This has a detrimental impact on farming since crop depredation by wildlife has become rampant. This not only affects crop yields, it has also led to farmers increasingly switching to crops such as coffee that are less prone to wildlife depredation. In turn this has negatively impacted the agrobiodiversity of the region. Traditional multilayered crop systems of millet, cereals, pulses, vegetable and oilseeds have been replaced by coffee and its companion plants like pepper and silver oak.

These combined changes in the forest and farm have inevitably impacted the traditional food systems of the Solega. Studies indicate that the shift from mixed food cropping to cash crops has reduced the diversity of nutritional basket, while forest degradation has reduced the supply of traditional forest foods. The reduced availability of fruit such as *amla* and green leafy vegetables, as well as tubers, mushrooms and bamboo shoots, has drastically reduced their dietary diversity. A significant outcome of these changes is the manifold increase in dependence on markets and the PDS for food grains, raising grave concerns about food sovereignty and nutritional security (Mundoli et al., 2016). While the changing food and dietary practices could also reflect improved access to markets, increased cash income from coffee cultivation and evolving cultural preferences, the role of the forest ecosystem transitions in this process through diverse routes is undeniable.

Many of the changes in forest ecosystems are long lasting and are not easily amendable, with several positive social-ecological feedbacks acting to trap forests in an unhealthy invasive-loaded state. Even if the rights to fire practices are restored under the FRA, with the current *Lantana*-dominated forest understorey, fires could be intense and damage the entire forest ecosystem (Sundaram et al., 2012). Similarly, even though land rights are ensured, revival of traditional mixed cropping would be challenging due to crop raiding by wildlife.

Weaving together insights from the exhaustive review of literature, we propose the concept of *flourishing* to flesh out linkages between the evolving food systems of the Solegas and their key contributors – forests and farming – and as the ultimate outcome for which they strive (Figure 11.2). Beyond narrow measures such as income or disease-free state, human flourishing consists in a much broader range of states, certainly including mental and physical health, but also encompassing happiness and life satisfaction, meaning and purpose, character and virtue, and close social relationships (VanderWheele, 2017). In Aristotelian ethics, human flourishing (eudaimonia) is the ultimate moral standard and involves the rational use of individual human potentialities in the pursuit of freely and rationally chosen values and goals.

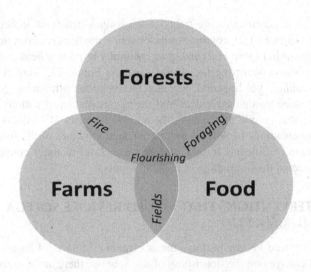

FIGURE 11.2 Interlinkages between forests, farms and food leading to flourishing.

Analyses using even reductionist indices of flourishing could throw light on the disadvantaged position of tribal communities. The global Child Flourishing Index (India ranks 131st) measures 'flourishing' as the geometric mean of child 'surviving' and 'thriving' (Clark et al., 2020). Child survival is measured by maternal survival, survival in children younger than 5 years of age, suicide, access to maternal and child health services, basic hygiene and sanitation, and lack of extreme poverty. Thriving is measured by educational achievement, growth and nutrition, reproductive freedom and protection from violence. While the index specifically refers to flourishing among children younger than 5 years of age, the idea of flourishing is nonetheless universal and one that could expand our understanding of what constitutes our sense of health and wellbeing.

Tribal flourishing has increasingly become a matter of concern. Sonowal (2010) highlights several reasons why this might be so: (1) tribal notions of health, nutrition and wellbeing are culturally mediated and not best captured by the usual metrics; (2) their physical, social and economic environment are evolving rapidly, impacting health and nutrition; (3) tribal life and sense of wellbeing and prosperity are embedded in their relationship with local ecology, which has transformed radically over time; and (4) access to basic public health services such as safe drinking water and sanitation, and health care for a range of services, is woefully inadequate in tribal areas, accompanied by widespread poverty which precludes private access. This is enough reason to examine whether the nutritional disadvantage already manifesting among tribal children is likely to worsen over time and what steps can be taken to prevent such problems in the future.

In the Solega context, besides health and nutritional parameters, flourishing appears to be intimately attached to forests and traditional farming and food practices. The freedom to forage freely in the forests (intersection between food and forests in Figure 11.2), continue traditional fire practices (intersection between forests and farms in Figure 11.2) and grow culturally important field crops in forest peripheries (fields connecting forests and farms in Figure 11.2) are all critical to Solega flourishing, yet impeded by state interventions attempting to conserve forests as pristine untouched spaces and developmental imaginations striving to mainstream tribal people by weaning them off the forests. BR hills is a place of deep cultural meanings to Solegas and the present structure of the forest itself is a manifestation of Solega's history of forest use. Loss of these connections has adversely affected the flourishing of the community.

11.5 INTERVENTIONS THAT COULD RESTORE SOLEGA FLOURISHING

While the literature vividly portrays the detrimental impacts of social-ecological and cultural changes on the flourishing of the Solegas, there are also narratives of responses that offer ways out of the crises. For instance, more recent research shows that recolonization by *Lantana*, which has proved so destructive to agroecology in BR hills, can be prevented through cutting and burning followed by post-removal monitoring and planting of alternate species (Hiremath et al., 2018). This both enhanced growth of native species of flora (trees and grasses) and fodder availability for wildlife (Madegowda & Rao, 2014). The employment of Solegas by the FD to weed out *Lantana* from forests under the Mahatma Gandhi National Rural Employment Guarantee Scheme (MGNREGS) in 2009 and 2011 also contributed to employment security, preempting distress migration.

Historically, competing claims over the forests between the Solegas and the state (represented by the FD) have often resulted in conflicts and contestations between them. This has led to a series of legal battles fought by the Solegas against the FD, culminating in the court recognizing their rights to habitat and NTFP collection in 2011 (Rajappa, 2018). The Solegas' campaign for their rights under FRA received major impetus with the formation of the Soliga Abhivruddhi Sagha (SAS). They have taken the Solega cause further, since even after the grant of forest rights, there have been conflicts on the control of NTFP trade which had earlier been regulated by LAMPS under the FD's supervision. The Solegas had fought a case in 2015 over marketing of honey, independently of LAMPs, and won it. With new channels of marketing now available and several NTFP value addition enterprises initiated by NGOs, LAMPs has also started offering higher prices to Solega collectors for NTFPs (Pallavi, 2015).

Interventions of FD and NGOs that adequately incorporate traditional perceptions and knowledge of Solegas have paved the way for win-win solutions for livelihood of the tribe and for biodiversity. For example, a participatory mapping exercise organized by ATREE with the community to mark sacred sites in BR hills was viewed by Solegas not only as a cultural and ecological process, but as a political one too. It asserted their association with the forests and provided spatial evidence of their historic presence, often ignored by state-driven forest governance and management processes (Mandal et al., 2010).

Based on a better understanding of the traditional harvesting practices of Solegas, participatory resource-monitoring activities for harvesting of *amla* (*Phyllanthus* spp.) were initiated following the establishment of Solega-run enterprises for the processing and value addition of NTFPs. Participatory monitoring protocols were evolved over a ten-year period from 1995 to 2005, including mapping and assessments of fruit production, harvest and regeneration combined with pre- and post-harvesting meetings for sharing information, and adaptive management (Setty et al., 2008). Visual estimates of fruit production made by harvesters at the forest level were found to be very similar to estimates obtained using standard scientific monitoring protocols, the reasons for the high congruence being the long-term and collective participation of experienced harvesters in the entire monitoring and evaluation program (Setty et al., 2008). Investigations on the independent and combined effects of NTFP harvest and two invasive species (*Lantana* and a mistletoe, *Taxillus tomentosus*) on *amla* populations illustrated that mistletoe and *Lantana*, not fruit harvest, were the main drivers of *amla* decline (Ticktin et al., 2012). Recent research and practice overwhelmingly suggest that traditional and participatory NTFP collection practices with appropriate monitoring and information sharing could preclude damage to forest ecosystems while ensuring livelihood benefits.

With their inimitable traditional knowledge, Solegas are eager to play a key role in managing the landscape and protecting the biodiversity. To assert their claims over forests, Solegas drafted and ratified area-specific community conservation plans with detailed proposals on weed control, fire, NTFP harvest and the prevention of poaching, timber smuggling, quarrying and so forth. These are proposed to be adopted through a collaborative institutional and governance model between the Solegas, the state and conservation groups (Rai & Madegowda, 2018; Rajappa, 2018). However, financial and state support for the plans is still awaited. The doubling of the tiger population in BR hills from 35 to 68 in 2011–2018 (Rajappa, 2018), a period coinciding with grant of forest rights, is ample proof that Solegas can coexist with and even conserve wildlife, debunking the popular conservation arguments that tigers should be protected in inviolate spaces devoid of tribal presence. The tiger, for Solegas, is the god *Huli Veerappa* who is praised in their songs and worshipped during festivals. The presence of Solegas in forest deters poachers and FD has employed some of them as tiger watchers (Benanav, 2017).

Farming in forest ecotones of BR hills is another wicked problem for which systemic adaptive solutions need to be devised. Bawa et al. (2007) analyzed the ways in which land use sustainability in forest–agriculture ecotones, such as Solega farmlands in BR hills, can be achieved. They identified three ways in which ecosystem services including provision of NTFPs, water, soils, pollinators and pest control from surrounding forests can be sustained: (1) reducing harvest of ecosystem products through diversification of livelihoods; (2) improvising and adapting traditional agricultural practices to incorporate local diversity; and

(3) providing economic incentives for maintenance of ecosystem services. Payment for Ecosystem Services (PES) mechanisms to incentivize biodiversity-friendly coffee, such as the initiative of Black Baza Coffee Company that guarantees a buy-back of produce at a 15% market premium for maintaining a certain abundance and diversity of indigenous trees and restricting chemical use on coffee farms, has benefitted 180 small growers in BR hills and Kodagu (Bose, 2017). Rich customs and rituals linked to crops and cultivation practices clearly signify the importance of cultivation of food crops for Solega subsistence and healthy life.

Other interventions in farm practices are aimed at strengthening on-farm cap-acities, improving sustainable traditional technologies for composting and seed conservation, conserving biodiversity, reducing soil losses and introducing value addition techniques. Preserving indigenous food crop diversity helps in commu-nity resilience (Mundoli et al., 2016) as well as landscape sustainability (Bawa et al., 2007). Shanker et al. (2005) and Setty and Mandal (2007) recommended strengthening traditional Solega institutions such as *kulas* with a pre-defined role in conservation to address the challenges of the biodiversity crisis. Interventions from NGOs like ATREE along with Solega farmers to increase agricultural prod-uctivity by enhancing on-farm diversity and conserving soil and water are note-worthy (Setty & Mandal, 2007). Such agricultural interventions are envisaged to be helping farmers to achieve greater on-farm contributions towards subsistence and cash needs, thereby reducing NTFP dependence.

In terms of ensuring food security, the PDS has played an important role by providing both basic and supplementary nutrition. The SAS directly discusses and negotiates the composition of this nutritional support with the district authorities. However, the more important issue is the lack of salience of health and nutrition in the lived reality of the Solegas. Recent research efforts such as the Towards Health Equity and Transformative Action (THETA) project have examined this issue and highlighted the social determinants of health and their role in determining the Solegas' health outcomes. They found that geographical remoteness, proximity to forest areas, cultural distance from the 'mainstream' population, historical iso-lation and social stratification are all important determinants that likely influence their perception of health and wellbeing overall (Prashanth et al., 2020). The par-ticipatory research, bringing together community members to discuss health issues, has helped to bring these concerns to the forefront and for the Solega community to recognize that this is an important aspect of their life.

11.6   SUGGESTIONS FOR FUTURE EXPLORATION

The review of literature also reveals certain critical knowledge gaps in understanding the links of agroecology of the Solegas with their food system and their role in flourishing. For example, quantitative assessments of the wild food component in the diet and the consequences of the decline in forest diversity on nutritional and health outcomes are scarce in the literature. In fact, quantifi-cation of agrobiodiversity is thin in the literature. Also, compared to forest–food interlinkages, the other two interfaces, i.e. forest–farm and farm–food, are relatively less explored. In particular, the process of transition to modern farming is a gap that is not addressed in the existing research from BR hills, though the later shift to coffee farming is well reported. Further, the flow of ecosystem benefits such as pollination and hydrological services from forests and their importance in supporting Solega farming and diets is an area requiring attention.

Regarding food availability, the relationship between food security-related policies and schemes (PDS, Food Security Act, etc.) on Solega food systems and relative importance of forest, farm and market sources in fulfilling food and nutritional requirements are poorly understood. A surprising finding of the review is the lack of evidence on community-initiated interventions for revival of traditional food systems among Solegas, in stark contrast to their active political assertion of claims over forest resources.

11.7 CONCLUSION

The experience of the Solegas demonstrates the interdependencies that are shaping traditional food systems everywhere. If the community is to flourish, in terms of their physical and mental health and sense of personal, social and economic wellbeing, then using a multi-pronged approach to address such interdependencies is essential. In the context of the BR hills, such an approach would need to closely link the forest and the farm to the food finally available to the Solega. The transformation of their relationship with the forest, due to policies and actions far beyond their control, has impacted the Solega diet fundamentally. For those who have been more seriously dislocated from the forest, this impact is more profound, in terms of the ways in which they access and consume food, and the ways in which they relate to the state and to markets (Mundoli et al., 2016).

The overall concern for food security has ensured some measure of food rights for the marginalized forest-dwelling community (Mundoli et al., 2016). Yet the discourse around food security largely leaves the challenges of malnutrition unaddressed. The main difference between food security schemes and traditional food systems is that of the balance, nutritional richness and variety of diet. Changes in forest governance, restrictions on access to forest, aspiration, migration and exposure to modern cultures have contributed significantly to changing food systems. This has jeopardized the nutritional security of the Solegas, who would earlier roam freely in the forest, collecting fruit, roots, green leaves and berries, as well as hunting wild boar and small game, that were central to their dietary diversity and nutritional adequacy.

The on-going quest of the Solegas for greater autonomy and ownership of their ancestral home – the forest – could perhaps be seen also as a quest for food sovereignty: for being able to gather and grow their own food rather than being dependent on government programs that are meant to compensate for their loss of access and control over their traditional food sources. We have argued in this chapter that the flourishing of the Solega community is intimately linked to the ways in which they produce, access and consume food; and the extent to which their connection to traditional food systems is supported. If the structural causes underlying this loss are not addressed urgently, the impacts may become permanent and irreversible.

NOTES

1   This tribe is variously referred to as "Solaga", "Sholagar", "Sholaga", "Sholiga" and "Soliga/ Soligaru". While the last term is the most used variant in popular and scientific literature, we use "Solega" following the observation of Si (2015) that the people emphasize their tribe's name as Solega and recognize Soliga as nomenclature used by outsiders.
2   https://harzing.com/resources/publish-or-perish.
3   www.zotero.org/.

REFERENCES

Bawa, K.S., Joseph, G., & Setty, S. (2007). Poverty, biodiversity and institutions in forest-agriculture ecotones in the Western Ghats and Eastern Himalaya ranges of India. *Agriculture, Ecosystems and Environment, 121*, 287–295.

Benanav, M. (2017). The tiger watchers. *Sierra, 102(4)*, 36–41.

Bhat, H.K. (1997). Socio-economic changes in a tribal settlement (1965–1990): a case study of Soliga of Karnataka. In Pfeffer, G., Behera, D.K. (eds.), *Contemporary Society: Tribal Society, Vol. II. Development Issues Transition and Change* (pp. 116–122). New Delhi: Concept.

Bose, A. (2006). Empowering Soliga tribes: 'Sudarshan model' of Karnataka. *Economic and Political Weekly, 84(7)*, 564–566.

Bose, A. (2017). Can a coffee company save forests? Seminar. Accessed on 5 May 2020 at www.india-seminar.com/2017/690/690_arshiya_bose.htm.

Buchanan, F. (1807). *A Journey from Madras Through the Countries of Mysore, Canara, and Malabar*, Vol II. London: The Honorable Directors of the East India Company, pp. 177–178.

Chatterjee, R. (2008). Dissociating people from nature. *Environmental Science & Technology, 42(20)*, 7552–7554.

Clark, H., Coll-Seck, A.M., Banerjee, A., Peterson, S., Dalglish, S.L., Ameratunga, S., Balabanova, D., Bhan, M.K., Bhutta, Z.A., Borrazzo, J., Claeson, M., Doherty, T., El-Jardali, F., George, A.S., Gichaga, A., Gram, L., Hipgrave, D.B., Kwamie, A., Meng, Q., ... Costello, A. (2020). A future for the world's children? A WHO–UNICEF–Lancet commission. *The Lancet, 395(10224)*, 605–658.

FAO, IFAD and WFP. (2014). The State of Food Insecurity in the World 2014. Strengthening the Enabling Environment for Food Security and Nutrition. Rome: FAO.

Ganesan, R., & Setty, R.S. (2004). Regeneration of Amla, an important non-timber forest product from Southern India. *Comment, Conservation and Society, 2(2)*, 365–375.

Ganeshaiah, K.N., Uma Shaanker, R., Murali, K.S., Shankar, U., & Bawa K.S. (1998). Extraction of non-timber forest products in the forests of Biligiri Rangan Hills, India. 5. Influence of dispersal mode on species response to anthropogenic pressures. *Economic Botany, 52(3)*, 316–319.

Ghosh, B., Barbhuiya, A.R., & Chowdhury, C. (2007). Changes in health status of the Soliga tribe at BRT due to modern interventions. *Current Science, 92(12)*, 1688–1689.

Harzing, A.W. (2010). *The Publish or Perish Book: Your Guide to Effective and Responsible Citation Analysis*. Australia: Tarma Software Research.

Hegde, R., Suryaprakash, S., Achoth, L., & Bawa, K.S. (1996). Extraction of non-timber forest products in the forests of Biligiri Rangan Hills, India. 1. Contribution to rural income. *Economic Botany, 50*, 243–251.

Hiremath, A.J., & Sundaram, B. (2005). The fire–Lantana cycle hypothesis in Indian forests. *Conservation and Society, 3(1)*, 26–42.

Hiremath, A.J., Prasad, A., & Sundaram, B. (2018). Restoring *Lantana camara* invaded tropical deciduous forest: the response of native plant regeneration to two common *Lantana* removal practices. *Indian Forester, 144*, 545–552.

Jadegowda, M., & Ramesh, M.N. (2008). Empowerment of Soliga tribes. *Leisa India*. http:// admin.indiaenvironmentportal.org.in/files/Empowerment%20of%20Soliga%20 tribes.pdf.

Kaggere, N. (2020). Soliga tribals brew a perfect success story. *Deccan Herald*, 29 June 2020.

Krishna Raj, V., Reddy, P.R., & Surendra, H.S. (2017). Assessment of nutrient consumption pattern among Soliga tribal adults in Chamaraja Nagar district of Karnataka state. *Trends in Biosciences, 10(30)*, 6325–6328.

Kuhnlein, H.V., & Receveur, O. (1996). Dietary change and traditional food systems of indigenous peoples. *Annual Review of Nutrition, 16*, 417–442.

Kuhnlein, H., Erasmus, B., Spigelski, D., & Burlingame, B. (2009). *Indigenous Peoples' Food Systems: The Many Dimensions of Culture, Diversity and Environment for Nutrition and Health*. Rome: Food and Agriculture Organization, p. 339.

Madegowda, C. (2009). Traditional knowledge and conservation. *Economic and Political Weekly, 44(21)*, 65–69.

Madegowda, C., & Rao, C. (2013). The sickle cell anemia health problems: traditional and modern treatment practices among the Soliga tribes at BR Hills, South India. *Antrocom Online Journal of Anthropology, 9(1)*, 105–114.

Madegowda, C. & Rao, C.U. (2014). The traditional ecological knowledge of Soliga tribe on eradication of *Lantana camara* and their livelihood through Mahatma Gandhi National Rural Employment Guarantee Act at Biligiri Rangaswamy Temple Wildlife Sanctuary, South India. *Antrocom: Online Journal of Anthropology, 10(2)*, 163–173.

Madegowda, C., & Rao, C.U. (2015). The health problems and health scenario of Soliga tribals at Biligiri Rangaswamy Temple Wildlife Sanctuary, Karnataka, South India. *International Journal of Research in Social Sciences, 5(3)*, 443–458.

Madegowda, C., & Rao, C.U. (2017). Impact of forest policies and the economy of the Soliga tribal's in Biligiri Rangaswamy Temple Wildlife Sanctuary, South India. *Journal of Historical Archeology & Anthropological Sciences, 1(4)*, 112–123.

Mallegowda, P., Ganesan, R., Krishnan, J., & Niphadkar, M. (2015). Assessing habitat quality of forest-corridors through NDVI analysis in dry tropical forests of South India: implications for conservation. *Remote Sensing, 7(2)*, 1619–1639.

Mandal, S., Rai, N.D., & Madegowda, C. (2010). Culture conservation and co-management: strengthening Soliga stake in biodiversity conservation in Biligiri Rangaswamy temple wildlife sanctuary, India. In Verschuuren, B., Wild, R., McNeely, J., Oviedo, G. (eds.), *Sacred Natural Sites: Conservation of Nature and Culture*. London: Earthscan.

Misra, T.K. (2006). Forest policy and deprivation of forest dwellers in independent India: the story of the Baidharas and other forest dependent communities. *Social Scientist, 34(7/8)*, 20–32.

Morab, S.G. (1977). The Soliga of Biligiri Rangana Hills. Memoir No. 45. Calcutta: Anthropological Survey of India, pp. 24–67.

Mundoli, S., Joseph, G., & Setty, S. (2016). "Shifting agriculture": the changing dynamics of Adivasi farming in the forest-fringes of a tiger reserve in south India. *Agroecology and Sustainable Food Systems, 40(8)*, 759–782.

Murali, K.S., Shankar, U., Uma Shaanker, R., Ganeshaiah, K.N., & Bawa, K.S. (1996). Extraction of non-timber forest products in the forests of Biligiri Rangan Hills, India. 2. Impact of NTFP extraction on regeneration, population structure, and species composition. *Economic Botany, 50(3)*, 252–269.

Narendran, M., Kumar, D.S., Kulkarni, P., Renuka, M., & Narayana Murthy, M.R. (2019). Treat the Troika: does depression and malnutrition affect activities of daily living? A study among elderly Soliga tribes, BR Hills, Karnataka. *Indian Journal of Public Health Research and Development, 10(5)*, 53–58.

Nautiyal, S., Sravani, M., Herald, K., & Rajasekaran, C. (2016). Plant diversity and associated traditional ecological knowledge of Soliga tribal community of Biligiriranga Swamy Temple Tiger Reserve (BRTTR): a biogeographic bridge of Western and Eastern Ghat, India. *Medicinal Plants – International Journal of Phytomedicines and Related Industries, 8(1)*, 1–17.

Naveena, N.L., Subramanya, S., & Setty, S. (2015). Diversity and distribution of stored grain insects among the Soliga tribal settlements of Biligirirangana Hills, Karnataka, India. *Journal of Stored Products Research, 62*, 84–92.

Naveena, N.L., Subramanya, S., Setty, S., & Palanimuthu, V. (2017). Grain storage losses in the traditional tribal settlements of Biligirirangana Hills, Karnataka, India. *Journal of Asia-Pacific Entomology, 20(2)*, 678–685.

Pallavi, A. (2015). Court upholds Soliga tribe's community forest rights. Down To Earth, July 4, 2015.

Patel, R. (2009). Food sovereignty. *The Journal of Peasant Studies, 36(3)*, 663–706.

Pimbert, M. (2019). Food sovereignty. In P. Ferranti, E. Berry, A. Jock (eds.), *Encyclopaedia of Food Security and Sustainability,* vol. *1(3)*. Elsevier: pp. 181–189.

Prabhakar, S.C.J., & Gangadhar, M.R. (2016). Hemoglobin level and prevalence of anemia in Soliga tribal children of Karnataka, India. *South East Asia Journal of Public Health, 6(2)*, 37–41.

Prashanth, N.S., Raman, V., Basappa, Y.C., & Nityasri, S.N. (2020). *Health Inequalities of Tribal Communities in India in Three Regions in Northeast, Central and South India.* Mid-term Progress & THETA Project Workshop Report. Bangalore: Institute of Public Health.

Rai, N.D., & Madegowda, C. (2018). The Social and Ecological Impacts of Conservation Policy: The Case of Biligiri Rangaswamy Temple Tiger Reserve, India. www.corneredbypas.com/india.

Rai, N.D., Benjaminsen, T.A., Krishnan, S., & Madegowda, C. (2019). Political ecology of tiger conservation in India: adverse effects of banning customary practices in a protected area. *Singapore Journal of Tropical Geography, 40(1)*, 1–17.

Rajappa, A. (2018). Soligas in tiger reserve win battle over forest rights. Village Square, Oct 1.

Ramesh, B.R. (1989). Evergreen Forests Biligiri Ranagan Hills (Ecology, Structure and Floristic Composition). Ph.D. thesis. University of Madras.

Ranganath, A.D. (2002). Identification of Indigenous Farm Practices Followed by Soliga Tribals. PhD thesis. Department of Extension, University of Agricultural

Sciences, Bangalore. Accessed on 27 May 2020: https://krishikosh.egranth.ac.in/displaybitstream?handle=1/5810016817.

Rathod, P., Swamy, K.R., & Charankumar, M.E. (2011). Studies on agro-biodiversity of Soliga tribes in BRT wildlife sanctuary. *International Journal of Forestry and Crop Management, 2(2)*, 158–162.

Roy, S., Hegde, H., Bhattacharya, D., Upadhya, V., & Kholkute, S. (2015). Tribes in Karnataka: status of health research. *The Indian Journal of Medical Research, 141*, 673–687.

Seshadri, T., Madegowda, C., Babu, G.R., & Prashanth, N.S. (2019). Implementation research with the Soliga indigenous community in southern India for local action on improving maternal health services. SSRN. Accessed on 5 May 2020 at: https://papers.ssrn.com/sol3/papers.cfm?abstract_id=3483650.

Setty, S., & Mandal, S. (2007). Tribal development and conservation in a wildlife sanctuary. In Swaminathan, M. (ed.), *Six Case Studies on Gender and Social Inclusion for Sustainable Livelihoods*. Chennai: M S Swaminathan Research Foundation and Food and Agriculture Organisation, Regional Office for Asia and the Pacific, pp. 7–17.

Setty, R.S., Bawa, K., Ticktin, T., & Gowda, C.M. (2008). Evaluation of a participatory resource monitoring system for nontimber forest products: the case of Amla (*Phyllanthus* spp.) fruit harvest by Soligas in South India. *Ecology & Society, 13(2)*, 1–16.

Shankar, U., Murali, K.S., Uma Shaanker, R., Ganeshaiah, K.N., & Bawa, K.S. (1996). Extraction of non-timber forest products in the forests of Biligiri Rangan Hills, India. 3. Productivity, extraction and prospects of sustainable harvest of Amla *Phyllanthus emblica* (Euphorbiaceae). *Economic Botany, 50(3)*, 270–279.

Shankar, U., Hegde, R., & Bawa, K.S. (1998). Extraction of non-timber forest products in the forests of Biligiri Rangan Hills, India. 6. Fuelwood pressure and management options. *Economic Botany, 52(3)*, 320–336.

Shanker, K., Hiremath, A., & Bawa, K. (2005). Linking biodiversity conservation and livelihoods in India. *PLoS Biology*, 3(11), e394.

Si, A. (2015). *The Traditional Ecological Knowledge of the Solega: A Linguistic Perspective*. Switzerland: Springer International Publishing.

Somagond, A.S., Patel, B.H.M., Singh, M., Basagoundanavar, S.H., Umapathi, V., Antil, M., Yadav, S., & Sanyal, A. (2019). Comparative study on the socio-economic profile of Soligas in core and buffer zone of Biligiri Rangana Hills (B.R. Hills) of Karnataka. *International Journal of Livestock Research, 9(1)*, 206–215.

Sonowal, C.J. (2010). Factors affecting the nutritional health of tribal children in Maharashtra. *Studies on Ethno-Medicine, 4*, 21–36.

Sundaram, B., & Hiremath A.J. (2012). *Lantana camara* invasion in a heterogeneous landscape: patterns of spread and correlation with changes in native vegetation. *Biological Invasion, 14(6)*, 1127–1141.

Sundaram, B., Krishnan, S., Hiremath, A., & Joseph, G. (2012). Ecology and impacts of the invasive species, *Lantana camara*, in a social-ecological system in South India: perspectives from local knowledge. *Human Ecology: An Interdisciplinary Journal, 40(6)*, 931–942.

Sundaram, B., Hiremath, A., & Krishnaswamy, J. (2015). Factors influencing the local scale colonisation and change in density of a widespread invasive plant species, *Lantana camara*, in South India. *NeoBiota, 25*, 27–46.

Ticktin, T., Ganesan, R., Paramesha, M., & Setty, S. (2012). Disentangling the effects of multiple anthropogenic drivers on the decline of two tropical dry forest trees. *Journal of Applied Ecology, 49(4)*, 774–784.

Uma Shaanker, R., Ganeshaiah, K.N., Nageswara Rao, M., & Arvind, N.A. (2004). Ecological consequences of forest use: from genes to ecosystem – a case study in the Biligiri Rangaswamy Temple Wildlife Sanctuary, South India. *Conservation and Society, 2(2)*, 345–363.

VanderWheele, T.J. (2017). On the promotion of human flourishing. *PNAS, 114(31)*, 8148–8156.

Yankanchi, G.M., & Channesh, T.S. (2017). Food habits and nutritional status in forest-based tribes: a case of Soligas of Chamarajanagar district in Karnataka. *International Journal of Humanities and Social Science Research, 3*(11), 40–43.

Zaraska, N.A. (1997). Health Behaviours of the Soliga Tribe Women (India). MSc thesis, Queen's University, Canada.

12 Evaluation of Arsenic Entry Routes into Rice Grain during Harvesting, Post-Harvesting of Paddy and Cooked Rice Preparation

Nilanjana Roy Chowdhury,
Madhurima Joardar, Antara Das and
Tarit Roychowdhury*

CONTENTS

* Corresponding author: Tarit Roychowdhury. rctarit@yahoo.com; tarit.roychowdhury@
jadavpuruniversity.in

DOI: 10.1201/9781003095422-12

12.1   INTRODUCTION

The geogenic arsenic pollutes the groundwater of over 107 countries across the world and has become a triggering issue (Polya and Charlet, 2009). Among these, south and south-east Asian countries like India and most parts of Bangladesh are more susceptible (Chakraborti et al., 2009; Roychowdhury, 2010). Studies have reported that groundwater of this region contains arsenic at levels much higher than the permissible limit laid down by the World Health Organization (WHO), i.e. 10 µg/l poses substantial risks to approximately 150 million people living worldwide (Brammer and Ravenscroft, 2009; Mondal et al., 2010). The Ganga–Meghna–Brahmaputra (GMB) river basin is remarkably an arsenic-affected province because of the occurrence of high concentrations of this lethal metalloid up to the upper 50 meters of aquifers when considering the depth (Singh, 2006). It is a common phenomenon that arsenic-tainted groundwater is significantly used for drinking and it is the principal route of entry in humans but when irrigational procedures harness the same water for their use, the problem is compounded (Brammer, 2009; Roychowdhury, 2008).

In eastern and southern India, rice forms a staple diet for people and a huge number of inhabitants live on a regular rice diet (Rahman et al., 2007). West Bengal as a state is one of the chief rice-producing areas in India, comprising a 5,900,000 ha area for exclusive rice cultivation (Signes et al., 2008). When such grains are consumed regularly in considerable quantities, the arsenic slowly creeps into the food chain. Arsenic accumulation in rice grain and its ongoing build-up in cooked rice leads to an increased risk factor for the Bengal delta where rice and its byproducts are the staple diet (Roychowdhury, 2008; Samal et al., 2011). Cumulatively, 88,750 km^2 in West Bengal form an arsenic-infested zone in which 38,861 km^2 separately scores as a highly affected zone, including major districts, viz. both North and South 24 Parganas, Nadia, Murshidabad and Maldah (Santra et al., 2013), where cultivation of rice is a regular practice.

However, prolonged use of arsenic-tainted water for cultivation procedures has eventually caused a resultant increased deposition of arsenic in irrigated areas (Meharg and Rahman, 2003; Roychowdhury et al., 2002, 2005). India and Bangladesh have a temperate pattern of rainfall and therefore paddy cultivation here is carried out in two seasons, i.e. Boro (pre-monsoon farming, chiefly done using groundwater) and Aman (monsoonal farming, which sometimes involves groundwater due to insufficient rain). Since 1970 pre-monsoonal Boro cultivation using irrigational supplementation of groundwater has found ways in parts of the Bengal delta (Harvey et al., 2005). Rice produced here is marketed in two forms: raw or sunned rice prepared by de-husking the paddy or parboiled rice that is prepared by light boiling of paddy and then mechanically de-husking the grains to collect the boiled rice grain. Processing parboiled rice with the use of arsenic-tainted water as a part of post-harvesting practice is a common action expected to increase the arsenic content of the rice grain. An earlier analysis amalgamating the comparison of drinking water, raw rice and cooked rice as general routes of arsenic entry elucidated a positive impact of arsenic gaining entry via cooked rice (Mondal et al., 2010). However, the interplay of arsenic between the food grain and water while cooking them together is barely known. Ongoing speculation fails to resolve whether the water used for cooking the rice has any role at all, either additive or synergistic, in building up the final arsenic content reflected in the final cooked rice.

This chapter will present and discuss arsenic accumulation and distribution throughout the paddy plant during the irrigation procedures of Boro and Aman cultivation. It also quantifies the detailed arsenic distribution in each plant part (paddy plant) with reference to their varying age. Concurrently, this chapter documents the role of post-harvesting measures involving arsenic-laden water, resulting in an increased arsenic load in parboiled rice. Besides, the passage of arsenic from rice grain to water and the other way round while cooking is yet to be studied in detail. As a complete study to answer all such queries, we focused on arsenic distribution patterns in various rice fractions isolated while cooking (viz. uncooked rice, water used for cooking, cooked rice and gruel/total discarded water) sunned and parboiled rice grain. Our endeavor helps to elucidate, classify and quantify the varying amounts of arsenic creeping into the food chain of the population in rural West Bengal.

12.2 MATERIALS AND METHODOLOGY

12.2.1 STUDY AREA

The work is mainly carried out in Deganga block, which is a community development area. Deganga block is an administrative domain of Barasat Sadar subdivision in North 24 Parganas district in West Bengal, India and is a part of the Gangetic delta, lying east of the River Hooghly. The aforementioned area is already known to be arsenic-contaminated (Chakraborti et al., 2001; Mandal et al., 1996).

12.2.2   Sample Collection, Preparation and Preservation

This work of paddy harvesting depicts the arsenic build-up, deposition and distribution in paddy plants, which are grown during pre-monsoonal and monsoon season. Our work encompasses analysis of paddy grown during Boro and Aman cultivation so that we could relate and document the consequences of irrigation with arsenic-containing groundwater and/or rainwater. Arsenic concentration in agricultural land soil reported from Deganga was in the range of 17,400–30,900 µg/kg (Ghosh et al., 2004; Stroud et al., 2011). The pre-monsoonal and monsoonal study samples were procured in the span of February–April and July–September of the year 2018, respectively. Subsequently, post-harvesting treatment is required to prepare the parboiled rice from raw paddy grain, which was harvested through Boro and Aman cultivation. Consequently, cooking with arsenic-free or contaminated water at 1:3 is a regular practice in rural Bengal. The excess water acts as gruel and became visible after cooking.

Groundwater samples from fields and domestic level were collected in sterile polyethylene containers and preserved with the addition of 0.1% (v/v) concentrated nitric acid, placed in a cool ice box during transportation and finally stored in a refrigerator prior to analysis. All the plant (paddy) and soil samples were collected from the field directly and processed in the laboratory, as mentioned in our earlier publications (Chowdhury et al., 2018a, 2020b). Wholegrain samples from all the stages of post-harvesting process were collected from different farmers and kept in sterile zip-lock packets. Detailed information on sample processing has been mentioned by Chowdhury et al. (2018b). All the sunned and parboiled rice grain samples for the cooking study were collected, preserved and processed as mentioned by Chowdhury et al. (2020a).

12.2.3   Chemicals and Reagents

All chemicals and reagents were of analytical grade. Double-distilled water was used for experimental and analytical purposes. Detailed information of the chemicals and reagents used for total digestion and arsenic analysis has been given previously (Chowdhury et al., 2020a, 2020b).

12.2.4   Digestion Protocol

No digestion protocol was maintained before estimation of arsenic in water samples. Solid samples such as soil, root, stem, leaf, pedicel, wholegrain and rice grain were processed using Teflon bomb digestion. The digestion was performed by a mixture of concentrated nitric acid and hydrogen peroxide (30%) at 2:1 ratio. Detailed information has been given in our other publications (Chowdhury et al., 2018a, 2018b, 2020a, 2020b).

12.2.5   Analysis

For all the digested (solid) and non-digested (water) samples, total arsenic was quantified using the hydride generation-atomic absorption spectrophotometric

(HG-AAS) method, as mentioned in our previous publications (Chowdhury et al., 2020a, 2020b; Samanta et al., 1999).

12.2.6 Data Analysis

To understand the interrelation and dependence among intake and output, regression analysis and correlation matrix were performed with the help of Microsoft Office Excel 2007. Risk thermometer is another rating scale which depicts a large picture of scaling according to risk (Chowdhury et al., 2020a).

12.2.7 Quality Control and Quality Assurance

Quality control study has been performed by standard reference material (SRM) analysis, duplicate analysis and spiking recovery of the digested samples and endorsed all the quality assurance strategy, according to Chowdhury et al. (2018a, 2018b, 2020a, 2020b).

12.3 RESULTS AND DISCUSSION

The arsenic accumulation and distribution pattern in rice grain was investigated thoroughly in this study during harvesting, post-harvesting of paddy grain and cooked rice preparation.

12.3.1 Pre-Monsoonal (Boro) and Monsoonal (Aman) Cultivation

Paddy plants were collected in the pre-monsoonal and monsoonal season for Boro and Aman cultivation, respectively. This cultivation period is of approximately 14 weeks or 90–120 days. The cultivation practice is mainly divided into three phases, viz. vegetative or plantation phase, reproductive or inflorescence phase and ripening phase, also known as the harvesting step. The first week is considered for field preparation in both cases. The pre-monsoonal season for paddy plant is mainly February to the middle of May. Simultaneously, for the monsoonal cultivation of paddy, the season is mid-July to October (Chowdhury et al., 2018a, 2020b).

12.3.1.1 Status of Irrigation Water at the Paddy Field

Groundwater (shallow depth) samples ($n = 5$) from 2016, which were used for cultivation of five agricultural fields of Deganga during the pre-monsoonal season, were analyzed for their arsenic estimation. The concentration ranged from 75.5 to 295.5 µg/l with a mean value of 178.5 ± 105 µg/l, which is above the WHO-recommended value in drinking water. The watering volume and conditions are highly dependent on seasons and rate of watering is decided upon by the average volume that the soil absorbs during summer. Water withdrawal rate from the shallow tube wells is about 20 m^3/h and amounts to approximately 20,000 l (Rahman et al., 2003). These tube wells provide water to the fields for 7 h/week, amassing about 1,40,000 l of water. However, this higher concentration of arsenic in five samples of collected groundwater shows a higher risk of exposure. Use of this highly tainted groundwater during irrigation leads to increased arsenic dissemination through the food chain.

Monsoon season mainly requires a sufficient amount of rainwater for Aman cultivation, but the scarcity of rainwater demands an ample amount of groundwater to continue the cultivation practice. The mean arsenic concentration in groundwater from shallow tube wells ($n = 5$) supplying water to the different contaminated fields of Deganga during 2016 was 13 ± 7 µg/l, with a range of 8–26 µg/l. Lesser amounts of arsenic have been observed in samples collected from water-logged conditions; this can be attributed to the co-precipitation of arsenic with iron and dilution by rainwater during monsoons. Alongside the groundwater used for irrigation, rainwater too has an important role during monsoonal cultivation towards lessening the basal soil arsenic concentration (Shrivastava et al., 2017).

12.3.1.2 Soil Arsenic Cohesion During the Cultivation of Paddy

The soil samples were collected from the fields of Deganga in the year of 2016 during pre-monsoonal season ($n = 5$) and monsoonal seasons ($n = 5$) respectively. Soil arsenic leads to an addition of the arsenic burden of paddy. The soil samples showed their individual entity at various phases of cultivation, i.e. vegetative, reproductive and ripening.

During the pre-monsoonal season, the arsenic concentration of root soil and surface soil of five paddy fields ($n = 5$) in vegetative phase showed a higher rate of arsenic accumulation in comparison to the other phases. After the end of the vegetative phase, a sharp decline in arsenic concentration was noted. After the reproductive phase, the concentration again increased with a steady build-up at the ripening phase. In root soil, the range of arsenic concentration was 29,362–54,645 µg/kg with a mean value of $38,108 \pm 9624$ µg/kg in the vegetative phase. Interestingly, a decreasing trend of 41% of arsenic was observed in the reproductive phase with a mean value of $22,451 \pm 6874$ µg/kg. Consequently, soil arsenic exhibited an average increase of approximately 3% in the ripening phase, amounting to $23,179 \pm 6321$ µg/kg (Figure 12.1a). Simultaneously in surface soil, the mean value of $37,410 \pm 7121$ µg/kg arsenic was observed during the vegetative phase. Mean arsenic concentration showed a sharp decrease (~36%) in the reproductive phase, i.e. $23,939 \pm 7016$ µg/kg. Also, an increase in arsenic concentration (4%) was observed in the ripening phase with mean concentration of $24,909 \pm 7579$ µg/kg (Figure 12.1b). The water-logged paddy fields in most of the cultivation period during pre-monsoon cultivation create an anaerobic condition which favors the conversion of pentavalent arsenic to its trivalent state.

The study revealed that, during the monsoon season, the root soil from the paddy fields ($n = 5$) contributed an average concentration of $14,687 \pm 7002$ µg/kg of arsenic in the vegetative phase, but with time, the concentration was increased by 74% with an average value of $25,544 \pm 18,872$ µg/kg in the reproductive phase. At the end of this phase, rainwater (flooding) is introduced into cultivation. As a result, the concentration decreases by 57%, with an average value of $16,267 \pm$

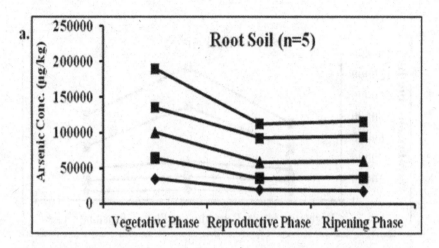

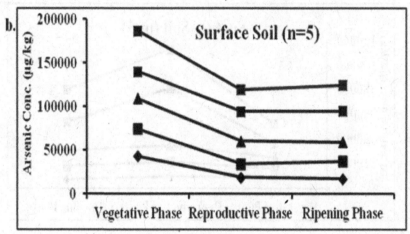

FIGURE 12.1 Arsenic accumulation and distribution pattern in soil. (a) Pre-monsoonal root soil; (b) pre-monsoonal surface soil; (c) monsoonal root soil; (d) monsoonal surface soil.

9284 µg/kg in the ripening phase (Figure 12.1c). Surface soil showed a substantial amount of arsenic in the vegetative phase at an average of 10,444 ± 3322 µg/kg. The mean arsenic concentration of 22,485 ± 15,720 µg/kg was abruptly increased in the reproductive phase and again fell in the ripening phase, with a mean value of 15,938 ± 8174 µg/kg (Figure 12.1d).

The initial vegetative-phase arsenic concentration is chiefly derived from irrigation water that further combines with soil arsenic (Ullah, 1998). This cumulative arsenic build-up is reflected in the final level for each field. So, soil arsenic and water arsenic both might cause a direct synergistic effect on arsenic accumulation

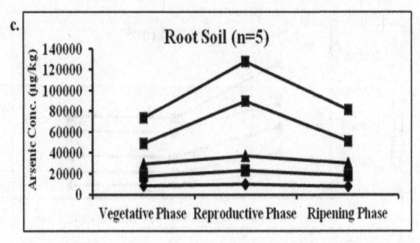

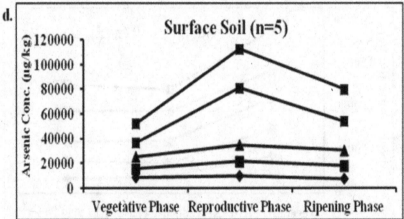

FIGURE 12.1 Continued

in paddy. In the field soil, arsenic mainly manifests in its oxidized form As(V). But monsoon flooding by irrigation water alongside rainwater leads to an anaerobic condition in the water-logged paddy field, as an outcome of which the pentavalent arsenic converts to its trivalent state. Arsenite is water-soluble and hence mixes with flood water and finally is removed as the water recedes (Liu et al., 2006).

Levels during the vegetative and reproductive phase are the resultant of arsenic dissolution and increased arsenic phytoavailability during the reproductive phase is thus observed. Arsenic diffusion into flood water is caused mainly by this variability (Roberts et al., 2010). Arsenic movement into the soil is mainly dependent upon the redox condition. As already known from earlier reports, the pentavalent form is predominantly seen in aerobic conditions and the trivalent form in anaerobic conditions (Fitz and Wenzel, 2002). Both the soil arsenic statuses depicted a completely opposite pattern of distribution between the two seasons due to the presence of rainwater.

12.3.1.3 Arsenic Translocation Throughout the Paddy Plant

The ability of arsenic to traverse from roots to the tiller of rice, with concentrations decreasing by several orders of magnitude on passage through the roots to the grain, is a known fact (Abedin et al., 2002; Welna et al., 2015). In this study, the translocation pattern of arsenic follows the trend in both seasons of cultivation: root > stem (bottom) > stem (mid) > stem (top) > leaf > pedicel > grain.

During the pre-monsoonal season average arsenic concentrations in grain, pedicel, leaves, stem (average of three different parts of the stem region with height) and root during the final ripening phase of paddy plant were 1121, 2350.5, 3885, 8838, 21,2139 µg/kg, respectively. Arsenic mobility was highest in roots and showed a decreasing trend with the height of the plant. It is a general perception that the root shows the greatest arsenic accumulation. Considering all the fields ($n = 5$) from Deganga of monsoonal season paddy, the average arsenic concentration showed a decreasing trend from root to grain: 61,894 > 6603 > 2803 > 1858 > 318 µg/kg.

12.3.1.4 The Pattern of Arsenic Distribution at Different Phases of Cultivation

During the pre-monsoon season, arsenic levels in plant parts from the paddy fields ($n = 5$) revealed a similar trend of arsenic accumulation. The samples were collected during the three phases of cultivation (vegetative, reproductive and ripening) (Figure 12.2a). Average arsenic concentrations in the plant parts in the vegetative phase (after 25 days) were 5374 ± 649, 592,447 ± 10,226, and 1,163,729 ± 917,917 µg/kg in leaves, stem, and root, respectively. Arsenic was found to be highest in the vegetative phase while it showed a sharp decline in the reproductive phase (55 days), i.e. 2549 ± 703, 5084 ± 2008 and 40,518 ± 10,867 µg/kg, respectively. Afterwards, a considerable increase in arsenic was observed during the ripening phase for all five fields. Average concentrations of arsenic observed in the ripening phase were 3884 ± 1446, 8838 ± 4735, and 212,139 ± 18,893 µg/kg, respectively. When compared to the vegetative phase the reproductive phase showed 52, 99 and 96% decrease of arsenic concentration in leaf, stem and root, respectively. An average increase of 52, 74 and 423% of arsenic was observed in leaf, stem and root parts, respectively, during the ripening phase compared to the reproductive phase (Figure 12.2a).

All paddy fields ($n = 5$) during the vegetative phase considering the monsoonal season showed an average arsenic concentration of 2461 ± 726, 6804 ± 5158 and 75,736 ± 61,052 µg/kg in leaf, stem and root, respectively. During this time the paddy plants reflected the increasing trend of 88, 58 and 33%, respectively in leaf, stem and root in the reproductive phase compared to vegetative phase. The reproductive phase showed an average arsenic concentration of 4646 ± 768, 10,788 ± 4724 and 101,101 ± 63,600 µg/kg in leaf, stem and root, respectively. An abrupt

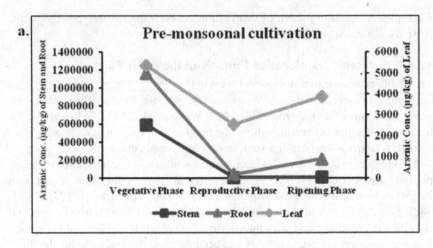

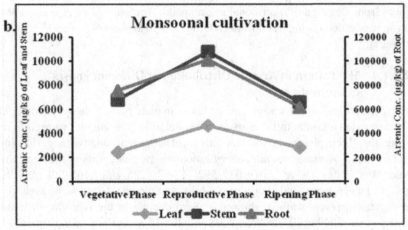

FIGURE 12.2 Pattern of arsenic distribution at different phases of cultivation. (a) Pre-monsoonal cultivation; (b) monsoonal cultivation.

decrease in arsenic concentration was observed in different paddy parts (approximately 39% in each case of leaf, stem and root) during the ripening phase compared to the reproductive phase. The ripening phase also showed an average arsenic concentration of 2803 ± 1107, 6603 ± 2335 and 61,894 ± 36,771 µg/kg in leaf, stem and root, respectively, at the time of harvesting (Figure 12.2b).

12.3.1.4.1 Vegetative Phase
During the pre-monsoonal season, surface deposition of arsenic occurred due to prolonged exposure of contaminated stagnant water. A water-logged situation creates an anaerobic condition, which encourages anaerobiosis. That facilitates the release of mobile arsenite from iron oxy hydroxide-bound arsenate. Simultaneously,

arsenic-reducing bacteria also release mobile arsenite which, as it is easily taken up by xylem tissue, mainly promotes a higher rate of translocation (Chowdhury et al., 2018a). But during the monsoonal season, dilution of arsenic creates a lower bioavailability of arsenic. Simultaneously, due to natural bio-methylation, the loss of volatile arsenic also decreases soil arsenic concentration. Both of them promote less translocation of arsenic (Chowdhury et al., 2020b).

12.3.1.4.2 Reproductive Phase

With a decrease of water-logged conditions in the pre-monsoonal season, the redox potential (E_h) increases in the field. This creates a reducing condition that leads to the formation of iron plaque. Iron plaque is an amorphous structure, which traps arsenate and inhibits its uptake. Iron plaques commonly form on roots of plants like paddy (Hansel et al., 2001), and help to control arsenic taken up by the same (Syu et al., 2013; Wu et al., 2012). Because of the strong affinity between iron oxides/hydroxides and arsenate, iron plaques are known to trap arsenic and trim down uptake by the root (Liu et al., 2004; Syu et al., 2013). Arsenic and iron concentrations in root plaques increase with maturity of the plant. Iron plaque in root soil sequesters arsenic, which lowers the translocation of arsenic in the reproductive phase. Sequential digestion studies reveal that arsenic is not directly available to the plant after its sequestration by iron plaques. However, during the monsoonal season the percolated arsenite from deeper layers became more bio-available and led to higher uptake in the reproductive phase compared to vegetative and ripening phases. No possibility of iron plaque formation was observed in root soils which sequestered arsenic (Chowdhury et al., 2020b).

12.3.1.4.3 Ripening Phase

At the time of the pre-monsoonal season, aging in iron plaque converts it into a crystalline form that decreases arsenate adsorption capacity and promotes translocation. Arsenic co-precipitates with iron in soil, increasing bioavailability in the ripening phase. But in the monsoonal season, the plant reaches saturation point and fails to accumulate arsenic. Simultaneously, the percolated arsenic stabilizes all the chemical reactions and promotes less translocation.

12.3.1.5 Comparative Study of Arsenic Accumulation and Distribution in Grain During Pre-Monsoonal and Monsoonal Cultivation

The mean arsenic concentration in rice grain cultivated from all the paddy fields ($n = 5$) during the pre-monsoon was 1121 ± 187 µg/kg. However, during monsoonal farming, the arsenic concentration observed in the grains cultivated from all the fields ($n = 5$) was 318 ± 56 µg/kg (Figure 12.3). However, the monsoonal grain arsenic concentration cultivated in an arsenic-exposed area was not below the acceptable limit (100 µg/kg), as suggested by Meharg et al. (2006). When compared to the accumulation patterns in paddy grains during pre- and post-monsoon periods, it was clear that arsenic accumulation in grain was nearly three times less during Aman (monsoonal) cultivation compared to Boro cultivation (pre-monsoon).

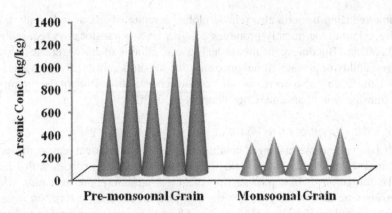

FIGURE 12.3 Distribution of arsenic in pre-monsoonal and monsoonal grain.

During pre-monsoon, the arsenic in paddy wholegrain was reported to depend on cultivar type as inferred – higher for "Minikit" and lower for the "Jaya" variety (Chowdhury et al., 2018a, 2020b). Similar findings were also documented by other studies (Bhattacharya et al., 2010; Rahman et al., 2007). But in the monsoon season, despite the variety in cultivars and cultivation area, the overall arsenic accumulation in rice grain amounted to only one-third that of pre-monsoonal cultivation.

12.3.2 POST-HARVESTING TECHNOLOGY

The sunned rice grain is prepared directly by de-husking the paddy grain. However, the paddy grain undergoes a light boiling followed by de-husking for the preparation of parboiled rice grain. Parboiling of matured wholegrains is a common post-harvesting technology carried out by farmers in rural Bengal. Parboiling is a process that involves soaking, steaming and drying of the grain with its intact hull (Goswami and Meghwal, 2015; Itoh et al., 1985).

The collected rice grains from Deganga market showed increased amounts of arsenic in parboiled rice in comparison to sunned rice grain. The mean arsenic concentrations of the collected sunned ($n = 5$) and parboiled rice grains ($n = 6$) were 75 ± 23 μg/kg (range: 52–102 μg/kg) and 169.5 ± 54 μg/kg (range: 97–259 μg/kg), respectively. Enhanced arsenic concentration in parboiled rice definitely indicates a role of the post-harvesting procedure being followed in these areas in the extraneous addition of arsenic to the rice samples after parboiling.

12.3.2.1 Arsenic Accumulation in Samples Collected During the Post-Harvesting Procedure

Groundwater samples used for parboiling of the paddy wholegrains were collected. The water samples were also collected at different stages of the post-harvesting (i.e. half and full-boiled water) and showed an overall increasing trend of arsenic concentration after each stage of parboiling (Table 12.1). The arsenic distribution in different parts of paddy/rice grain showed a substantial increase of arsenic concentration in parboiled rice compared to sunned rice grain.

12.3.2.1.1 Water Arsenic Scenario During Post-Harvesting

The mean arsenic concentration in groundwater samples collected from farmers in the studied areas used to parboil paddy grain at domestic level was 184 ± 100 µg/l (range: 61–308.5 µg/l, $n = 5$) (Table 12.1). Arsenic concentrations in water samples showed an increasing trend due to two ways of parboiling process of paddy grain. The regression analysis clearly indicates a positive correlation between arsenic concentrations in raw groundwater and half-boiled water ($r^2 = 0.967$), and full-boiled water ($r^2 = 0.929$), respectively (Figure 12.4). The half-boiled and full-boiled water showed a mean value of arsenic 204 ± 75 µg/l and 236 ± 87 µg/l, respectively. However, the water sample that had the lowest arsenic concentration (61 µg/l) showed the highest increase in arsenic concentration during boiling, mainly at half boiling stage. An increment of 96% arsenic was observed in half-boiled water with respect to raw water arsenic concentration, whereas the increased arsenic was 9% in full-boiled water with respect to the half-boiled water (Table 12.1). An increasing trend of arsenic was observed in both the boiling stages, including an average addition of 27% and 15% for half-boiled and full-boiled water, respectively.

12.3.2.1.2 Variation in Arsenic Concentration in Paddy Wholegrains During Different Stages of Post-Harvesting

Arsenic concentrations in paddy grains ($n = 5$) during different stages of post-harvesting procedures (i.e. parboiling) with arsenic-tainted groundwater showed a holistic increase in arsenic concentration of parboiled paddy grain. Initially, the paddy grains showed the arsenic concentration in the range of 229–412 µg/kg with a mean value of 297 ± 73 µg/kg. Consequently, half-boiled wholegrains ($n = 5$) showed an average increase of 33% compared to paddy wholegrains after first boiling (Figure 12.5). Samples showing high arsenic concentration in paddy grain boiled in low/moderately arsenic-tainted water did not show much increase in arsenic concentration for half-boiled rice. The overall increase of arsenic concentration in full-boiled water samples with simultaneous average increase of 3% in arsenic concentration of full-boiled grains can be explained on the basis of reduction of volume of water after the parboiling process (Figure 12.5). The final volume of water became reduced due to gelatinization and evaporation; hence the final concentration of full-boiled water increased (Mondal et al., 2010; Ohno et al., 2009).

Bae et al. (2002) reported analogous observations for cooked rice with the parallel effect of chelation of arsenic through water evaporation and rice grains at the time of cooking to cause addition of arsenic in cooked rice. This primary theory also applies for these two-way boiling procedures, where the concentration gradient among the raw water and the wholegrain being used for post-harvesting is an indispensable factor to evaluate flow of arsenic from water to grain or vice versa.

TABLE 12.1
Arsenic concentrations for samples collected throughout post-harvesting procedure of paddy (µg/kg) and water (µg/l)

| Sample no. | Water | | | Paddy | | | | Parboiled condition | |
	Raw water	Half boiled water	Full boiled water	Paddy grain (whole)	Sunned rice	Half-boiled paddy grain (whole)	Full-boiled paddy grain (whole)	Parboiled paddy grain (whole)	Parboiled rice
1	61	119.5	130	229	240	316.5	303	318	236
2	113.5	156	195.5	412.5	303	350.5	447.5	348.5	345
3	185.5	195.5	226.5	311.5	297	375.5	309	323	258
4	251	236.5	260.5	294	219.5	430	398	379.5	311.5
5	308.5	313	366.5	238	252.5	411.5	472	393	461.5
Mean	184	204	236	297	262	377	386	352	322

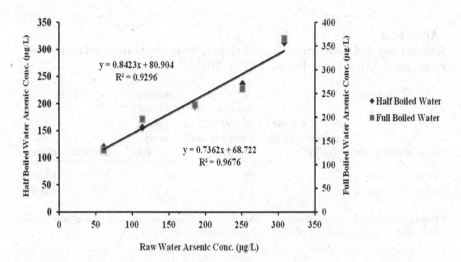

FIGURE 12.4   Regression analysis for arsenic concentration of three types of water samples (raw, half-boiled and full-boiled).

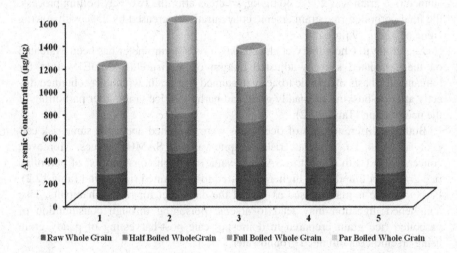

FIGURE 12.5   Stacked cylinder showing arsenic concentration of individual wholegrain samples at various stages of parboiling.

Finally, the parboiled wholegrains depicted an average increase of 24% than the raw paddy grain after the entire procedure of two-way boiling (Figure 12.5).

12.3.2.1.3   Risk Quotient of Sunned and Parboiled Rice Grain

This study focuses on one of the major steps where the arsenic concentration of rice increases dramatically. Parboiling of the paddy grain with arsenic-contaminated

TABLE 12.2
Risk of class and concern level with respect to severity-adjusted margin of exposure (SAMOE) (Sand et al., 2015a, 2015b)

Types of rice grain	Mean arsenic concentration (µg/kg)	Average rate of arsenic consumption* (µg/day)	Exposure factor ** (µg/kg body wt/day)	SAMOE	Risk class
Sunned rice grain	262	96	1.37	0.02	Class 4
Parboiled rice grain	322	118	1.69	0.01	Class 4

* Regular intake of raw rice grain (weight) = 366 g (for all age groups, median value) (Halder et al., 2013).
** For adults, assuming a weight of 70 kg (Torres-Escribano et al., 2008).

groundwater during post-harvesting procedures contributes to enrichment of arsenic concentration in parboiled rice grain. The mean arsenic concentration of sunned rice grain was 262 ± 36 µg/kg, whereas after the two-way boiling process, the final parboiled rice grain arsenic concentration increased by 25% with a mean value of 322 ± 89 µg/kg.

According to Chowdhury et al. (2020a), a risk thermometer has been evaluated on the calculated severity-adjusted margin of exposure (SAMOE) values for humans on a basis of arsenic toxicity in sunned rice grain, which was obtained directly after de-husking the paddy grain and parboiled rice grain, after parboiling of the paddy grain (Table 12.2).

Both the different types of rice grains were classified under the same risk category (class 4, i.e. moderate risk), despite variable SAMOE values. Moreover, concern level (with respect to SAMOE value) through consumption of parboiled rice grain was found to be higher compared to the sunned rice grain (Table 12.2). Parboiled rice is mainly used as part of the daily diet for rural inhabitants. This lengthened ingestion may lead to arsenic poisoning through consumption of parboiled rice grain prepared in domestic-scale post-harvesting of paddy grain using arsenic-contaminated groundwater.

12.3.3   COOKING OF RICE GRAIN

During cooked rice preparation for both sunned and parboiled rice grain with arsenic-tainted and untainted water, the flow of arsenic from rice grain to water and vice versa was elucidated in this study.

12.3.3.1   Sunned Rice Grains

Arsenic distribution in different fractions of cooked rice using sunned rice grain is shown in Table 12.3. The mean arsenic concentration of the sunned rice grains

TABLE 12.3
Arsenic status in uncooked and cooked rice grains of sunned variety

No. of rice grains	Arsenic concentration of uncooked rice grains (µg/kg)	Arsenic concentration of cooking water (µg/l)	Arsenic concentration of cooked rice grains (µg/kg)	Arsenic concentration of total discarded water (µg/l)
1	114	3	32	19
		30	105	81
		80	165	145
2	148	3	20	45
		30	121	119
		80	185	86
3	170	3	78	30
		30	130	69
		80	219	49
4	239	3	43	55
		30	124	134
		80	253	94
5	265	3	25	58
		30	205	155
		80	364	245

was 187 ± 63 µg/kg (range: 114–265 µg/kg, $n = 5$). Post-cooking with arsenic-free water (3 µg/l), the arsenic concentrations in the cooked rice grains showed a mean value of 40 ± 23 µg/kg (range: 20–78 µg/kg), which was decreased by 54–90% with respect to raw rice grain (Figure 12.6). The average arsenic concentration of the gruel was 41 ± 16 µg/kg, ranging from 19 to 58 µg/kg (Table 12.3). When the same rice grains were cooked with moderately arsenic-contaminated water (30 µg/l), the cooked rice grain showed a remarkable drop of 7–48% arsenic with a mean value of 137 ± 39 µg/kg (range: 105–205 µg/kg), compared to the raw rice grain. In this case, the average arsenic concentration of gruel was 112 ± 36 µg/kg, ranging from 69 to 155 µg/kg (Table 12.3). The subsequent cooked rice grains depicted an increasing trend of 6–45% arsenic when the same rice grains were cooked with highly arsenic-contaminated water (80 µg/l) with a mean arsenic concentration of 237 ± 78 µg/kg, ranging from 165 to 364 µg/kg (Figure 12.6). Here, the average arsenic concentration of gruel was 124 ± 75 µg/kg (Table 12.3).

Arsenic content of cooked rice is a variable entity whose nature can be attributed to factors like geographic origin of the grain, cultivar, water used for cooking and the cooking procedure followed (Mondal and Polya, 2008; Mondal et al., 2010; Pal et al., 2009). While low-arsenic water (<3 µg/l) has been used for cooking, cooked

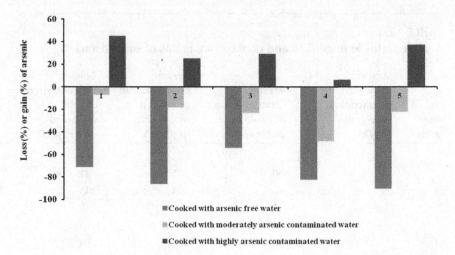

FIGURE 12.6 Percentage of arsenic increase or decrease in cooked rice in comparison with raw rice grain (sunned) when cooked with arsenic-free, moderately contaminated and highly arsenic-contaminated water.

rice arsenic concentrations decreased constantly during the course of this study. Therefore, a unidirectional flow of arsenic from rice grain to water was observed. Concurrently, a higher amount of arsenic was found in the supernatant liquid compared to the raw water used for cooking. When water arsenic concentration ~30 μg/l was used for cooking, a flow of arsenic from rice grain to water was also observed but the decreasing trend of arsenic in cooked rice was lesser compared to low-arsenic water. This condition changes with increasing water arsenic concentration and water arsenic ~80 μg/l inverses the arsenic flow, where an opposite flow of arsenic was observed. Therefore, apart from water arsenic concentration, variety of rice grain is also a significant feature behind discharge or loading of arsenic in cooked rice.

12.3.3.2 Parboiled Rice Grains

Arsenic distribution in different fractions of cooked rice using parboiled rice grain is shown in Table 12.4. An increased amount of arsenic was observed in parboiled rice grain in comparison with a sunned rice variety due to parboiling of paddy grain with arsenic-contaminated water on a domestic scale for parboiled rice preparation (Chowdhury et al., 2018b; Rahman et al., 2007). It is of principal importance to perform the steaming process in low-arsenic water when preparing parboiled rice, although this often becomes difficult at domestic level in arsenic-infested zones. In the dearth of such water, it is important to determine the threshold arsenic content in cooking water above which parboiled rice grain accumulates water arsenic.

In the first case, when the parboiled rice grains (mean: 198 ± 82 μg/kg, range: 95–305 μg/kg, $n = 5$) were cooked with arsenic-free water (3 μg/l), the

TABLE 12.4
Arsenic status in uncooked and cooked rice grains of parboiled variety

No. of conditions	Arsenic concentration of cooking water (µg/l)	Arsenic concentration of uncooked rice grains (µg/kg)	Arsenic concentration of cooked rice grains (µg/kg)	Arsenic concentration of total discarded water (µg/l)
1	3	95	18	28
		149	110,	32
		195	99	66
		247	109	28
		305	135	60
2	35	165	88	116
		155	129	75
		128	65	55
		160	95	45
		210	155	75
3	55	322	143	88
		309	135	90
		295	129	110
4	100	65	120	124
		115	191	135
		229	331	105

arsenic concentrations in the cooked rice grains (mean: 94 ± 45 µg/kg, range: 18–135 µg/kg) showed a remarkable drop of 26–81% (Figure 12.7). The average arsenic concentration of the gruel was 43 ± 18 µg/kg, ranging from 28 to 66 µg/kg (Table 12.4). In the second case, when the parboiled rice grains (mean: 164 ± 29 µg/kg, range: 128–210 µg/kg, $n = 5$) were cooked with moderately arsenic-contaminated water (35 µg/l), the cooked rice grain (mean: 106 ± 35 µg/kg, range: 65–155 µg/kg) showed a remarkable drop of 17–49% (Figure 12.7). In this case, the average arsenic concentration of gruel was 73 ± 27 µg/kg, ranging from 45 to 116 µg/kg (Table 12.4). Concurrently, when another set of rice grains (mean: 309 ± 13 µg/kg, range: 295–322 µg/kg, $n = 3$) were cooked with moderately arsenic-contaminated water (55 µg/l), the cooked rice grains (mean: 136 ± 7 µg/kg, range: 129–143 µg/kg) demonstrated a decreasing trend of 55–56% (Figure 12.7). The average arsenic concentration of gruel was 96 ± 12 µg/kg (Table 12.4). In the final set, when the rice grains (mean: 136 ± 84 µg/kg, range: 65–229 µg/kg, $n = 3$) were cooked with highly arsenic-contaminated water (100 µg/l), the cooked rice grains (mean: 214 ± 107 µg/kg, range: 120–331 µg/kg) showed an increasing trend of 44–84% (Figure 12.7). In this case, the mean arsenic concentration of gruel was 121 ± 15 µg/kg, ranging from 105 to 135 µg/kg (Table 12.4).

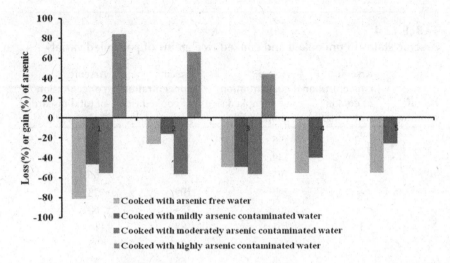

FIGURE 12.7 Percentage of arsenic increase or decrease in cooked rice in comparison with raw rice grain (parboiled) when cooked with arsenic-free, mildly contaminated, moderately contaminated and highly arsenic-contaminated water.

Similarly to sunned rice grain, a unidirectional flow of arsenic from rice grain to water was observed for parboiled rice grain when cooked with low or moderately arsenic-contaminated water. In contrast, an opposite flow of arsenic was observed from water to rice grain when cooked with highly arsenic-contaminated water.

12.3.3.3 Arsenic Flow Determination

Arsenic flow direction between rice grain and cooking water during preparation of cooked rice accounts for several factors like initial rice grain arsenic concentration, cooking method, cooking water arsenic concentration, presence of micronutrients like selenium and zinc, and the rice cultivar (Chowdhury et al., 2020a).

12.3.3.3.1 Initial Arsenic Concentration in Uncooked Rice Grain

Initial rice grain arsenic concentration influences the percentage of increase or decrease of arsenic in cooked rice prepared with arsenic-contaminated water. The higher the initial arsenic in in raw rice, the lower is the percentage increase in cooked rice, even cooked with contaminated water. Similarly, the lower the initial arsenic in rice grain, the higher is the percentage increase in cooked rice.

12.3.3.3.2 The Method of Cooked Rice Preparation

In rural Bengal, access to uncontaminated water is limited, especially in arsenic-exposed zones. Our study demonstrates that a moderate volume of water can be utilized for cooked rice preparation. Initially, the rice grain was washed several times until clear; a rice-to-water ratio of 1:2 was maintained each time. This was followed by soaking in water, maintaining the same ratio for some time, and the soaked rice was cooked with water at 1:3. The gruel that was discarded resulted in a 77% dip in average arsenic in cooked rice grain (sunned variety) when prepared using arsenic-free water. While cooking with moderately arsenic-laden water (30 μg/l), cooked rice arsenic in sunned variety decreased by 24% (Figure 12.6). For parboiled rice grain, about 53% of arsenic was decreased in cooked rice while cooking with arsenic-free water. Concurrently, on cooking with mild to moderately arsenic-tainted water (35 μg/l and 55 μg/l), about a 46% dip in average arsenic was observed in parboiled cooked rice (Figure 12.7). The protocol followed in this study for cooked rice preparation was able to decrease the arsenic load approximately 50% when cooked in arsenic-free or moderately arsenic-tainted water.

12.3.3.3.3 Impact of Arsenic-Concentrated Cooking Water on Rice Cultivar

The flow of arsenic has been observed from rice grain to water when cooked with arsenic-free, low or moderately arsenic-contaminated water for most of the rice grains of both varieties, i.e. sunned or parboiled rice grain with different cultivars. But the flow of arsenic has been reversed from water to rice grain when cooked with highly contaminated water. The percentage of increase or decrease of arsenic in wet cooked rice from uncooked grain (both sunned and parboiled) according to changing water arsenic concentration being utilized for cooked rice preparation is shown in Figures 12.6 and 12.7, respectively. A strong correlation between water arsenic and percentage of arsenic increase or decrease from raw rice grain to wet cooked rice has been shown through regression analysis ($y = 1.1959x - 72.063$, $R^2 = 0.7458$) (Figure 12.8).

12.3.3.3.4 Function of Micronutrients

Micronutrients such as selenium have been evaluated in this study since they are known to regulate arsenic flow in rice (Das et al., 2005; Malik et al., 2012). Varieties of rice grains with different range of arsenic concentrations have been examined in this study. Hence, it is difficult to control the movement of arsenic concentration, especially the uptake of arsenic in raw rice grain and its flow in cooked rice with cooking water when both the soil and irrigation water have alarming levels of arsenic in the areas studied (Chowdhury et al., 2018a).

Arsenic contents of uncooked sunned rice grains (five different cultivars) depicted a significantly strong negative correlation with selenium ($r = -0.91$, $p < 0.05$), as the average concentration of selenium was 27 ± 8 μg/kg. The uncooked parboiled rice too displays a strong negative correlation of arsenic with selenium ($r = -0.86$, $p < 0.05$), where the average selenium concentration was 35 ± 20 μg/ kg. Distribution of selenium has been further examined in cooked rice along with uncooked rice grain from both the varieties. The individual uncooked rice grain (sunned and parboiled) was prepared with three to four types of different arsenic-tainted water (arsenic-free water, mildly contaminated, moderately contaminated

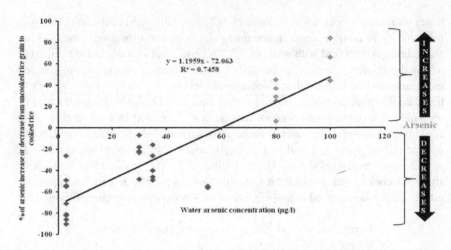

FIGURE 12.8 Regression analysis for percentage of arsenic increase or decrease in cooked rice from uncooked rice grain with respect to the change of water arsenic used for cooking.

and highly arsenic-contaminated water). The arsenic and selenium content in either forms of rice grain (uncooked/cooked) showed an inversely proportional relation. On cooking with arsenic-free or moderately arsenic-containing water, the arsenic concentration was found to decrease in cooked rice while inversely, increasing selenium content was observed. While cooking with highly tainted water, the arsenic and selenium concentration was observed to be reversed. A profound negative correlation was observed between the percentage changeover of arsenic and selenium from uncooked to cooked rice grain for both varieties ($r = -0.30$ and -0.94).

12.3.3.3.5 Arsenic Species Diversity

The distribution pattern of arsenic species in rice grain (before and after cooking) with arsenic-free or low-arsenic-contaminated water was evaluated in this study. The average arsenite concentration was 64 and 35 µg/kg in uncooked and cooked rice, respectively. But dimethylarsinic acid (DMA) was present only in cooked rice grain. There was no prevalence of methylarsonic acid anywhere. The average arsenate concentration was 215 and 88 µg/kg in uncooked and cooked rice grain, respectively. The extraction of As(III) and As(V) was 22% and 75%, respectively with respect to total arsenic (285 µg/kg) in uncooked rice grain. But in cooked rice grain the extraction was 27% and 68%, respectively; with 5% of DMA compared to total arsenic (128 µg/kg). The occurrence of DMA in cooked rice grain was also reported by Halder et al. (2014). In this study, approximately 45% of As(III) and 59% of As(V) decreased from uncooked rice grain to cooked rice. Amusingly, the decreasing trend of both As(III) and As(V) were relative to that of decreasing trend of total concentration of arsenic (55%) in this study. The increasing trend of total arsenic concentration in cooked rice compared to uncooked rice grain has been seen evidently because highly arsenic contaminated water used for cooking might contribute additional arsenic in cooked rice grain (Laparra et al., 2005).

12.4 CONCLUSION

Arsenic movement in paddy plant and molecular mechanistic pathway of assimilation and build-up in the grain is not properly demarcated. The specific work of cultivation sheds light on the processes of arsenic movement in rice from tainted irrigation water. Arsenic uptake by paddy plant reduced from root to grain. The decreased translocation of arsenic in the reproductive phase of the pre-monsoonal season (Boro) was endorsed by the development of amorphous iron plaques in the region of the root (rhizosphere), which lowers arsenic translocation capacity through sequestration of arsenic and iron. During Aman cultivation, along with groundwater used for irrigation, rainwater has a pivotal role in diluting the existing arsenic for translocation. Here, both types of cultivation practice exclusively determine that monsoonal rice grain also holds a load of arsenic concentration, which is much safer than the high-arsenic-containing Boro rice grain (different cultivars). Paddy plants of Boro and Aman variety displayed the same translocation capacity but the arsenic accumulation pattern in different parts of paddy plant at different phases of cultivation (vegetative, reproductive and ripening) in monsoon (Aman) is completely opposite to that of pre-monsoon (Boro). Consequently, the role of the post-harvesting (parboiling) procedure of whole paddy grain being processed in arsenic-contaminated regions recommended that two-way boiling (parboiling) with arsenic-tainted groundwater majorly promotes greater arsenic content in parboiled rice. The study analyzed that different strains of parboiled rice depicted a huge amount of arsenic concentrations in comparison to sunned rice strains. Hence, the consumption of parboiled rice grain is a serious health concern for the inhabitants of the Bengal delta.

Subsequently, the study of cooked rice preparation encourages careful thought about arsenic accumulation, movement and distribution in each portion of rice whilst cooking, leading to an improved elucidation of arsenic flow between water and rice grain. A noteworthy decrease in arsenic has been observed in cooked rice when it is cooked with arsenic-free, low-arsenic and moderately arsenic-contaminated water with increasing selenium concentration. Conversely, this scenario changes with increased water arsenic concentration (80–100 µg/l) and its flow became reversed from cooking water to rice grain along with declining selenium concentration.

The speciation study of arsenic highlights the fact of the analogous decreasing pattern of arsenite, arsenate and total arsenic in wet cooked rice when cooked with arsenic-free water. From the overall observations, it is recommended to keep away from arsenic-tainted groundwater for the irrigation, procurement of parboiled rice and regular cooking and conversely employ new methods like rainwater harvesting or surface water channeling to supply arsenic-free water.

ACKNOWLEDGMENTS

Financial support from the Department of Science and Technology, Government of West Bengal in providing research project grant (Memo No. 262(Sanc.)/ST/P/ S&T/1G-64/2017, dated 25/3/2018) and Inter University Research Project, RUSA (R-11/1092/19, dated 06/08/2019) is gratefully acknowledged.

REFERENCES

Abedin, M. J., Cotter-Howells, J., & Meharg, A. A. (2002). Arsenic uptake and accumulation in rice (*Oryza sativa* L.) irrigated with contaminated water. Plant and Soil, 240(2), 311–319.

Bae, M., Watanabe, C., Inaoka, T., Sekiyama, M., Sudo, N., Bokul, M. H., & Ohtsuka, R. (2002). Arsenic in cooked rice in Bangladesh. The Lancet, 360(9348), 1839–1840. doi.org/10.1016/S0140-6736(02)11738-7.

Bhattacharya, P., Samal, A. C., Majumdar, J., & Santra, S. C. (2010). Arsenic contamination in rice, wheat, pulses, and vegetables: a study in an arsenic affected area of West Bengal, India. Water, Air, & Soil Pollution, 213(1–4), 3–13.

Brammer, H. (2009). Mitigation of arsenic contamination in irrigated paddy soils in South and South-east Asia. Environment International, 35(6), 856–863.

Brammer, H., & Ravenscroft, P. (2009). Arsenic in groundwater: a threat to sustainable agriculture in South and South-east Asia. Environment International, 35(3), 647–654.

Chakraborti, D., Basu, G. K., Biswas, B. K., Chowdhury, U. K., Rahman, M. M., Paul, K., Roychowdhury, T., et al. (2001). Characterization of arsenic bearing sediments in Gangetic delta of West Bengal-India. In Arsenic Exposure and Health Effects. New York: Elsevier Science, pp. 27–52.

Chakraborti, D., Das, B., Rahman, M. M., Chowdhury, U. K., Biswas, B., Goswami, A. B., & Hossain, A. (2009). Status of groundwater arsenic contamination in the state of West Bengal, India: a 20-year study report. Molecular Nutrition and Food Research, 53(5), 542–551. 10.1002/mnfr.200700517.

Chowdhury, N. R., Das, R., Joardar, M., Ghosh, S., Bhowmick, S., & Roychowdhury, T. (2018a). Arsenic accumulation in paddy plants at different phases of pre-monsoon cultivation. Chemosphere, 210, 987–997.

Chowdhury, N. R., Ghosh, S., Joardar, M., Kar, D., & Roychowdhury, T. (2018b). Impact of arsenic contaminated groundwater used during domestic scale post harvesting of paddy crop in West Bengal: arsenic partitioning in raw and parboiled whole grain. Chemosphere, 211, 173–184.

Chowdhury, N. R., Das, A., Joardar, M., De, A., Mridha, D., Das, R., Rahman, M. M., & Roychowdhury, T. (2020a). Flow of arsenic between rice grain and water: its interaction, accumulation and distribution in different fractions of cooked rice. Science of the Total Environment, 731, 138937. https://doi.org/10.1016/j.scitotenv.2020. 138937.

Chowdhury, N. R., Das, A., Mukherjee, M., Swain, S., Joardar, M., De, A., Mridha, D., & Roychowdhury, T. (2020b). Monsoonal paddy cultivation with phase-wise arsenic distribution in exposed and control sites of West Bengal, alongside its assimilation in rice grain. Journal of Hazardous Materials, 400, 123206. https://doi.org/10.1016/j. jhazmat.2020.123206.

Das, D. K., Garai, T. K., Sarkar, S., & Sur, P. (2005). Interaction of arsenic with zinc and organics in a rice (*Oryza sativa* L.)-cultivated field in India. The Scientific World Journal, 5, 646–651.

Fitz, W. J., & Wenzel, W. W. (2002). Arsenic transformations in the soil–rhizosphere–plant system: fundamentals and potential application to phytoremediation. Journal of Biotechnology, 99(3), 259–278.

Ghosh, A. K., Bhattacharyya, P., & Pal, R. (2004). Effect of arsenic contamination on microbial biomass and its activities in arsenic contaminated soils of Gangetic West Bengal, India. Environment International, 30(4), 491–499.

Goswami, T. K., & Meghwal, M. (2015). Quick parboiling, drying and milling of paddy. Research Review Journal of Food and Dairy Technology, 3(2), 37–43.

Halder, D., Bhowmick, S., Biswas, A., Chatterjee, D., Nriagu, J., Guha Mazumder D. N., Le Kovec, Z., Jacks, G., & Bhattacharya, P. (2013). Risk of arsenic exposure from drinking water and dietary components: implications for risk management in rural Bengal. Environmental Science and Technology, 47, 1120–1127.

Halder, D., Biswas, A., Le Kovec, Z., Chatterjee, D., Nriagu, J., Jacks, G., & Bhattacharya, P. (2014). Arsenic species in raw and cooked rice: implications for human health in rural Bengal. Science of the Total Environment, 497, 200–208.

Hansel, C. M., Fendorf, S., Sutton, S., & Newville, M. (2001). Characterization of Fe plaque and associated metals on the roots of mine-waste impacted aquatic plants. Environmental Science and Technology, 35(19), 3863–3868.

Harvey, C. F., Swartz, C. H., Badruzzaman, A. B. M., Keon-Blute, N., Yu, W., Ali, M. A., Jay, J., Beckie, R., Niedan, V., Brabander, D., & Oates, P. M. (2005). Groundwater arsenic contamination on the Ganges Delta: biogeochemistry, hydrology, human perturbations, and human suffering on a large scale. Comptes Rendus Geoscience, 337(1–2), 285–296.

Itoh, K., Kawamura, S., & Ikeuchi, Y. (1985). Processing and milling of parboiled rice. Journal of the Faculty of Agriculture of Hokkaido University, 62(3), 312–324.

Laparra, J. M., Vélez, D., Barberá, R., Farré, R., & Montoro, R. (2005). Bioavailability of inorganic arsenic in cooked rice: practical aspects for human health risk assessments. Journal of Agricultural and Food Chemistry, 53(22), 8829–8833.

Liu, W. J., Zhu, Y. G., Smith, F. A., & Smith, S. E. (2004). Do iron plaque and genotypes affect arsenate uptake and translocation by rice seedlings (*Oryza sativa* L.) grown in solution culture? Journal of Experimental Botany, 55(403), 1707–1713.

Liu, W. J., Zhu, Y. G., Hu, Y., Williams, P. N., Gault, A. G., Meharg, A. A., Charnock, J. M., & Smith, F.A. (2006). Arsenic sequestration in iron plaque, its accumulation and speciation in mature rice plants (*Oryza sativa* L.). Environmental Science & Technology, 40(18), 5730–5736.

Malik, J. A., Goel, S., Kaur, N., Sharma, S., Singh, I., & Nayyar, H. (2012). Selenium antagonises the toxic effects of arsenic on mungbean (*Phaseolus aureus* Roxb.) plants by restricting its uptake and enhancing the antioxidative and detoxification mechanisms. Environmental and Experimental Botany, 77, 242–248.

Mandal, B. K., Roychowdhury, T., Samanta, G., Basu, G. K., Chowdhury, P. P., Chanda, C. R., Lodh, D., Karan, N. K., Dhar, R. K., Tamili, D. K., Saha, K. C., & Chakraborti, D. (1996). Arsenic in groundwater in seven districts of West Bengal, India – the biggest arsenic calamity in the world. Current Science, 70(11), 976e986.

Meharg, A. A., & Rahman, M. M. (2003). Arsenic contamination of Bangladesh paddy field soils: implications for rice contribution to arsenic consumption. Environmental Science & Technology, 37(2), 229–234. DOI: 10.1021/es0259842.

Meharg, A. A., Adomaco, E., Lawgali, Y., Deacon, C., & Williams, P. (2006). Food Standards Agency Contract C101045: Levels of Arsenic in Rice – Literature Review. www. food.gov.uk/sites/defauit/files/169-1-605.

Mondal, D., & Polya, D. A. (2008). Rice is a major exposure route for arsenic in Chakdaha block, Nadia district, West Bengal, India: a probabilistic risk assessment. Applied Geochemistry, 23(11), 2987–2998.

Mondal, D., Banerjee, M., Kundu, M., Banerjee, N., Bhattacharya, U., Giri, A. K., & Polya, D. A. (2010). Comparison of drinking water, raw rice and cooking of rice as arsenic exposure routes in three contrasting areas of West Bengal, India. Environmental Geochemistry and Health, 32(6), 463–477.

Ohno, K., Matsuo, Y., Kimura, T., Yanase, T., Rahman, M. H., Magara, Y., & Matsui, Y. (2009). Effect of rice-cooking water to the daily arsenic intake in Bangladesh: results of field surveys and rice-cooking experiments. Water Science and Technology, 59(2), 195–201. DOI: 10.2166/wst.2009.844.

Pal, A., Chowdhury, U. K., Mondal, D., Das, B., Nayak, B., Ghosh, A., Maity, S., & Chakraborti, D. (2009). Arsenic burden from cooked rice in the populations of arsenic affected and non-affected areas and Kolkata City in West-Bengal, India. Environmental Science and Technology, 43(9), 3349–3355.

Polya, D., & Charlet, L. (2009). Rising arsenic risk? Nature Geoscience, 2(6), 383–384.

Rahman, M. M., Mandal, B. K., Chowdhury, T. R., Sengupta, M. K., Chowdhury, U. K., Lodh, D., Chanda, C. R., Basu, G. K., Mukherjee, S. C., Saha, K. C., & Chakraborti, D. (2003). Arsenic groundwater contamination and sufferings of people in North 24-Parganas, one of the nine arsenic affected districts of West Bengal, India. Journal of Environmental Science and Health, Part A, 38(1), 25–59.

Rahman, M. A., Hasegawa, H., Rahman, M. M., Rahman, M. A., & Miah, M. A. M. (2007). Accumulation of arsenic in tissues of rice plant (*Oryza sativa* L.) and its distribution in fractions of rice grain. Chemosphere, 69(6), 942–948.

Roberts, L. C., Hug, S. J., Dittmar, J., Voegelin, A., Kretzschmar, R., Wehrli, B., Cirpka, O. A., Saha, G. C., Ali, M. A., & Badruzzaman, A. B. M. (2010). Arsenic release from paddy soils during monsoon flooding. Nature Geoscience, 3(1), 53.

Roychowdhury, T. (2008). Impact of sedimentary arsenic through irrigated groundwater on soil, plant, crops and human continuum from Bengal delta: special reference to raw and cooked rice. Food and Chemical Toxicology, 46(8), 2856–2864.

Roychowdhury, T. (2010). Groundwater arsenic contamination in one of the 107 arsenic-affected blocks in West Bengal, India: status, distribution, health effects and factors responsible for arsenic poisoning. International Journal of Hygiene and Environmental Health, 213, 414–427. doi:10.1016/j.ijheh.2010.09.003.

Roychowdhury, T., Uchino, T., Tokunaga, H., & Ando, M. (2002). Arsenic and other heavy metals in soils from an arsenic-affected area of West Bengal, India. Chemosphere, 49(6), 605–618.

Roychowdhury, T., Tokunaga, H., Uchino, T., & Ando, M. (2005). Effect of arsenic contaminated irrigation water on agricultural land soil and plants in West Bengal, India. Chemosphere, 58(6), 799–810. https://doi.org/10.1016/j.chemosphere.2004.08.098.

Samal, A. C., Kar, S., Bhattacharya, P., & Santra, S. C. (2011). Human exposure to arsenic through foodstuffs cultivated using arsenic contaminated groundwater in areas of West Bengal, India. Journal of Environmental Science and Health, Part A, 46(11), 1259–1265.

Samanta, G., Chowdhury, T. R., Mandal, B. K., Biswas, B. K., Chowdhury, U. K., Basu, G. K., Chanda, C. R., Lodh, D., & Chakraborti, D. (1999). Flow injection hydride generation atomic absorption spectrometry for determination of arsenic in water and biological samples from arsenic-affected districts of West Bengal, India, and Bangladesh. Microchemical Journal, 62(1), 174–191.

Sand, S., Concha, G., Öhrvik, V., & Abramsson, L. (2015a). Inorganic arsenic in rice and rice products on the Swedish market 2015. Part 2 – risk assessment, Livsmedelsverket: National Food Agency, report no. 16/2015.

Sand, S., Bjerselius, R., Busk, L., Eneroth, H., Sanner-Färnstrand, J., & Lindqvist, R. (2015b). The risk thermometer – a tool for risk comparison. Swedish National Food Agency Report Serial Number 8.

Santra, S. C., Samal, A. C., Bhattacharya, P., Banerjee, S., Biswas, A., & Majumdar, J. (2013). Arsenic in food chain and community health risk: a study in Gangetic West Bengal. Procedia Environmental Sciences, 18, 2–13. https://doi.org/10.1016/j.proenv.2013.04.002.

Shrivastava, A., Barla, A., Singh, S., Mandraha, S., & Bose, S. (2017). Arsenic contamination in agricultural soils of Bengal deltaic region of West Bengal and its higher assimilation in monsoon rice. Journal of Hazardous Materials, 324, 526–534.

Signes, A., Mitra, K., Burló, F., & Carbonell-Barrachina, A. A. (2008). Effect of two different rice dehusking procedures on total arsenic concentration in rice. European Food Research and Technology, 226(3), 561–567. https://doi.org/10.1007/s00217-007-0571-6.

Singh, A. K. (2006). Chemistry of arsenic in groundwater of Ganges–Brahmaputra river basin. Current Science, 91, 599–606.

Stroud, J. L., Norton, G. J., Islam, M. R., Dasgupta, T., White, R. P., Price, A. H., Meharg, A. A., McGrath, S. P., & Zhao, F. J. (2011). The dynamics of arsenic in four paddy fields in the Bengal delta. Environmental Pollution, 159(4), 947–953.

Syu, C. H., Jiang, P. Y., Huang, H. H., Chen, W. T., Lin, T. H., & Lee, D. Y. (2013). Arsenic sequestration in iron plaque and its effect on As uptake by rice plants grown in paddy soils with high contents of As, iron oxides, and organic matter. Soil Science and Plant Nutrition, 59(3), 463–471.

Torres-Escribano, S., Leal, M., Vélez, D., & Montoro, R. (2008). Total and inorganic arsenic concentrations in rice sold in Spain, effect of cooking, and risk assessments. Environmental Science and Technology, 42(10), 3867–3872.

Ullah, S. M. (1998). Arsenic contamination of groundwater and irrigated soils of Bangladesh. In International Conference on Arsenic Pollution of Groundwater in Bangladesh: Causes, Effects and Remedies. Dhaka: Dhaka Community Hospital.

Welna, M., Szymczycha-Madeja, A., & Pohl, P. (2015). Comparison of strategies for sample preparation prior to spectrometric measurements for determination and speciation of arsenic in rice. TrAC Trends in Analytical Chemistry, 65, 122–136.

Wu, C., Ye, Z., Li, H., Wu, S., Deng, D., Zhu, Y., & Wong, M. (2012). Do radial oxygen loss and external aeration affect iron plaque formation and arsenic accumulation and speciation in rice? Journal of Experimental Botany, 63(8), 2961–2970.

13 Ill Effects of Untreated Household Grey Water used in Agricultural Irrigation

Sushma* and Chandra Shekhar Sanwal

CONTENTS

13.1 INTRODUCTION

Use of wastewater from households, i.e. grey water for irrigation, has become a common practice, especially in Indian villages. Due to the Swach Bharat mission, in every house one can see a toilet but as there is no proper drainage the other wastewater apart from the toilet drains outside the house unattended or drained to the fields, which are generally planted with vegetables and fruit. Over the last two decades, as a result of a decline in annual rainfall, such practice has been intentionally adopted by farmers in arid and semi-arid regions. Such practice in India is called "blackwater farming", as it is also in other countries like Australia, France, Germany, the UK and the USA.

It is estimated that about 10% of the world population consumes food that has been irrigated with wastewater (WHO, 2006). According to an estimate by

* Corresponding author: Sushma. sushmabhel@gmail.com

DOI: 10.1201/9781003095422-13

the World Health Organization (WHO), 7% of all irrigated land, i.e. 20 million hectares, is irrigated by wastewater. The world has entered into a situation where it is must use water judicially and manage it. Various studies have revealed that an individual uses water on a daily basis between 15–55 L and 90–120 L/day per capita and reuse of this water not only reduces the pressure on fresh water requirement but also saves the water from entering unnecessarily into septic tanks (Nolde, 1999).

The recycling or reuse of such waste water not only reduces the pressure on fresh water requirements but also saves the water from entering unnecessarily into septic tanks. The use of this grey water seems an economically feasible method but it needs to be monitored because of its ill effects. Without any treatment this water has been reported to create several ill effects.

Grey water can be used for a variety of purposes, such as irrigating lawns/gardens (college and school campuses, sports fields, golf grounds, parks and, domestic gardens), for ornamental use in fountains and waterfalls, landscaping, to develop and preserve wetlands, to infiltrate into the ground, in agriculture/horticulture, fire protection, brick/concrete production, car washing and toilet flushing, and so on.

13.2 CHARACTERISTICS OF GREY WATER

Grey water is defined as the water collected from waste water discharge of bath, shower, cloth washers, washing machines and kitchen sinks excluding the waste water from the toilets.

(Al-Jayyousi, 2003)

It is known as grey water because when it is stored for even very short periods of time, the water turns turbid and is grey in colour (Emmerson, 1998). The exact sources of grey water sometimes vary; according to countries and organizations some definitions include water sourced from the kitchen and dishwasher and some do not. This chapter includes both kitchen and dishwasher as source of grey water. The major factors affecting the characteristics of grey water generally depends on the following:

- Quality of water supply (tap water or bore water/ground water)
- Quantity of water used in relation to the discharged pollutants
- Household activities (use of chemical products like soap, shampoo, washing powder etc.)
- Source from which the grey water is drawn (kitchen sink, bathroom, hand basin or washing machine/laundry)
- Type of source (household or commercial laundries).

The composition of grey water varies greatly throughout the world. Various studies, detailed in Tables 13.1–13.4 demonstrate that grey-water composition

TABLE 13.1

General hydrochemical characteristics of grey water (modified from Ledin et al., 2001)

Serial no.	Chemical properties	Laundry	Bathroom	Kitchen sink	References
1	pH	9.3–10[3]	5–8.1[2,3,8,9]	6.5[4]	1. Almeida
		8.2[12]	6.7–7.4[4]	6.3–7.4[10]	et al. 1999
		7.5–10[4]	7.6[12]		2. Burrows
2	EC [µS/cm]	190–1400[3]	82–20000[3,9]		et al. 1991
3	Alkalinity [mg/l]	83–200 as CaCO$_3$[3]	24–136 as CaCO$_3$[2,3]	20.0–340.0[10]	3. Christova-Boal et al. 1996
4	Hardness [mg/l]	–	18–52 as CaCO$_3$[2]	-	4. Friedler 2004
5	BOD$_5$ [mg/l]	48–290[3]	76–200[3]	536[3]	5. Hargelius et al. 1995
		280-470[4]	424[4]	530–1450[4]	6. Laak 1974
		282[6]	192[6]	2762[6]	7. Nolde 1999
		150-380[11]	170[11]	1460[11]	8. Rose et al. 1991
		472[12]	216[12]		9. Santala
6	BOD$_7$ [mg/l]	150[5]	170[5]	387–1000[5]	et al. 1998
7	COD [mg/ l]	1815[1]	210–501[1]	1079[1]	10. Shin et al. 1998
		725[3,6]	645[4]	936[3]	11. Siegrist
		1339[4]	280[5]	644–1340[4]	et al. 1976
		375[5]	282[6]	26–1600[5,10]1380[6]	12. Surendran and Wheatley 1998
			100–633[7]		
8	TOC [mg/l]	381[4]	15–225[2]	318[4]	
		100–280[11]	30–120[4]	100–280[11]	
			100[11]		
			104[12]		
9	Dissolved oxygen [mg/l]	–	0.4–4.6[9]	2.2–5.8[10]	
10	Sulphate [mg/l]	–	12–40[8]	-	
11	Chloride (as Cl) [mg/l]	9.0–88[3]	3.1–18[3,8]	-	
12	Oil and grease [mg/l]	8.0–35[3]	37–78[3]	-	

EC, electrical conductivity; BOD5, biological oxygen demand 5-day test; BOD7, biological oxygen demand 7-day test; COD, chemical oxygen demand; TOC, total organic carbon.

TABLE 13.2
Nutrient components in grey water (modified from Ledin et al., 2001)

Serial no.	Nutrients [mg/l]	Laundry	Bathroom	Kitchen sink	References
1	Ammonia (NH$_3$-N)	2.0[1] <0.1–0.9[3] 4.9–11.0[4] 11.3[6] <0.1–3.47[5,9] 0.06–3.5[8] 0.4–0.7[11] 10.7[12]	1.1–1.2[1] <0.1–25[3,9] 1.2[4] 1.3[5] 0.1–0.4[8] 2.0[11] 1.6[12]	0.3[1] 0.6–6.0[4] 5.4[6] 0.2–23.0[10] 6.0[11] 4.6[12]	1. Almeida et al. 1999 2. Burrows et al. 1991 3. Christova-Boal et al. 1996 4. Friedler 2004 5. Hargelius et al. 1995
2	Nitrate and nitrite as N per 100 ml	2.0[1] 0.1–0.3[3] 1.3[6] 0.4–0.6[11] 1.6[12]	4.2–6.3[1] <0.05–0.20[3] 0.4[5,11] 0.9[12]	0.6[6] 5.8[8] 0.3[11] 0.5[12]	6. Laak 1974 7. Nolde 1999 8. Rose et al. 1991 9. Santala et al. 1998
3	Nitrate (NO$_3$-N)	0.4–0.6[11]	0–4.9[8]	-	10. Shin et al. 1998 11. Siegrist et al. 1976
4	Phosphorus as PO$_4$	4.0–15[11]	4–35[8,9]	0.4–4.7[10]	12. Surendran and Wheatley 1998
5	Total nitrogen	1–40[3] 6–21[5,11]	0.6–7.3[5,8] 5–10[7] 17[11]	13–60[5] 15.4–42.5[10] 74[11]	
6	Total phosphorus	0.06–42[3] 0.062–57[5] 21–57[11]	0.11–2.2[3,5] 0.2–0.6[6] 2.0[11]	74.0[11] 3.1–10[5]	

varies according to its origin. A variety of pollutants are present in grey water, including acidic and alkaline products, dissolved and suspended particle fats and oil and heavy metals (Eriksson and Donner, 2009). The chemical components may be toxic to crops and the biological (i.e. pathogens) components which are of main concern to public health in general require treatment before the water can be used for irrigation.

13.3 EFFECT OF UNTREATED GREY-WATER IRRIGATION

13.3.1 IN HUMANS

Studies have shown a diverse effect of untreated grey water for irrigation. In humans it is reported that diseases or illnesses which are food-borne are directly related to the pathogen present in the irrigation water (Finley et al., 2008). However, there is an urgent need for detailed research work related to risk and identification of indicators.

TABLE 13.3
Microbiological parameters in grey water (modified from Ledin et al., 2001)

Serial no.	Microbiological parameters	Laundry	Bathroom	Kitchen sink	References
1	*Escherichia coli* (per 100 ml)	$8.3 \times 10^{6(2)}$	$3.2 \times 10^{7(2)}$	1.3×10^5–$2.5 \times 10^{8(2)}$	1. Christova-Boal et al. 1996
2	Faecal coliforms (per 100 ml)	9–$1.6 \times 10^{4\,(1,3,5)}$	1–$8 \times 10^{6\,(1,3,5)}$		2. Hargelius et al. 1995
3	Faecal streptococci (per 100 ml)	23–$1.3 \times 10^{6(1,2,3,5,)}$	1–$5.4 \times 10^{6\,(1,2,5)}$	5.15×10^3–$5.5 \times 10^{8(2)}$	3. Rose et al. 1991 4. Santala et al., 1998
4	Thermotolerant coli (per 100 ml)	$8.4 \times 10^{6(2)}$	Up to $8.9 \times 10^{6(2,5)}$	0.2×10^6–$3.75 \times 10^{8(2)}$	5. Siegrist et al., 1976
5	Total coliform (per 100 ml)	56–$8.9 \times 10^{5(1,3,5,)}$	70–$2.8 \times 10^{7(1,3,5)}$		
6	Total bacterial population (cfu/100ml)	300–$6.4 \times 10^{8(3)}$			

The presence of organic and chemical pollutants in grey water makes it a potential health hazard and the risk can increase if microbial contamination is increased (Dixon et al., 1999) It is important to understand that grey water does have the potential to transmit disease. Fatta-Kassinos et al. (2011) reported that xenobiotic compounds (XOCs), which are the synthetic organic compounds present in the household chemicals like bleaches, softeners and other beauty products and are also formed by partial modifications during treatment, can easily accumulate in plants and animals, causing risks to the ecosystem and therefore the environment. These are also formed by partial modifications during treatment and can easily accumulate in plants and animals, causing risks to the ecosystem and therefore the environment. Eriksson et al. (2002) identified 900 such potential XOCs which are known to originate from beauty cosmetics and detergents in Denmark. The presence of antibiotics is also reported, and this has the potential to create proliferation of resistant bacteria strains (Le-Minh et al., 2010).

According to Ludwig (2000) the transmission of pathogens can occur in ways such as:

- Through direct contact with grey water
- Through contaminated drinking water
- Through food products which are in direct contact with contaminated water or soil, such as vegetables, shellfish
- By inhalation of aerosols during irrigation with grey water

TABLE 13.4
Trace elements and heavy metals in grey water (modified from Ledin et al., 2001)

Serial no.	Trace elements/heavy metals [mg/l]	Laundry	Bathroom	Kitchen sink	References
1	Aluminium (Al)	<0.1–21[1]	<1.0[1]–1.7[3]	0.67–1.8[3]	1. Christova-
2	Arsenic (As)	0.001–<0.038[1,3]	0.001[1]–<0.0038[3]	<0.038[3]	Boal et al. 1996
3	Barium (Ba)	0.019[3]	0.032[3]	0.018–0.028[3]	2. Friedler 2004
4	Boron (B)	<0.1–0.51	<0.11	-	3. Hargelius
5	Cadmium (Cd)	<0.01–<0.038[1,3]	<0.01[1,3]	<0.007[3]	et al. 1995
6	Calcium (Ca)	3.9–14[1,3]	3.5–21[1,3]	13–30[3]	4. Surendran and Wheatley
7	Chromium (Cr)	<0.025[3]	0.036[3]	<0.025-0.072[3]	1998
8	Cobalt (Co)	<0.012[3]	<0.012[3]	<0.013[3]	
9	Copper (Cu)	<0.05–0.27[1,3]	0.06–0.12[1,3]	0.068–0.26[3]	
10	Iron (Fe)	0.29–1.0[1,3]	0.34–1.4[1,3]	0.6–1.2[3]	
11	Lead (Pb)	<0.063[3]	<0.063[3]	<0.062–0.14[3]	
12	Magnesium (Mg)	1.1–3.1[1,3]	1.4–6.6[1,3]	3.3–7.3[3]	
13	Manganese (Mg)	0.029[3]	0.061[3]	0.031–0.075[3]	
14	Mercury (Hg)	0.0029[3]	<0.0003[3]	<0.0003–0.00047[3]	
15	Nickel (Ni)	<0.025[3]	<0.025[3]	<0.025[3]	
16	Potassium (K)	1.1–17[1,3] 1.63–101[4]	1.5–6.6[1,3]	19–59[3]	
17	Selenium (Se)	<0.001[1]	<0.001[1]	-	
18	Silicon (Si)	3.8–49[1]	3.2–4.1[1]	-	
19	Silver (Ag)	0.002[3]	<0.002[3]	<0.002–0.013[3]	
20	Sodium (Na)	44–480[1,3] 151–530[2]	7.4–21[1,3]	29–180[3]	
21	Sulphur (S)	9.5–40[1]	0.14–3.3[1,3]	0.12	
22	Zinc (Zn)	0.09–0.44[1,3]	0.01–6.3[1,3]	0.0007–1.8[3]	

- By vector-borne transmission where the vectors are the intermediate host that breeds in water
- By secondary transmission through contact with an infected person.

The health risk from untreated grey water can never be eliminated; however it can be minimized by appropriate treatment, careful risk management and responsible use. The WHO guidelines and suggestions include a risk management approach in order to protect public health and sustainable utilization of grey water. Many countries throughout the world have followed the standards but very few were able to enforce them. The WHO risk management approach is a systematic management tool that consistently ensures the safety and acceptability of water reuse practices. A central feature is that it is sufficiently flexible to be applied to all types of water reuse systems, irrespective of size and complexity (WHO, 2004, 2011).

13.3.2 IN PLANTS AND SOIL

The use of grey water for irrigation can cause an adverse effect in both plants and soil, such as development of soil hydrophobicity and reduction of soil hydraulic conductivity. The presence of cadmium decreases agricultural productivity even in very low concentrations, while increases in the pH of soil can reduce the availability of some micronutrients for plants and pH above 9 is reported to reduce the transpiration rate in plants, as shown in Table 13.5. There is a misconception regarding grey water that it is cleaner than blackwater and therefore it can be reused with minimal or no treatment (Gross et al., 2007). On the contrary, many recent investigations have emphasized the need for grey-water treatment before it is used in irrigation (Friedler & Gilboa, 2010).

13.4 WORLDWIDE MAJOR MILESTONE IN WASTEWATER REUSE-RELATED STRATEGIES

- 1933: California was the first to issue a strict health regulation regarding use of wastewater among developed countries. According to the guidelines the effluent standard requires 2.2 coliforms/100 mL to be used for irrigation of crops that are eaten uncooked, indicating concern about the risk related to water-borne vectors. The health authorities noted that pathogens can survive long enough to contaminate crops even if their populations are very low (Ongerth and Jopling, 1977).
- 1973: WHO published general guidelines in order to protect public health and reuse wastewater in agriculture and aquaculture under the title *Guidelines for the Safe Use of Wastewater and Excreta in Agriculture and Aquaculture* (WHO, 1973).
- 1989: WHO updated the previous guidelines under the title *Health Guidelines for the Use of Wastewater in Agriculture and Aquaculture* (WHO, 1989b).

  In 1989 the United Nations Environment Program (UNEP) and WHO also jointly published guidelines under the title *Guidelines for the Safe Use of Wastewater and Excreta in Agriculture and Aquaculture*, with emphasis on environmental and public health protection (WHO, 1989a). Following this the third edition was published under the title *Guidelines for the Safe*

TABLE 13.5
Effect of untreated grey water in soil and plants as reported

Serial no.	Effect of grey water irrigation on plants and soil	References
1	Development of soil hydrophobicity	Chen et al. 2003; Tarchitzky et al. 2007; Wallach et al. 2005
2	Reduction of soil hydraulic conductivity by surfactants or food-based oils	Travis et al. 2008
3	Synthetic compounds commonly found in grey water may accumulate in soils which ultimately lead to water-repellent soils which causes decrease in agricultural productivity like cadmium, reported to be toxic at low concentrations as 0.1 mg/l in nutrient solutions.	Wiel-Shafran et al. 2006
4	Increases pH of soils which reduces availability of some micronutrients for plants	Christova-Boal et al. 1996
5	When pH is above 9 the transpiration rate reduces	Eriksson et al. 2006
6	Possibilities of accumulation of sodium and boron in soil, that affects soil properties and plant growth adversely	Misra & Sivongxay 2009; Gross et al. 2005
7	Soil aggregate dispersion from sodium accumulation	Misra & Sivongxay 2009
8	Aluminium can cause non-productivity in acid soils (pH < 5.5), although if more alkaline soils at pH > 7.0 it will precipitate the ion and eliminate any toxicity	National Academy of Sciences 1972; Pratt 1972
9	Arsenic and beryllium cause toxicity to plants which varies widely, ranging from 12 mg/l for Sudan grass to less than 0.05 mg/l for rice and ranging from 5 mg/l for kale to 0.5 mg/l for bush beans respectively. Its recommended concentration for both is 0.10 mg/l	National Academy of Sciences 1972; Pratt 1972
10	Lead can inhibit plant cell growth at very high concentrations. Its recommended concentration is 5.0 mg/l	National Academy of Sciences 1972; Pratt 1972

TABLE 13.5 Continued
Effect of untreated grey water in soil and plants as reported

Serial no.	Effect of grey water irrigation on plants and soil	References
11	Selenium is toxic to plants at concentrations as low as 0.025 mg/l and toxic to livestock also if forage is grown in soils with relatively high levels of added selenium. Although it is a necessary element for animals it is required in very low concentrations so its recommended concentration is 0.02 mg/l	National Academy of Sciences 1972; Pratt 1972
12	Phytotoxicity due to anionic surfactant content that alters the microbial communities associated with rhizosphere	Eriksson et al. 2006
13	Microbial risks	Gross et al. 2007
14	Enhanced contamination transport	Graber et al. 2001

Use of Wastewater, Excreta and Grey Water (WHO 2006) and presented in four separate volumes: volume 1: policy and regulatory experts; volume 2: wastewater used in agriculture; volume 3: wastewater and excreta used in aquaculture; and volume 4: excreta and grey-water use in agriculture.

- 1991: UNEP and the Food and Agriculture Organization (FAO) jointly published Environmental Guidelines for Wastewater Reuse in the Mediterranean Region (UNEP, 1991).
- 1992: FAO published Wastewater Treatment and Use in Agriculture (Pescod, 1992).
- 1995: FAO Regional Office in Cairo produced a publication on *Wastewater Reuse in the Near East Region* (Bazza, 2002) and during 1991–93 it also published seven technical bulletins with the aim of promoting use of wastewater sustainably in agriculture.
- 2000: The United Nation General Assembly adopted the Millennium Development Goals (MDGs) on 8 September 2000; these included reuse of wastewater in agriculture.
- 2003: FAO and WHO jointly published *User Manual for Irrigation with Treated Wastewater* (FAO, 2003) which was intended to help farmers, irrigation operators and the extensionists who are in close contact with farmers, irrigationists, other forestry users and those involved in landscaping.
- 2012: The United States Environmental Protection Agency (USEPA) issued *Guidelines for Water Reuse* (USEPA, 2012) which address a wide range of reuse applications (e.g. agricultural irrigation and aquifer recharge).

- 2015: The International Organization for Standardization (ISO) published *Guidelines for Treated Wastewater Use for Irrigation Projects* which include use of grey water in agriculture irrigation (ISO 16075-2, 2015). These guidelines addressed health, environment, hydrology and monitoring and maintenance of water reuse for restricted irrigation of agricultural crops, use in community places such as parks, gardens and schools. The guidelines are divided into four parts:
  Part 1: Based on reuse project for irrigation, relating to climate, soils, design, materials, construction and performance;
  Part 2: Development of the project, including water quality requirements like microbiological and chemical parameters, potential barriers and potential corresponding water treatments.
  Part 3: Based on components of a reuse project for irrigation.
  Part 4: Including recommendations for irrigation systems, distribution and storage facilities, and monitoring. To ensure health and environmental safety ISO guidelines endorsed parameters similar to WHO and USEPA guidelines.

13.5   GREY-WATER TREATMENT

Grey-water treatment not only reduces health risk but also increases its usability. Once proper treatment has been undertaken, the water thus obtained will be clean and safe for use. It is basically required to reduce the organic load of potential pathogenic microorganisms which poses health risks. Treatment options vary from low-cost to a very sophisticated expensive treatment system which involves disinfection and conversion to a standard required for irrigation. In general the treatment systems reduce the level of contamination in grey water before reuse or final disposal. They are contaminant-specific, and each system adopts either physicochemical or biological means of treatment. Physicochemical means a combination of physical and/or chemical methods of treatment which may include filtration, adsorption and reverse osmosis.

13.5.1   PHYSICAL TREATMENT

Physical treatment includes coarse filtration and purification with the help of various materials like sand, pebbles, marble chips, activated carbon, jute coir, coconut shell, sawdust, charcoal, zeolite, wood chips, bricks, rice husk, and so forth (Parjane and Sane, 2011) and even organic mulch (leaves, tree bark, etc.) is being used to treat grey water (Ludwig, 2000). Physical treatment is reported to achieve varied levels of treatment efficiency. The removal efficiencies reported by Noutsopoulos et al. (2018) are as follows: 53–93% total suspended solids (TSS), 89–98% biological oxygen demand (BOD_5), 37–94% chemical oxygen demand (COD), 5–98% total nitrogen, 17–73% ammonium + -N, 0–100% total phosphorus, 12–99% methylene blue active substances (MBAS), 100% *Escherichia coli*, 100% calcium, 100% magnesium, 47% sodium and 56.2% potassium.

13.5.2 BIOLOGICAL TREATMENT

In biological method the grey-water treatment can be divided into aerobic and anaerobic treatment methods. Commonly partially submerged rotating biological contractors (RBCs) are used for BOD_5 removal and combined carbon oxidation/nitrification of secondary effluents and completely submerged RBCs are used for the same applications with additional de-nitrification (Wu, 2019). Moving bed bio-film reactor (MBBR) is another technology which is widely used to treat grey water; it is based on organic matter oxidation and nitrogen removal. The removal efficiencies of BOD_5 and COD are reported to be 59% and 70% respectively (Chrispim and Nolasco, 2017).

13.5.3 CHEMICAL TREATMENT

The most adopted chemical grey-water treatment processes are coagulation and flocculation; these are reported to achieve the following removal percentages: 85–89% BOD_5, 64% COD, 13% total nitrogen, >99% total organic carbon (TOC) and >99% *E. coli* (Ghaitidak and Yadav, 2013).

13.6 GRAPHICAL ABSTRACT

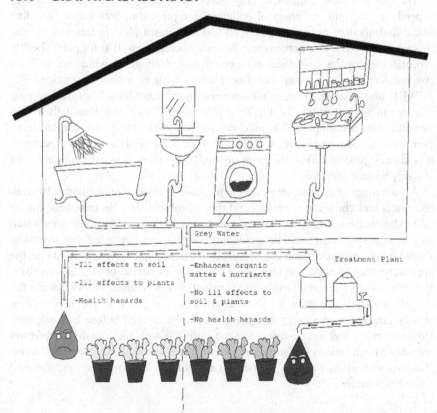

13.7 CONCLUSION

Grey water, which is the discharge from bath, shower, washing machine and kitchen sink, is a potential resource to meet the needs of present water-scarce conditions. Furthermore, irrigation of grey water in the agricultural sector enhances the availability of organic matter and nutrients in the soil. The only drawback related to grey-water reuse is the inherent microbial risks and the presence of toxic heavy metals and micropollutants. With reuse of grey water wastewater is used sustainably and it also prevents water entering into septic tanks unnecessarily. The overall benefits of reuse of wastewater/grey water can be summarized as follows:

- It reduces pressure on potable water use for irrigation.
- Environmental degradation, eutrophication and health hazards because of pooling of wastewater can be resolved.
- Potentially lost nutrients can be reclaimed.
- It results in overty alleviation and food security.

Thus although grey-water reuse poses health risk and environmental concerns which can never be eliminated, they can be minimized by following the guidelines issued by different agencies such as WHO and using grey water safely.

The characteristic features of grey water vary throughout the world as they depend on its origin. A variety of pollutants are present in grey water, including acidic and alkaline products, dissolved and suspended particle fats and oil and heavy metals. These components may be toxic to crops as well as for public health, especially as regards biological components (i.e. pathogens) which are of main concern, so grey water requires treatment before it can be used for irrigation.

WHO and other such organizations have issued guidelines from time to time in order to protect public health. Several countries have also issued their own guidelines and are adopting the guidelines issued by WHO and other entities; however some developing countries, including India, have not issued such guidelines. It is always good to follow the great saying, "prevention is better than cure" and use grey water judicially.

A wide range of grey-water treatment methods are available involving physical, biological and chemical processes and their combinations. No treatment can be said to be the best method as the choice depends on the end use of the grey water, its contaminants and economic availability. WHO recommended that treatment should reduce pollutants and contaminants to usable limits or else if used raw, the grey water should not come into direct contact with people or pose health risks. If required to irrigate plants subsurface irrigation can be used as this reduces the risk of contact. If the crops are to be used for consumption, irrigation should be strictly directed to the crops and these should be cooked before consumption. However crops that are in direct contact with the soil, like potatoes (*Solanum tuberosum*) and onions (*Allium cepa*) or eaten raw as salad, for example, lettuce (*Lactuca sativa*), carrot (*Daucas carota*) and tomato (*Lycopersicon esculentum*) should be avoided.

REFERENCES

Al-Jayyousi, O. R. (2003). Greywater reuse, towards sustainable water management. *Desalination*, 156(1): 181–192.

Almeida, M. C., Butler, D. & Friedler, E. (1999). At-source domestic wastewater quality. *Urban Water*, 1: 49–55.

Bazza, Md. (2002). Wastewater Reuse in the Near East Region: Experience and Issues. Regional Symposium on Water Recycling in the Mediterranean Region, Iraklio, Crete, Greece.

Burrows, W. D., Schmidt, M. O., Carnevale, R. M. & Shaub, S. A. (1991). Nonpotable reuse: development of health criteria and technologies for shower water recycle. *Water Science Technology*, 24(9): 81–88.

Chen, Y., Lerner, O., Shani, U. & Tarchitzky, J. (2003). Hydraulic conductivity and soil hydrophobicity: effect of irrigation with reclaimed wastewater. In: Lundstrum U (edr.), Nordic IHSS Symposium on Abundance and Function of Natural Organic Matter Species in Soil and Water. Sweden: Sundsvall.

Chrispim, M. & Nolasco, M. A. (2017). Greywater treatment using a moving bed biofilm reactor at a university campus in Brazil. *Journal of Cleaner Products*, 142: 290–296.

Christova-Boal, D., Eden, R. E. & McFarlane, S. (1996). An investigation into greywater reuse for urban residential properties. *Desalination*, 106: 391–397.

Dixon, A., Butler, D. & Fewkes, A. (1999). Guidelines for greywater re-use: health issues. *Journal of the Chartered Institution of Water and Environmental Management*, 13(October): 322–326.

Emmerson, G. (1998). Every Drop is Precious: Greywater as an Alternative Water Source. Research Bulletin No. 4/98. Brisbane: Queensland Parliamentary Library.

Eriksson, E. & Donner, E. (2009). Metals in greywater: sources, presence and removal efficiencies. *Desalination*, 248(1–3): 271–278.

Eriksson, E., Auffarth, K., Henze, M. & Ledin, A. (2002). Characteristics of grey wastewater. *Urban Water*, 4(1): 85–104.

Eriksson, E., Baun, A., Henze, M. & Ledin, A. (2006). Phytotoxicity of grey wastewater evaluated by toxicity tests. *Urban Water*, 3(1): 13–20. doi:10.1080/ Z15730620600 578645.

FAO. (2003). User Manual for Irrigation with Treated Wastewater. Cairo, Egypt: FAO Regional Office for the Near East and North Africa, p. 73.

FAO. (2010). Global Water Statistics of the Land and Water Division of the Food and Agricultural Organisation, United Nations. www.fao.org/nr/water.

Fatta-Kassinos, D., Kalavrouziotis, I. K., Koukoulakis, P. H. & Vasquez, M. I. (2011). The risks associated with wastewater reuse and xenobiotics in the agroecological environment. *Science of the Total Environment*, 409: 3555–3563.

Finley, S., Barrington, S. & Lyew, D. (2008). Reuse of domestic greywater for the irrigation of food crops. *Water Air Soil Pollution*, 199(1): 235–245.

Friedler, E. (2004). Quality of individual domestic greywater streams and its implication on on-site treatment and reuse possibilities. *Environmental Technology*, 25(9): 997–1008.

Friedler, E. & Gilboa, Y. (2010). Performance of UV disinfection and the microbial quality of greywater effluent along a reuse system for toilet flushing. *Science of the Total Environment*, 408: 2109–2117.

Ghaitidak, D. M. & Yadav, K. D. (2013). Characteristics and treatment of greywater – a review. *Environmental Science Pollution Research*, 20(5): 2795–2809.

Graber, E. R., Dror, I., Bercovich, F. C. & Rosner, M. (2001). Enhanced transport of pesticides in a field trial with treated sewage sludge. *Chemosphere*, 44: 805–811.

Gross, A., Azulai, N., Oron, G., Ronen, Z. & Arnold, M. (2005). Environmental impact and health risks associated with greywater irrigation: a case study. *Water Science and Technology*, 52(8): 161–169.

Gross, A., Kaplan, D. & Baker, K. (2007). Removal of chemical and microbiological contaminants from domestic greywater using a recycled vertical flow bioreactor (RVFB). *Ecological Engineering*, 31: 107–114.

Hargelius, K., Holmstrand, O. & Karlsson, L. (1995). Hushallsspillvatten. Framstagande avnyaschablonvärdenför BDT-vatten. In Vadinnehalleravloppfranhushall? Närin gochmetalleriurinochfekaliersamti disk-, tvätt, bad- & duschvatten. Stockholm: Naturvardsverket.

ISO 16075-2. (2015). Guidelines for treated wastewater use for irrigation projects. Available online: www.iso.org/standard/62758.html.

Ledin, A., Eriksson, E. & Henze, M. (2001). Aspects of groundwater recharge using grey wastewater. In Lettinga G. (ed.), Decentralised Sanitation and Reuse. London: p. 650.

Le-Minh, N., Khan, S. J., Drewes, J. E. & Stuetz, R. M. (2010). Fate of antibiotics during municipal water recycling treatment processes. *Water Research*, 44: 4295–4323.

Ludwig, A. (2000). Create an Oasis with Greywater. Santa Barbara: Oasis Design.

Misra, R. K. & Sivongxay, A. (2009). Reuse of laundry greywater as affected by its interaction with saturated soil. *Journal of Hydrology*, 366: 55–61.

National Academy of Sciences and National Academy of Engineering. (1972). Water Quality Criteria. Report No. EPA-R373-033. 592. Washington, DC: US Environmental Protection Agency.

Nolde, E. (1999). Greywater reuse system for toilet flushing in multi-storey buildings – over ten years experience in Berlin. *Urban Water*, 1: 275–284.

Noutsopoulos, C. et al. (2018). Greywater characterization and loadings – physico-chemical treatment to promote onsite reuse. *Journal of Environmental Management*, 216: 337–346.

Ongerth, H. J. & Jopling, W. F. (1977). Water reuse in California. In Shuval, H. I. (ed.), *Water Renovation and Reuse*. New York: Academic Press, pp. 219–256.

Parjane, S. & Sane, M. (2011). Performance of grey water treatment plant by economical way for Indian rural development. *International Journal of Chemical and Technical Research*, 3(4): 1808–1815.

Pescod, M. (1992). Wastewater Treatment and Use in Agriculture – FAO Irrigation and Drainage Paper 47. Rome: Food and Agriculture Organization of the United Nations.

Pratt, P. F. (1972). Quality Criteria for Trace Elements in Irrigation Waters. USA: California Agricultural Experiment Station.

Rose, J. B., Sun, G-S., Gerba, C. P. & Sinclair, N. A. (1991). Microbial quality and persistence of enteric pathogens in greywater from various household sources. *Water Research*, 25(1): 37–42.

Santala, E., Uotila, J., Zaitsev, G., Alasiurua, R., Tikka, R. & Tengvall, J. (1998). Microbiological greywater treatment and recycling in an apartment building. AWT98 Advanced Wastewater Treatment, Recycling and Reuse Milan, 14–16 September 1998, pp. 319–324.

Shin, H. S., Lee, S. M., Seo, I. S., Kim, G. O., Lim, K. H. & Song, J. S. (1998). Pilot scale SBR and MF operation for the removal of organic and nitrogen compounds from greywater. *Water Science Technology*, 38(6): 79–88.

Siegrist, H., Witt, M. & Boyle, W. C. (1976). Characteristics of rural household wastewater. *Journal of the Environmental Engineering Division,* 102(EE3): 533–548.

Surendran, S. & Wheatley, A. D. (1998). Grey-water reclamation for non-potable reuse. *Journal of the Chartered Institution of Water and Environmental Management,* 6: 406–413.

Tarchitzky J., Lerner, O., Shani, U., Arye, G., Lowengart-Aycicegi, A., Brener, A. & Chen, Y. (2007). Water distribution pattern in treated wastewater irrigated soils: hydrophobicity effect. *European Journal of Soil Science,* 58(3): 573–588.

Travis, M. J., Weisbrod, N. & Gross, A. (2008). Accumulation of oil and grease in soils irrigated with greywater and their potential role in soil water repellency. *Science of the Total Environment,* 394(1): 68–74.

UNEP. (1991). Environmental guidelines for municipal wastewater reuse in the Mediterranean region. In: Tedeschi, S. and Pescod, M. B. (eds.) Mediterranean Action Plan – Priority Actions Programme. Split, Yugoslavia: Regional Activity Centre.

USEPA. (2012). Guidelines for Water Reuse. EPA/600/R-12/618. Washington, DC: United States Environmental Protection Agency.

Wallach, R., Ben-Arie, O. & Graber, E. R. (2005). Soil water repellency induced by long-term irrigation with treated sewage effluent. *Journal of Environmental Quality,* 34(5): 1910–1920.

WHO. (1973). Guidelines for the Safe Use of Wastewater and Excreta in Agriculture and Aquaculture. Technical Report Series, No. 517. Geneva: WHO.

WHO. (1989a). Guidelines for the Safe Use of Wastewater and Excreta in Agriculture and Aquaculture. Measures for Public Health Protection. Geneva: WHO.

WHO. (1989b). Health Guidelines for the Use of Wastewater in Agriculture and Aquaculture. Technical Report Series, No. 776. Geneva: WHO.

WHO. (2004). Guidelines for Drinking-Water Quality. Geneva: WHO.

WHO. (2006). Guidelines for the Safe Use of Wastewater, Excreta and Greywater, Volume I: Policy and Regulatory Aspects. Geneva: WHO, UNEP.

WHO. (2011). Guidelines for Drinking-Water Quality. Geneva: WHO.

Wiel-Shafran, A., Ronen, Z., Weisbrod, N., Adar, E. & Gross, A. (2006). Potential changes in soil properties following irrigation with surfactant-rich greywater. *Ecological Engineering,* 26(4): 348–354.

Wu, B. (2019). Membrane-based technology in greywater reclamation: a review. *Science and Total Environment,* 656: 184–200.

14 Impact of Genetically Modified Organisms on Environment and Health

Bingshati Sarkar, Ushmita Gupta Bakshi,
Chandini Sayeed and Srijan Goswami*

CONTENTS

14.1 INTRODUCTION

The father of medicine, the great Hippocrates, said that food is our medicine. He also indicated that, just as food can be used as medicine, it can also engender chronic diseases. While we are talking about "food," the hot budding issues these days are genetically modified foods. When we go to the market to buy fruit, vegetables, dairy, and meat we find two sections: one for genetically modified food and the other for organic food. The question arises: why this differentiation? Are there any genuine differences between the two? The honest answer is that there is a huge difference because the food has been genetically modified, which academically means it is different at a molecular level compared to its natural form. Now what that actually means nobody knows for sure – are the genetically modified foods going to help us lead a healthy life or make us prone to chronic illnesses? We have to understand that God and Mother Nature are smarter than humans and manmade technologies, and historically whenever we have attempted to manipulate nature, it hasn't really worked out that well. So if we had to make a decision

* Corresponding author: Bingshati Sarkar. bingshati980@gmail.com

DOI: 10.1201/9781003095422-14

based on (the holistic point of view) the nature of existence of the human body and its relationship to planet Earth (because we are part of the environment we live in), it is essential that we respect Mother Nature as it is meant to be. But the problem is our arrogance based on the knowledge that we have and the assumption that we can challenge and change Nature according to our own will. So the genuine evidence-based scientific research about whether genetically modified food is making us healthy or making us prone to chronic illnesses has not been done, and as a result we cannot objectively say yes or no. So we have to figure out intuitively which way to go (Smith, 2003, 2007; Null and Polonetsky, 2016; Shiva, 2016). This brings us to a statement made by Dr. David Suzuki:

> Anyone who says that GMOs are perfectly safe, is either unbelievably stupid, or deliberately lying. The reality is we don't know because the experiments simply haven't been done, and now we have become the guinea pigs.
>
> **Dr. David Suzuki**[1]

The present paper covers some aspects that indicate the possible and unpredictable dangers of genetically modified foods or organisms. It sheds light on the aspects that are generally ignored by mainstream researchers. The aim of the scientific community should be to point out the prevailing concerns regarding GMO (or any scientific and technological aspects) and address them in an evidence-based manner through thorough and in-depth research globally, instead of completely ignoring them and forcefully assuming that the science of GMO is 100% perfect.

14.2   GENETICALLY MODIFIED ORGANISMS

GMOs are those organisms whose genetic materials are forcefully modified (in a procedure that is not in tune with the environment we live in) using certain genetic engineering method. The basic motive behind this is to introduce a new trait to that very organism which otherwise cannot occur naturally. So basically genetic modification is a technology that involves changing an organism's DNA by altering an existing natural or native sequence(s) of the DNA or by inserting new genes altogether. The insertion of a desired gene to the organism is facilitated by several laboratory techniques such as gene cloning, DNA splicing, and insertion of genes into cells; collectively this is termed recombinant DNA technology. Once genetically modified, the organisms (be it plants or animals) receive the characteristics held within the genetic code of the desired gene. And in this way we, the humans, manipulate Nature by introducing new traits into a living organism.

> *Science is all about understanding how Nature works. But unfortunately with science we are trying to teach Nature, a lesson or two.*
>
> **Dr. B. M. Hegde**[2]

For example, introducing a pesticide-producing gene from *Bacillus thuringiensis* (a bacteria commonly found in the soil) into the genome of the cotton plant will result in production of a toxin by the genetically modified cotton plant (not found in native form) that destroys the intestinal lining of the insect that feeds upon the plant, making the plant pest-resistant.

> You cannot insert a gene you took from a bacteria into a seed and call it life. You haven't created a life, instead you have polluted it.
>
> **Dr. Vandana Shiva**

In order to produce a GMO certain steps need to be followed (Figure 14.1).

- Step 1: The gene of interest is identified and isolated.
- Step 2: The gene of interest is amplified into multiple copies.
- Step 3: Specific promoter and poly A tail are joined to the gene of interest, followed by insertion into plasmids.
- Step 4: The plasmid is inserted in bacteria, multiplied, and a cloned construct is recovered for injection.
- Step 5: The recovered cloned construct is transferred into recipient tissue.
- Step 6: The cloned gene is integrated into the recipient genome.
- Step 7: The inserted gene is expressed in the recipient genome.
- Step 8: The inserted gene is inherited in subsequent generations.

There are mainly 10 common genetically modified crops available commercially: alfa alfa, corn, sugar beet, papaya, canola, soybeans, squash, cotton, apple, potato.

In 2007, for the 12th consecutive year, the global area used for genetically modified crops continued to increase up to 12% across 23 countries. Principal crops

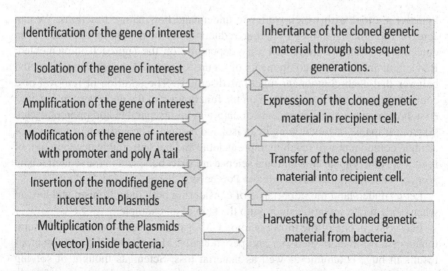

FIGURE 14.1 Steps involved in the production of genetically modified organisms (Beardmore and Porter 2003).

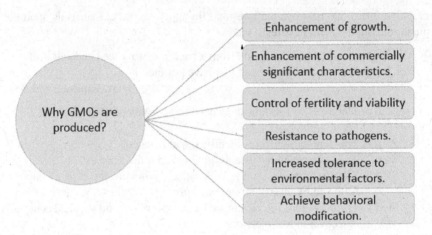

FIGURE 14.2   Reasons for producing genetically modified organisms (GMOs) (Beardmore and Porter 2003).

such as soybean and maize along with other crops such as cotton, canola, and rice showed a subsequent increment. Genetically modified salmon, which grows twice as fast as normal fish, will be marketed soon globally (Beardmore and Porter, 2003). The major reasons for producing GMOs are presented in Figure 14.2.

14.3   GENETIC MODIFICATION: THE REDUCTIONISTIC AND HOLISTIC VIEW POINT

Science is a tool with which we try to understand how nature functions. We can achieve this understanding by either reductionistic or a holistic approach. The outcome of scientific study will vary depending on the approach implemented. Reductionism views the components of nature as arts making up a mashine, and believes that each component functions discretely. The addition or removal of a component part will have no effect on the functioning of the entire system. In contrast, holism views the components of nature as an inseparable and interconnected system incapable of functioning in an isolated manner. The addition or removal of a single component will result in unpredictable and uncontrollable degeneration of function. Adherents to conventional science are strict believers in the reductionistic point of view (Lipton, 2016; Null and Polonetsky, 2016).

Let us understand the importance of considering both reductionism and holism when designing a scientific study with the help of an example.

Flavr Savr is one of the most common GMOs developed by Monsanto. Natural tomatoes have a short shelf life and perish easily. This fast spoilage of tomatoes results in huge economic as well as material loss. Scientists thought of solving this real-life problem using genetic engineering technology. If observed from a reductionistic point of view, the short shelf life of the tomato is a weakness of nature and modifying its genetic makeup using modern technology and replacing the undesirable gene with a gene that enables a longer shelf life sounds like a great scientific achievement. Because of sophisticated genetic engineering technology, the modern-day Flavr Savr tomatoes of Monsanto not only have a longer shelf life but also have enhanced flavor as well as antibiotic resistance compared to natural tomatoes.

But when analyzed from a holistic perspective, changing the genetic characteristic of the organism converts it to a form that is not compatible with the normal ecological web. The GMO can be seen as a misfit in the surrounding environment and leads to ecological incompatibility. Such ecological incompatibility has the potential to cause unpredictable and uncontrollable disruption of ecological balance, leading to deterioration of health and environment. By genetically modifying one particular organism we are breaking the pathways through which organisms were meant to function naturally (Smith, 2007; Druker, 2015; Perro and Adams, 2017).

In the past few years the scientific community has acknowledged that human health and environment are related and cannot be isolated from each other. So they felt the need to integrate various aspects related to health and the environment. The scientific term is the "One Health" concept. The One Health concept recognizes that the health of people is connected to the health of animals and the environment (Figure 14.3).

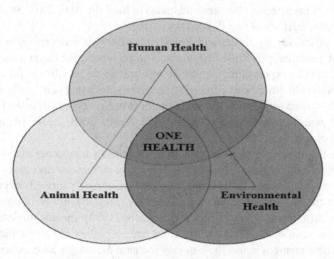

FIGURE 14.3 Relation between human health, animal health, and environmental health (Holistic Perspective – One Health Concept).

14.4 GENETICALLY MODIFIED FOOD AND AGRICULTURAL OUTCOME

In recent times genetically modified crops have proved themselves handy and useful enough if being judged superficially. They provide us with a much wider selection of traits for improvement (that is, not only pest, disease and herbicide resistance – which had already been achieved – but also potentially drought resistance, increased nutritional content, and improved sensory properties). These methods are fast and cost-effective, they help to bring about a desired change within very few generations, and they reduce the risk of occurrence of undesirable traits. It is widely claimed that an increase in genetically modified crops will satiate world hunger of the ever-growing population. However, if we delve deeper into this matter we will realize that "all that glitters is not gold." GMOs do more harm than good (Pusztai, 2003; Smith, 2003; Adams, 2016; Gillam, 2017; Cohen, 2019). Below a few examples will prove how unpredictable and devastating genetically modified crops can be for a human body.

First, though genetically modified crops have to date had a great deal of media attention, most of the general public remain largely unaware of what a genetically modified crop is or how it harms us in the cruelest of cruel ways. Scientists have speculated that rises in reproductive problems, infertility, and low-birth-weight babies since the mid-1990s may be due to the introduction of genetically modified crops (Pusztai, 2003; Smith, 2003, 2007; Adams, 2016; Null and Polonetsky, 2016).

Second, according to Fagan et al. (2014) genetic engineering processes and recombinant DNA technology may cause potential changes in either naturally occurring proteins produced by plants or metabolic pathways which result in the production of unexpected allergens and toxins in food (Pusztai, 2003; Smith, 2003, 2007; Adams, 2016; Null and Polonetsky, 2016).

Third, in a study by Butler and Reichhardt (1999) it was proposed that production of genetically modified bean plants to increase cysteine and methionine content results in expression of a protein of a transgene which was proved to be highly reactive. In other cases certain studies have shown that genetically modified soy contains seven times more trypsin inhibitor (a certain type of allergen) than soy that is not genetically modified (Pusztai, 2003; Smith, 2003, 2007; Adams, 2016; Null and Polonetsky, 2016).

Fourth, the number of enzymes which are encoded by transgenes may disrupt or alter biochemical pathways, possibly resulting in an increase or decrease of certain biochemical components. Besides this, the presence of newly formed enzymes may disturb the enzyme–substrate balance, which may result in build-up of unnecessary chemicals. Also, according to Conner and Jacobs (1999), the enzymes expressed by transgenes can diverge metabolites from one secondary metabolic pathway to another. These changes in metabolism may increase the body's toxin concentration (Pusztai, 2003; Smith, 2003, 2007; Adams, 2016; Null and Polonetsky, 2016).

Fifth, the forceful and random insertion of mutagenesis may result in many catastrophes. It may disrupt or change the pre-existing gene expression of a host plant, then it may cause changes in the endogenous gene, and it may even produce fusion protein from plant DNA and inserted DNA. This may in turn lead to the expression of protein and toxic compounds in the edible portion of the plant (Pusztai, 2003; Smith, 2007; Adams, 2016; Perro and Adams, 2017; Cohen, 2019).

Sixth, the involvement of antibiotic-resistant genes as selectable markers may lead to the production of antibiotic-resistant bacterial strains, and this is potentially problematic for health. According to Steinbrecher (1996), as a disease-resistant plant mostly deals with viral disease, it may produce a viral strain which in turn will lead to new disease. According to certain reports the recombination of naturally occurring viral nucleic acid with the new viral fragment may create many new variations which can be potentially problematic for health (Pusztai, 2003; Smith, 2003, 2007; Adams, 2016; Null and Polonetsky, 2016).

> Researchers say the Bt toxin insecticides in the DNA of the GMO crops are safe for human consumption. But independent scientific evidence disagrees. There are evidence that these endotoxins, so called Cry Proteins, are both allergens and have adverse effects on immune system and gut. And it should also be pointed out that there are sequence similarities between some of these Cry Proteins and known human allergens.
>
> **Dr. Michael Hansen**[3]

In other studies it has been noticed that the introduction of recombinant DNA technology reduces the nutritional value of food material instead of increasing it. Nowadays, although genetically modified soybean is gradually replacing conventional soybean, a study notes that herbicide-resistant soybean has a 12–14% reduced phytoestrogen level in comparison to its conventional counterpart. In these genetically modified plants two key ingredients, genistin and diadzin (the main source of phytoestrogen), are present in much reduced quantities. As a result it can be presumed that genetically modified soybean is a less potent source of clinically relevant phytoestrogen.

When tested on other animals genetically modified crops had an adverse effect. One study showed that when rats or salmon were fed genetically modified crops they showed symptoms such as increased weight gain, changes in immune system, and changes in intestinal structure (Ewen and Pusztai, 1999). Moreover in this study by Ewen and Pusztai (1999), when rats were fed with genetically modified potatoes expressing genes for lectin *Glanthus nivalis*, they suffered damage to gut mucosa. This is why more and more doctors are prescribing a diet free from genetic modification (Pusztai, 2003; Druker, 2015; Adams, 2016).

14.5 GENETICALLY MODIFIED MEAT AND DAIRY

Genetic modification has also had a huge impact on the meat and dairy industry. In addition to the ethical issues there are various points people are overlooking while consuming these foods. The genetic modification which enhances the growth rate of certain animals results in some of the most devastating side effects. As a result of the genetic modification these animals suffer from deformities, feeding and breathing difficulties, and have a low tolerance for disease. Unregulated gene expression along with high copy number may result in over- or underproduction of gene products. Possible side effects can be seen; examples include growth hormone transgenic swine that developed arthritis, altered skeletal growth, cardiomegaly, dermatitis, gastric ulcers, and renal disease. As a result of insertional mutations some of the essential biological pathways can be altered, disrupting metabolism. There is a risk that new disease formed due to the genetic engineering process can spread from transgenic animals to normal animals and even to humans. Many genetically modified embryos cannot thrive for long.

Genetically engineered meat or dairy products usually result in similar harmful side effects in the human body as do genetically modified crops. In humans hey mainly cause obesity, immunological disorder, autoimmune disease, and organ dysfunction. Genetically modified food may push human beings towards a new disease (Adams, 2016; Druker, 2015; Null and Polonetsky, 2016; Gillam, 2017; Perro and Adams, 2017; Cohen, 2019).

14.5.1 ETHICAL ISSUE

Genetic engineering violates the basic rights of animals and it modifies them in such a way that, instead of being beneficial, results in pain and discomfort.

14.6 GENETICALLY MODIFIED FOOD: HEALTH CONCERNS

GMOs were introduced in agriculture globally to maximize crop yield and ensure sufficient quality food for the ever-growing population. Companies like Monsanto, Eli Lilly, and DuPont among many others sell about 90% of genetically modified crops all over the world. Ever since the first genetically modified plant was produced in 1983, the technology has boomed with each passing years. After marketing approval of transgenic Flavr Savr tomato was granted by the US Food and Drug Administration (FDA) in 1994, a number of transgenic crops received marketing approval in 1995. These crops include canola with modified oil composition (Calgene), cotton resistant to the herbicide bromoxynil (Calgene), Bt cotton (Monsanto), Bt potatoes (Monsanto), soy bean resistant to glyphosate (Calgene), virus-resistant squash (Asgrow), and many more. Despite such a huge response, genetically modified crops were accepted by everyone. Scientists and activists have raised certain points against genetically modified crops which cannot be completely ignored. In this segment such points are mentioned for the sake of clarity.

According to the report of certain environmental activists, companies like Monsanto, Eli Lilly, and DuPont had long been producing fertilizers, pesticides, and other chemical-based farming supplements. With the introduction of GMOs in the market they initiated promotion of mass production of these artificial crops, seeds, and other organisms and/or "organic" product at a huge rate. This is because they turned out to be a huge money spinner with their apparent disease resistance, high yield, and labor-saving cultivation. However this came at a staggering cost.

To begin with, the health threats and dangers posed by these novel organisms are tremendous (Null and Polonetsky, 2016).

A chemical herbicide Roundup, produced by the US-based organization Monsanto, contains glyphosate as its active ingredient and has been the number-one selling herbicide worldwide since at least 1980. But glyphosate was patented in 1964 not as a herbicide but as a broad-spectrum chelator which reacts with a lot of soil minerals together, thereby blocking the plant's access to vital soil nutrients. This also kills the beneficial soil's microorganisms and promotes pathogenic growth in the soil, resulting in weaker plants and stronger disease, which ultimately kills the plant. Now, Monsanto scientists found these bacteria growing in a chemical waste dump in the presence of Roundup herbicide, which was highly irregular. Genes from these bacteria were used to create Roundup Ready soybean which, when spread with herbicide didn't die, although the remaining plant diversity in the field disintegrated. Roundup Ready crops like corn, soy, and canola are primary fodder for US livestock. With the ingestion of such nutrient-deficient food the livestock are growing weaker. One of the top researchers in this field, Dr. Arpad Pusztai of Rowett Research Institute, had to take a lot of flak for his work on these aspects of genetically modified crops.

Activists and researchers like Mr. Jeffrey Smith and Dr. Rima Laibow also found out that these crops are directly responsible for allergies, toxins, new diseases, and nutritional problems among test subjects in a lab, such as rats or other rodents. In his book *Genetic Roulette* Mr. Jeffery Smith, an activist against genetically modified food and the founder of the Institute of Responsible Technology, campaigned fiercely against US food safety policies and revealed the *entente cordiale* between biotechnology giants like Monsanto and the FDA (Smith, 2007; Null and Polonetsky, 2016). According to Smith, when the US government ignored repeated warnings by its own scientists and allowed untested genetically modified crops into our environment and food supply, this was a gamble of unprecedented proportions. The health of all living things and all future generations was put at risk by an infant technology. After two decades physicians and scientists have uncovered a grave trend. The same serious health problems found in lab animals, livestocks, and pets that have been consuming genetically modified foods are now on the rise in the US population, as Smith claims. He also added that when people stopped eating genetically modified foods their heath improved.

> Monsanto's roundup has been linked to over 29 diseases according to peer-reviewed research, including: DNA damage, liver cancer, lymphoma, skin cancer, hormonal disorders, kidney damage, infertility etc. …
>
> **Dr. Stephanie Seneff (Samsel and Seneff, 2013)**

Drug evaluator of Health Canada Dr. Shiv Chopra says that 90% of all our foods are the result of such genetic modifications or at least they are contaminated.[4] In a study by Professor Gillis Eric Seralini it was shown that when rats are fed with genetically modified crops (genetically modified maize NK603, MON 810, MON 863) and Roundup Ready diet in all possible combinations the kidney and liver, the dietary detoxifying organs, were affected.[5] In this case other effects were also noticed in the heart, adrenal glands, spleen, and hematopoietic system. The data highlights from that study led researchers to the conclusion that the rats were primarily showing hepato-renal toxicity and metabolic consequences due to genetic modifications. Many other similar studies showed that animals fed with genetically modified crops exhibit symptoms such as cancer of the mammary glands in females (equivalent to breast cancer in humans), cancer of the renal tract, reproductive failure, triggering of autoimmune disease, accelerated aging, organ damage, and gastrointestinal distress.

> Our gut bacteria contains same metabolic pathway found in plants that is targeted and disrupted by roundup. Is it any wonder that leaky gut syndrome, IBD [inflammatory bowel disease], colitis and other gastrointestinal diseases have spiked since the onset of Roundup Ready GMO crops?
>
> **Dr. Stephanie Seneff (Samsel and Seneff, 2013)**

14.7 CONCLUSION

> Judging by the absence of published data in peer-reviewed scientific literature, apparently no human clinical trials with GM foods have ever been conducted.
>
> **Dr. Arpad Pusztai (Ewen and Pusztai, 1999)**

Through the course of evolution humans have learned how to rationalize every aspect of their life. With this analytical power people should evaluate the pros and cons of all new technologies presented before them. Instead of blindly following, they should ask for proper details about the food they are consuming in their daily life. Moreover people should ask for proper validation and claims for a label in regard to genetically modified crops. In addition there should be properly validated and substantiated seminal research which will provide compelling evidence to help explain the deteriorating health of people worldwide, especially children, and the entire global population feeding on transgenic crops, to offer a plan to protect ourselves and our future.

> The food you eat can either be safest & most powerful form of medicine or the slowest form of poison
>
> **Ann Wigmore[6]**

NOTES

1   www.betterworld.net/quotes/GMO.htm.
2   www.youtube.com/watch?v=r0rRgvhNy1U.
3   https://foodrevolution.org/blog/former-pro-gmo-scientist/.
4   https://filmsfortheearth.org/en/films/seeds-of-death.
5   https://filmsfortheearth.org/en/films/seeds-of-death.
6   www.goodreads.com/author/quotes/385454.Ann_Wigmore.

REFERENCES

Adams, M. (2016). Food Forensics: The Hidden Toxins Lurking in Your Food and How You Can Avoid Them for Lifelong Health. USA: BenBella Books.

Beardmore, J.A. and Porter, J.S. (2003). Genetically modified organisms and aquaculture. *FAO Fisheries Circular* no. 989. Rome: FAO.

Butler, D. and Reichhardt, T. (1999). Long-term effect of GM crops serves up food for thought. Nature, 98(6729): 651–656.

Cohen, M. (2019). The Fight Against Monsanto's Roundup: The Politics of Pesticides. USA: Skyhorse Publishing.

Conner, A.J. and Jacobs, J.M. (1999). Genetic engineering of crops as potential source of genetic hazard in the human diet. Mutation Research, 443(1–2): 223–234.

Druker, S. (2015). Altered Genes, Twisted Truth: How the Venture to Genetically Engineer Our Food Has Subverted Science, Corrupted Government, and Systematically Deceived the Public. USA: Clear River Press.

Ewen, S.W.B. and Pusztai, A. (1999). Effect of diets containing genetically modified potatoes expressing *Galanthus nivalis* lectin on rat small intestine. Lancet, 354(9187): 1353–1354.

Fagan, J., Antoniou, M. and Robinson, C. (2014). GMO Myths and Truths, 2nd edition, version 1.0. Great Britain: Earth Open Source. https://earthopensource.org/wordpress/downloads/GMO-Myths-and-Truths-edition2.pdf.

Gillam, C. (2017). Whitewash: The Story of a Weed Killer, Cancer and the Corruption of Science, 3rd ed. USA: Island Press.

Lipton, B.H. (2016) The Biology of Belief. Unleashing the Power of Consciousness, Matter & Miracles, 18th reprint. India: Hay House Publishers.

Null, G. and Polonetsky, R. [Maxious NL]. (2016, July, 28) Seeds of Death: Unveiling the Lies of GMO [Video]. YouTube. www.youtube.com/watch?v=z64syQoixyk, accessed on November 15, 2020.

Perro, M. and Adams, V. (2017). What's Making Our Children Sick?: How Industrial Food is Causing an Epidemic of Chronic Illness, and What Parents (and their Doctors) Can Do About It, 1st ed. USA: Chelsea Green Publishing.

Pusztai, A. (2003). Genetically Modified Foods: Potential Human Health Effects. In Food Safety: Contaminants and Toxins (ed. J.P.F. D'Mello). USA: CAB International.

Samsel, A. and Seneff, S. (2013). Glyphosate, pathways to modern diseases II: celiac sprue and gluten intolerance. Interdisciplinary Toxicology, 6(4): 159–184. https://doi.org/10.2478/intox-2013-0026.

Shiva, V. (2016). Seed Sovereignty, Food Security. Women in the Vanguard of the Fight against GMOs and Corporate Agriculture. North Atlantic Books.

Smith, J. (2003). Seeds of Deception: Exposing Industry and Government Lies About the Safety of the Genetically Engineered Foods You're Eating. Yes! Books.

Smith, J. (2007). Genetic Roulette: The Documented Health Risks of Genetically Engineered Foods. Yes! Books.

Steinbrecher, R.A. (1996). From green to gene revolution. The environmental risks of genetically engineered crops, vol. 26, issue 6, pp. 273–281. London: Test Tube Harvest Campaign, Women's Environmental Network.

Unit VI

Successful Models of Waste Management

15 Solid Waste Management Models
Past, Present and Future

Rojita Mishra, Amrita Kumari Panda* and Satpal Singh Bisht

CONTENTS

15.1 INTRODUCTION

Solid waste management is a multifaceted process comprising various steps, such as source separation, recycling and treatment (Xiao et al., 2020). Population growth, urban densification and industrialization are the three primary reasons for the increased generation of solid waste (Zhang et al., 2010). Reduction of waste at source by recycling is continuously encouraged to lessen the load on incineration and landfill (Hearn and Ballard, 2005). Conventional waste disposal techniques cause a great deal of harm, such as groundwater and soil contamination, air pollution, harm to ecosystem, greenhouse gas (GHG) emissions, loss of biodiversity and human health loss. The ideal waste management methods decrease waste production and environmental and social problems and increase energy production (Yousefloo & Babazadeh, 2020). The hierarchy of waste management comprises various steps, i.e. waste minimization, recycling, waste-to-energy conversion and disposal.

Waste treatment strategies have gained more attention during the last decade due to their impact on economic growth, environmental protection and human health (Soltani et al., 2015). Maximum waste management models consider

* Corresponding author: Amrita Kumari Panda. itu.linu@gmail.com

DOI: 10.1201/9781003095422-15

environmental and economic aspects, but very few consider social features. A sustainable waste management model needs to be economically reasonable, environmentally safe and socially tolerable. Petts (2000) said that "the most effective management of solid waste has to relate to local environmental, economic and social priorities" and must go for the conventional approaches that require active community involvement. Recent waste management models imitate a change in policy where integrated solid waste management is applied instead of landfill and incineration (Behzad et al., 2020; Hosseinalizadeh et al., 2020; Hrabec et al., 2020; Oh and Hettiarachchi, 2020; Olapiriyakul et al., 2019; Perteghella et al., 2020). The present chapter covers various models designed for integrated solid waste management.

15.2 SOLID WASTE GENERATION AND IMPACTS ON ENVIRONMENT

Solid waste comprises various kinds of waste (sorted waste, mixed urban waste, waste from public spaces and hospital waste) collected from residential, industrial, institutional, commercial, destruction, land dissipating or construction sources through numerous means, including door-to-door, curb side pick-up, community bins, self-delivered and contracted service (Hoornweg and Bhada-Tata, 2012). During the last decade significant improvements and innovations have been made in waste management methodologies to combat social and environmental impacts (de Oliveira, 2019). Incineration is one of the most popular methods of solid waste management when there is no option of reusing the waste (Brunner and Rechberger, 2015). Incineration methods reduce land utilization as well as avoid detrimental impacts on the environment but generate byproducts such as 25–30% bottom ash and 1–3% fly ash (Quina et al., 2018). Leachable volatile heavy metals (Ni, Zn, Cu, Hg, As, Cr and Cd) are found in fly ash, thus fly ash generated from solid waste incineration plants is treated as toxic waste and intended for landfill. Due to an upsurge in landfill costs and decrease in landfill sites acceptable treatment of fly ash and its recycling is more likely to be the option rather than landfill (Assi et al., 2020). There has been a drive towards altering solid waste management from landfill to zero-waste programs due to the rising significance of space and urban densification in the largest cities of the world. The regulations and unquestionable exhaustion of some materials endorse the benefits of conversion of waste from anthropogenic sources into efforts that should be reintegrated into their unique production cycles or into other consumer goods (Paes et al., 2019). Toxic waste such as e-waste from electronic equipment was estimated to have increased by 200–500% in countries like China, India, Brazil and South Africa according to a study from the United Nations Environment Program (UNEP). *The Global E-waste Monitor* report stated that 1.5 million tons of electronic waste (7.1 kg per citizen) was generated in Brazil during the year 2016. This amount is almost similar to that of other developing countries like India, Indonesia and Russia (Balde et al., 2017).

15.3   SOLID WASTE MANAGEMENT APPROACHES

Solid waste is defined as any waste or garbage produced either from a waste water plant in the form of sludge, or any discarded solid from industrial, agricultural activities, water treatment plant operations, mining residues, municipal garbage, commercial waste and waste generated from animal husbandary activities (OECD 2001). The rate of waste production rises in the world from day to day at an alarming rate. There are reports that cities throughout the world produced 2.01 billion tonnes of solid waste in 2016; that is equivalent to 0.74 kg/day per person. This yearly waste generation is projected to increase from 2.01 to 3.40 billion tonnes in the year 2050 (Kaza et al., 2018).

Failure to manage solid waste properly creates serious environmental pollution and degradation in many metropolitan cities of the world (Obi, 2016; Haraguchi et al., 2019). Poor waste disposal processes produce GHGs that emit and absorb infrared energy, leading to the greenhouse effect (Banyai et al., 2019). An incineration approach emits a diversity of pollutants such as furans and dioxins (Tchobanoglous and Kreith, 2002), tenacious organic pollutants that harm human and ecological health. A landfill waste management approach emits GHGs, for example, methane, as organic waste decomposes. Badly managed waste functions as a propagation ground for many pathogenic microorganisms and disease vectors, adds to global climate change through methane production and promotes metropolitan violence.

Waste management is costly and uses around 20–50% of municipal funds. Operating this indispensable municipal amenity needs integrated systems that must be sustainable, efficient and socially sustained. Innovative waste management methods are required for effective execution of waste-to-energy technology.

Solid waste is divided into diverse kinds of waste, e.g. industrial waste, municipal waste, hazardous waste, etc. Over the years, waste disposal has been processed; however, in recent decades the handling and disposal of waste have been addressed differently with an energy recovery drive. Various organizations such as the World Bank, Asian Development Bank and the Asia-Pacific Economic Cooperation (APEC) play key roles in sustainable green energy development in the Southeast Asian region by using appropriate business models (Tun et al., 2020). The percentage of landfill is noticeably decreased, while the percentage of eco-friendly waste treatment technologies such as composting, biogas and electricity plants has increased dramatically in recent years (Figure 15.1). During the 1970s the first solid waste management models were optimization models and were directed at a specific problem, for example, vehicle routing. Vehicle routing mainly depends on the vehicle capacity and collection points. Fuel consumption by such vehicles leads to carbon emission and fuel cost.

A recent model developed by Sarmah et al. (2019) helped policy makers to make decisions on waste collection and vehicle routing. They considered two factors for this model: (1) ward clustering; and (2) variation in waste production. Sarmah et al. (2019) applied Wright's algorithm to cluster wards on the basis of vehicle capability and cost-saving matrix.

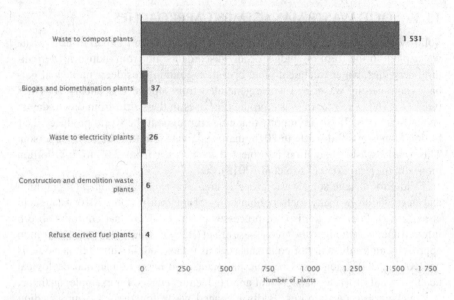

FIGURE 15.1   Types of solid waste treatment plants in India as of December 2019 (www.statista.com/statistics/1061462/india-solid-waste-treatment-plants-by-type/).

The models established during the 1980s stretched the system boundaries of the previously developed models and covered solid waste management at system level. Rogers (2001) categorized waste management models into two categories: (1) models that use optimizing methods; and (2) those that practice compromising methods. The models looked at the interactions between various factors rather than at each individually in the waste management system (Morissey and Browne 2004). These models were mainly designed to reduce the costs of mixed waste management and recycling was involved to some extent.

15.4   MIXED-INTEGER LINEAR PROGRAMMING MODEL

Mohammadi et al. (2018) designed a general mixed-integer linear programming (MILP) model that covers collection of waste from several cities, separation at separation points/dump sites, waste treatment and recycling in plants and lastly selling the end products to the market. This model was directed to dispense the optimal quantity of waste to all supply chain organizations and also to distribute the products to consumers, in addition to exploiting the total net yield of the supply chain network in terms of shipping, storage, packing and production capacity restrictions imposed by separation centers, distribution centers and waste-processing plants. The MILP model also controls the magnitude of waste delivered from cities to separation centers and further to recycling plants, the quantity of waste relocated to varied processing technologies and amount and the types of products directed from processing plants to distribution centers and lastly to market places in cities.

15.5 COST–BENEFIT ANALYSIS MODELS

Cost–benefit analysis models are framed by considering monetary terms (Finnveden and Moberg, 2005; Hansjurgens, 2004; Morrissey and Browne, 2004). Cost–benefit analysis models follow six basic steps (EC, 2008), depicted in Figure 15.2, where losses are presented as costs and benefits as gains in environment. Benefits and costs are how an individual wants to pay to obtain gains or how much an individual is willing to accept as a loss (Pearce et al., 2006). Cost–benefit analysis is preferred as it takes into account all positive and negative impacts. The uncertainty can be overcome by risk assessment.

In this model selection of discount rate and analysis are critical factors. A cost–benefit analysis model compares various solid waste recycling strategies to determine their cost-effectiveness. A recent study by Hsu (2021) reported a cost–benefit analysis evaluating the cost-effectiveness between three feasible recycling methods – composting, biogas power generation and biomass fuel – for agricultural waste management in Taiwan. Hsu (2021) suggested creating co-processing centers within the agricultural industry and using biogas slurry on the farm to improve the cost-effectiveness of agricultural waste recycling in comparison to current waste-recycling measures.

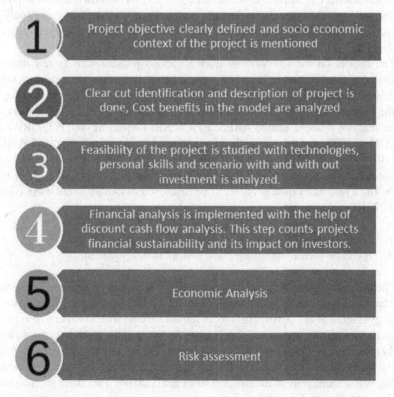

1. Project objective clearly defined and socio economic context of the project is mentioned

2. Clear cut identification and description of project is done, Cost benefits in the model are analyzed

3. Feasibility of the project is studied with technologies, personal skills and scenario with and with out investment is analyzed.

4. Financial analysis is implemented with the help of discount cash flow analysis. This step counts projects financial sustainability and its impact on investors.

5. Economic Analysis

6. Risk assessment

FIGURE 15.2 Diagrammatic representation of cost–benefit analysis models.

A recent study reported a new quantitative decision support model: the Waste to Energy Recovery Assessment (WERA) framework, to assess diverse thermo-chemical treatment methods of municipal wastes (Haraguchi et al., 2019). This framework interrelates benefits through electricity generation, emissions and also the related social cost of carbon.

The cost–benefit analysis model has a shortcoming in the analysis of costs and benefits, and comparative analysis (Gasparatos et al., 2008). Discounting is the most significant part of this model in which comparative analysis of future and present cost–benefit assembly is done (Hansjurgens, 2004).

15.6   LIFE CYCLE ANALYSIS MODELS

Management of solid waste and the effects of solid waste minimization to the environment can be analyzed using life cycle analysis models (Chubbs and Steiner, 1998). This model mainly helps assess the utilization of raw materials and energy sources (Marano and Rogers, 1999). It analyzes the impact of the waste manage-ment process on the receptor surface, like land, water and air and transfer of envir-onmental burdens to another stage of the life cycle (Young-Jin and Rousseaux, 2001). Life cycle analysis is broadly divided into four different phases following the International Organization for Standardization (ISO) standard and these phases are interrelated. The four phases include goal and scope phase, inventory analysis, impact assessment and interpretation (ISO, 2006). A typical life cycle analysis model can be divided into three parts, as shown in Figure 15.3.

The impact on the environment during various phases, such as raw material acquisition, manufacturing, use and reuse of material, transportation and waste treatment, is calculated in the second important phase of model design and finally all the products released can be estimated (Ramakrishna, 2013). There are six life cycle analysis models, named ARES, EPIC/CSR, IWM2, MSW-DST, ORWARE and UMBERTO, and these models were analyzed by Winkler (2004) and Winkler and Bilitewski (2007). These researchers attempted to compare quantitatively the six models and discuss in detail their similarities and differences. The application of the life cycle analysis approach can be discussed in two different ways (Gentil et al., 2010):

1. It can be used for technology development.
2. It can be used in monitoring and historical development.

The life cycle analysis model has improved but it requires more time and money. One has to choose carefully the process to meet the need and fit the life cycle meth-odology (Gentil et al., 2010). This model requires technological experts; it is best if it can be hired from an external source as in such a case the stake holders are more likely to believe in the model. This model has developed a more user-friendly meth-odology to make it easy for common people to understand and interpret the data during waste management treatment (Gentil et al., 2010). Two main shortcomings

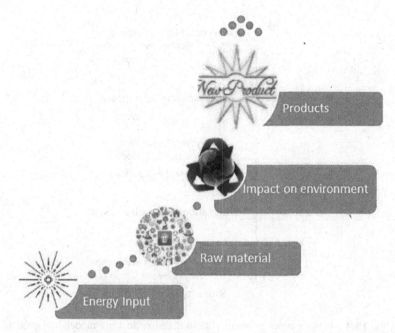

FIGURE 15.3 Diagrammatic representation of life cycle analysis models (adapted from Ramakrishna, 2013).

of life cycle analysis include difficulties in collecting marginal data accurately and that the prediction of a final result is not certain because of huge data requirement.

15.7 MULTI-CRITERIA DECISION ANALYSIS MODELS

Multi-criteria decision analysis models involve three basic steps. First it identifies the problem and organizes it properly; secondly the model is made and evaluated; and thirdly a well-planned action plan is developed based on the model (Belton and Stewart, 2002). The main advantage of this method is that decision makers are free to choose according to the application performance scores, measurement is quantified using various units and there are ample alternatives for selection. Each alternative can be easily compared and it is applicable for each criterion (Achillas et al., 2013). This method is effective in complex analysis; it has provided a plasticity irrespective of using quantitative data and qualitative data. The most important thing is this can satisfy a wider range of stakeholders (Mendoza and Martins, 2006). There are five multicriteria decision analysis models, discussed further for better understanding in Figure 15.4.

There are two main shortcomings of multicriteria analysis models (Table 15.1). These models do not take consideration of risks and their impacts (Karmperis et al.,

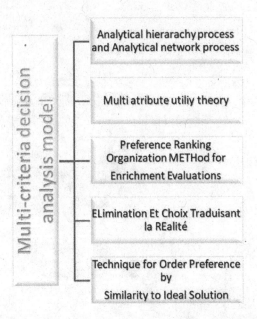

FIGURE 15.4 Various types of multi-criteria decision analysis models (adapted from Soltani et al., 2015).

2012). They do not provide information regarding waste management like waste minimization and waste prevention (Morissey and Browne, 2004).

15.8 MATHEMATICAL MODELING-BASED MODELS

Development of new software technologies and internet leads to frame more useful modeling system for waste management (Rada et al., 2013). Moutavtchi et al. (2010) developed a model named WAMED, which helps model solid waste management on a regional scale. This model aims in the development of an integrated approach to decrease harmful effects on the environment and brings economic benefits. A few common steps are followed in various types of mathematical modeling, including: (1) collection of solid waste data; (2) database creation; (3) expansion of the database; (4) data input; (5) waste management modeling design and implementation; (6) analysis of output data; and (7) final model validation (Singh, 2019).

Mathematical modeling and its application in solid waste management can be categorized in four ways: (1) optimization models; (2) multi-objective approach; (3) multi-criteria decision analysis; and (4) artificial neural networks (Singh, 2019). The use and utilization of different mathematical modeling techniques are listed in Table 15.2.

TABLE 15.1
Comparative chart of multi-criteria decision analysis methods

Name of method	Approach	Advantage	Disadvantage	Available software	References
AHP and ANP (utility-based)	Pairwise comparisons of criteria to find out which criteria are more important than others. All individual criteria must be paired against all others and the results compiled in matrix form	1. Produce scores for each criterion 2. Generate inconsistency index relative to decision maker's inconsistency index	1. Loss of information 2. No possibility of using thresholds	• DECERNS • Criterium decision plus • Super decisions • Expert choice	Soltani et al., 2015 Kiker et al., 2005
MAUT (utility-based)	Convert the criteria units into the 0–1 utility scale. Single-attribute value and utility functions range from 0 (worst case) to 1 (best case), and multi-attribute value and utility functions, also ranging from 0 to 1, are constructed as sums or other aggregation of the single-attribute utility functions	1. Deal with uncertain information 2. Manage random and probabilistic input criteria values	1. No possibility of using thresholds 2. Bad performance on some criteria can be offset by good performance on others	• DecideIT • DECERNS	Cegan et al., 2017 Antunes et al., 2012
PROMETHEE (outranking)	Determine a preference function for each criterion, expressing the difference in performance of alternative a over alternative b	1. Higher compensation 2. Handle effectively different thresholds	1. Time-intensive threshold identification	• Visual PROMETHEE • D-Sight	Cinelli et al., 2014

(continued)

TABLE 15.1 Continued
Comparative chart of multi-criteria decision analysis methods

Name of method	Approach	Advantage	Disadvantage	Available software	References
ELECTRE (outranking)	Determine whether criteria of alternative a are the same as or better than those of b and also where criteria of a are not as good as those of b	1. Consider uncertainty and vagueness 2. Highly non-compensatory 3. Eliminate alternatives that perform excessively badly in any criteria	1. Outcomes are difficult to explain in lay terms 2. Lowest performances under certain criteria are not displayed	• ELECTRE IS • ELECTRE III-IV	Velasquez and Hester, 2013 Cinelli et al., 2014
TOPSIS	Selects the alternative that is the closest to the ideal solution and farthest from the negative ideal alternative	1. Weights of criteria are determined by means of entropy weight method 2. Ranking of waste treatment methods possible on the basis of distance of each waste treatment strategy from the overall best alternative treatment strategy and the overall worst alternative treatment strategy	1. Identify the preferable method of waste conversion, based on their respective performance in terms of pollutant production	• PyTOPS	Kaneesamkandi et al., 2020 Yadav et al., 2019

TABLE 15.2
Various types of mathematical models with advantages and disadvantages

Types of model	Mathematical approach	Outcome	Drawbacks	References
Optimization model	This model uses sequential quadratic programming (SQP) optimizer of ASPEN PLUS 12.1. Environment impact is evaluated by a waste reduction algorithm	This is an optimal economic and waste treatment process. The factors that mostly affect the waste treatment process are temperature, pressure and the residence time of the reactor along with the inlet feed flow rates	Not specified	Shadiya et al., 2012
Multi-objective approach	It uses multi-objective mixed-integer linear program along with optimization	This model is designed in such a way as to optimize six different environmental objectives inclusively	The critical factor for the outcome is determined by results of the sensitivity analysis	Vadenbo et al., 2014
Multi-criteria decision analysis	This model uses material flow analysis and multi-criteria decision analysis	Material flow analysis added an extra advantage when it is applied with multi-criteria decision analysis for solid waste management	This model can be successful based on the decision maker's performance. It requires an integrative approach for solid waste management	Makarichi et al., 2018
Artificial neural network analysis	Feed-forward non-linear autoregressive network with exogenous inputs is used in this model. It uses Fletcher–Powell's conjugate gradient as the algorithm	This model produced lowest testing mean square error and highest coefficient of determination in solid waste management	Appropriate input variable selection is essential to increase the modeling process	Younes et al. (2015)

15.9   CONCLUSIONS AND FUTURE PERSPECTIVES

The progress of solid waste management models during the last decade are mainly focused on integrated waste management approach with the conception of sustainable waste management. Five categories of models have been explained: cost–benefit analysis models, MILP models, life cycle analysis models, multi-criteria decision analysis models and mathematical modelling-based models. The non-involvement of all the stakeholders such as general public, local authorities, government and technical experts is the primary drawback of all the existing models. All the models discussed have advantages and limitations and none of the models individually can be considered as complete for sustainable waste management rather the combination of more than one model will be best option for sustainability. Integrated optimization modeling methodologies should be established for waste collection, transport and disposal. It is very important to explore how the amount and type of waste, logistic costs affect the sustainability metrics. Further research must be concentrated on design of effective algorithm based mathematical models to gain solutions on waste disposal by considering economic, environmental and social facets.

REFERENCES

Achillas, C., Moussiopoulos, N., Karagiannidis, A., Banias, G., & Perkoulidis, G. (2013). The use of multi-criteria decision analysis to tackle waste management problems: a literature review. Waste Management Research, 31(2), 115–129. http://dx.doi.org/10.1177/0734242X12470203.

Antunes, P., Santos, R., Videira, N., Colaco, F., Szanto, R., Dobos, E. R., Kovacs, S. J., & Vari, A. (2012). Approaches to integration in sustainability assessment of technologies. PROSUITE project. http://prosuite.org/c/document_library/get_-file?uuid=c378cd69-f785-40f2-b23e-ae676b939212&groupId=12772 (accessed on February 4, 2014).

Assi, A., Bilo, F., Zanoletti, A., Ponti, J., Valsesia, A., La Spina, R., ... & Bontempi, E. (2020). Zero-waste approach in municipal solid waste incineration: reuse of bottom ash to stabilize fly ash. Journal of Cleaner Production, 245, 118779.

Balde, C. P., Forti, V., Gray, V., Kuehr, R., & Stegmann, P. (2017). The Global E-waste Monitor. United Nations University (UNU), International Telecommunication Union (ITU) & International Solid Waste Association (ISWA), Bonn/Geneva/Vienna. 2017. Available online: https://collections.unu.edu/eserv/UNU:6341/GlobalEwaste_Monitor_2017__electronic_single_pages_.pdf (accessed on 17 September 2018).

Banyai, T., Tamás, P., Illés, B., Stankevičiūtė, Ž., & Bányai, Á. (2019). Optimization of municipal waste collection routing: impact of industry 4.0 technologies on environmental awareness and sustainability. International Journal of Environmental Research and Public Health, 16(4), 634.

Behzad, M., Zolfani, S. H., Pamucar, D., & Behzad, M. (2020). A comparative assessment of solid waste management performance in the Nordic countries based on BWM-EDAS. Journal of Cleaner Production, 266, 122008. https://doi.org/10.1016/j.jclepro.2020.122008.

Belton, V., & Stewart, T. (2002). Multiple Criteria Decision Analysis: An Integrated Approach. Dordrecht: Springer Science and Business Media.

Brunner, P. H., & Rechberger, H. (2015). Waste to energy e key element for sustainable waste management. Waste Management, 37, 3e12. https://doi.org/10.1016/J.WASMAN.2014.02.003.

Cegan, J. C., Filion, A. M., Keisler, J. M., et al. (2017). Trends and applications of multicriteria decision analysis in environmental sciences: literature review. Environment Systems and Decisions, 37, 123–133. https://doi.org/10.1007/s10669-017-9642-9.

Chubbs, S. T., & Steiner, B. A. (1998). Life cycle assessment in the steel industry. Environmental Progress, 17(2), 92–95.

Cinelli, M., Coles, S. R., & Kirwan, K. (2014). Analysis of the potentials of multi criteria decision analysis methods to conduct sustainability assessment. *Ecological Indicators*, 46, 138–148.

de Oliveira, J. A. P. (2019). Intergovernmental relations for environmental governance: cases of solid waste management and climate change in two Malaysian states. Journal of Environmental Management, 233, 481–488.

EC. (2008). Guide to Cost–Benefit Analysis of Investment Projects. Brussels: European Commission, Directorate General Regional Policy, pp. 13–15, 41–42, 99, 233–239.

Finnveden, G., & Moberg, A. (2005). Environmental systems analysis tools: an overview, Journal of Cleaner Production, 13, 1165–1173.

Gasparatos, A., El-Haram, M., & Horner, M. (2008). A critical review of reductionist approaches for assessing the progress towards sustainability. Environmental Impact Assessment Review, 28, 286–311.

Gentil, C. E., Damgaard, A., Hauschild, M., Finnveden, G., Eriksson, O., Thorneloe, S., Kaplan, P. O., Barlaz, M., Muller, O., Matsui, Y., Ii, R., & Christensen, T. H. (2010). Models for waste life cycle assessment: review of technical assumptions. Waste Management, 30(12), 2636–2648. https://doi.org/10.1016/j.wasman.2010.06.004.

Hansjurgens, B. (2004). Economic valuation through cost benefit analysis – possibilities and limitations. Toxicology, 205, 241–252.

Haraguchi, M., Siddiqi, A., & Narayanamurti, V. (2019). Stochastic cost–benefit analysis of urban waste-to-energy systems. *Journal of Cleaner Production*, 224, 751–765.

Hearn, G. L., & Ballard, J. R. (2005). The use of electrostatic techniques for the identification and sorting of waste packaging materials. Resources, Conservation and Recycling, 44(1), 91–98.

Hoornweg, D., & Bhada-Tata, P. (2012). What a Waste: A Global Review of Solid Waste Management. Washington, DC: World Bank.

Hosseinalizadeh, R., Izadbakhsh, H., & Shakouri, H. (2020). A planning model for using municipal solid waste management technologies – considering energy, economic, and environmental impacts in Tehran-Iran. Sustainable Cities and Society, 65, 102566. https://doi.org/10.1016/j.scs.2020.102566.

Hrabec, D., Šomplák, R., Nevrlý, V., Viktorin, A., Pluháček, M., & Popela, P. (2020). Sustainable waste-to-energy facility location: influence of demand on energy sales. Energy, 207, 118257.

Hsu, E. (2021). Cost–benefit analysis for recycling of agricultural wastes in Taiwan. Waste Management, 120, 424–432.

ISO. (2006). Environmental Management – Life Cycle Assessment – Principles and Framework (ISO 14040: 2006). European Standard EN ISO 14040. Geneva: International Organization for Standardization.

Kaneesamkandi, Z., Rehman, A. U., Usmani, Y. S., & Umer, U. (2020). Methodology for assessment of alternative waste treatment strategies using entropy weights. Sustainability, 12(16), 6689.

Karmperis, A. C., Sotirchos, A., Aravossis, K., & Tatsiopoulos, I. P. (2012). Waste management project's alternatives: a risk-based multi-criteria assessment (RBMCA) approach. Waste Management, 32, 194–212.

Kaza, S., Yao, L., Bhada-Tata, P. & Van Woerden, F. (2018). What a Waste 2.0: A Global Snapshot of Solid Waste Management to 2050. Urban Development. Washington, DC: World Bank.

Kiker, G. A., Bridges, T. S., Varghese, A., Seager, T. P., & Linkov, I. (2005). Application of multicriteria decision analysis in environmental decision making. Integrated Environmental Assessment and Management: An International Journal, 1(2), 95–108.

Makarichi, L., Techato, K., & Jutidamrongphan, W. (2018). Material flow analysis as a support tool for multi-criteria analysis in solid waste management decision-making. Resources, Conservation and Recycling, 139, 351–365.

Marano, J. J., & Rogers, S. (1999). Process system optimization for life cycle improvement. Environmental Progress, 18(4), 267–272.

Mendoza, G. A., & Martins, H. (2006). Multi-criteria decision analysis in natural resource management: a critical review of methods and new modelling paradigms. Forest Ecology and Management, 230(1–3), 1–22. http://dx.doi.org/10.1016/j.foreco.2006.03.023.

Mohammadi, M., Harjunkoski, I., Mikkola, S., & Jämsä-Jounela, S. L. (2018). Optimal planning of a waste management supply chain. In Computer Aided Chemical Engineering, Vol. 44, pp. 1609–1614. The Netherlands: Elsevier.

Morissey, A. J., & Browne, J. (2004). Waste management models and their application to sustainable waste management. Waste Management, 24, 297–308.

Moutavtchi, V., et al. (2010). Solid waste management by application of the WAMEDA model. Journal of Material Cycles and Waste Management, 12, 169–183.

Obi, E. U. (2016). Environmental xenobiotics and the use of natural products to minimize and/or counteract their risk of exposure. Doctoral dissertation, Texas Southern University.

OECD. (2001). OECD Annual Report 2001. Paris: OECD Publishing. https://doi.org/10.1787/annrep-2001-en.

Oh, J., & Hettiarachchi, H. (2020). Collective action in waste management: a comparative study of recycling and recovery initiatives from Brazil, Indonesia, and Nigeria using the institutional analysis and development framework. Recycling, 5(1), 4.

Olapiriyakul, S., Pannakkong, W., Kachapanya, W., & Starita, S. (2019). Multiobjective optimization model for sustainable waste management network design. Journal of Advanced Transportation, 2019. https://doi.org/10.1155/2019/3612809.

Paes, M. X., Medeiros, G. A., Mancini, S. D., Ribeiro, F. M., Puppim De Oliveira, J. A. (2019). Transition to circular economy in Brazil: a look at the municipal solid waste management in the state of Sao Paulo. Management Decisions. https://doi.org/10.1108/ MD-09-2018-1053.

Pearce, D., Atkinson, G., & Mourato, S. (2006). Cost–Benefit Analysis and the Environment: Recent Developments. Paris: OECD Publishing, pp. 253–267.

Perteghella, A., Gilioli, G., Tudor, T., & Vaccari, M. (2020). Utilizing an integrated assessment scheme for sustainable waste management in low and middle-income countries: case studies from Bosnia-Herzegovina and Mozambique. Waste Management, 113, 176–185.

Petts, J. (2000). Municipal waste management: inequities and the role of deliberation. Risk Analysis, 20(6), 821–832.

Quina, M. J., Bontempi, E., Bogush, A., Schlumberger, S., Weibel, G., Braga, R., Funari, V., Hyks, J., Rasmussen, E., & Lederer, J. (2018). Technologies for the management of MSW incineration ashes from gas cleaning: new perspectives on recovery of secondary raw materials and circular economy. Science of the Total Environment, 635, 526e542. https://doi.org/10.1016/J.SCITOTENV.2018.04.150.

Rada, E. C., et al. (2013). Web-GIS oriented systems viability for municipal solid waste selective collection optimization in developed and transient economies. Waste Management, 33(4), 785–792.

Ramakrishna, V. (2013). Life cycle assessment model for integrated solid waste management. International Journal of Engineering Research & Technology, 2(9), 1742–1748.

Rogers, M. (2001). Engineering Project Appraisal. London: Blackwell Science.

Sarmah, S. P., Yadav, R., & Rathore, P. (2019). Development of vehicle routing model in urban solid waste management system under periodic variation: a case study. IFAC-Papers On Line, 52(13), 1961–1965.

Shadiya, O. O., et al. (2012). Process enhancement through waste minimization and multi objective optimization. Journal of Cleaning Products, 31(1), 137–149.

Singh, A. (2019). Solid waste management through the applications of mathematical models. Resources, Conservation and Recycling, 151. https://doi.org/10.1016/j.resconrec.2019.104503.

Soltani, A., Hewage, K., Reza, B., & Sadiq, R. (2015). Multiple stakeholders in multi-criteria decision-making in the context of municipal solid waste management: a review. Waste Management, 35, 318–328. https://doi.org/10.1016/j.wasman.2014.09.010.

Tchobanoglous, G., & Kreith, F. (2002). Handbook of Solid Waste Management, 2nd ed. New York: McGraw-Hill.

Tun, M. M., Palacky, P., Juchelkova, D., & Síťař, V. (2020). Renewable waste-to-energy in Southeast Asia: status, challenges, opportunities, and selection of waste-to-energy technologies. Applied Sciences, 10(20), 7312.

Vadenbo, C., et al. (2014). Multi-objective optimization of waste and resource management in industrial networks. Part II: model application to the treatment of sewage sludge. Resources Conservation and Recycling, 89, 41–51.

Velasquez, M., & Hester, P. T. (2013). An analysis of multi-criteria decision making methods. International Journal of Operations Research, 10(2), 56–66.

Winkler, J. (2004). Comparative Evaluation of Life Cycle Assessment Models for Solid Waste Management. PhD thesis. Dresden: TU Dresden, p. 127.

Winkler, J., & Bilitewski, B. (2007). Comparative evaluation of life cycle assessment models for solid waste management. Waste Management, 27(8), 1021–1031.

Xiao, S., Dong, H., Geng, Y., Tian, X., Liu, C., & Li, H. (2020). Policy impacts on municipal solid waste management in Shanghai: a system dynamics model analysis. Journal of Cleaner Production, 262, 121366. https://doi.org/10.1016/j.jclepro.2020.121366.

Yadav, V., Karmakar, S., Kalbar, P. P., & Dikshit, A. K. (2019). PyTOPS: a Python based tool for TOPSIS. SoftwareX, 9, 217–222.

Younes, M. K., et al. (2015). Prediction of municipal solid waste generation using nonlinear autoregressive network. Environment Monitoring and Assessment, 187, 753. https://doi.org/10.1007/s10661-015-4977-5.

Young-Jin, S., & Rousseaux, P. (2001). Considerations in Life Cycle Inventory Analysis of Municipal Wastewater Systems. Presented at COST 624 WG Meeting, April 26–27.

Yousefloo, A., & Babazadeh, R. (2020). Designing an integrated municipal solid waste man-
    agement network: a case study. Journal of Cleaner Production, 244, 118824. https://
    doi.org/10.1016/j.jclepro.2019.118824.
Zhang, D. Q., Tan, S. K., & Gersberg, R. M. (2010). Municipal solid waste management
    in China: status, problems and challenges. Journal of Environmental Management,
    91(8), 1623–1633.

16 Biomedical Waste Management in Healthcare

Rehab A. Rayan, Moharana Choudhury,
Mohamed Kamal, Arghya Chakravorty,
Rinku Moni Devi and Jyoti Mehta*

CONTENTS

16.1 INTRODUCTION

Recently, BWM management has grown as a leading problem for both healthcare facilities and the ecosystem. The BWM produced by healthcare facilities relies on many elements, for example, the type, specialty, and occupancy of the healthcare facility, the technique for managing waste, rate of reused objects, the availability of supplies, and infrastructure, among others (Pasupathi, 2011). Adequately managing BWM has turned into a global public health concern. However, inadequately managing BWM worldwide endangers both the ecosystem and health (Singh et al., 2007).

Today, it has been proved that waste produced by healthcare facilities has several negative and hazardous influences on health and the ecosystem. The waste

* Corresponding author: Rehab A. Rayan. raynr@alexu.edu.eg

DOI: 10.1201/9781003095422-16

from healthcare facilities is a prospective risk for the health and well-being of healthcare personnel, the community, animals, and plants in the neighborhood. Disposal of waste in healthcare facilities has become a major worry (Windfeld & Brooks, 2015). This chapter presents definitions, types, and issues related to BMW. It examines methods of handling, disposing of, and managing BMW, BMW in low-income countries, and regulating laws. It displays some challenges and some future insights. It ends by raising awareness among healthcare workers that more research is needed given the increased generation of BMW.

16.2 BIOMEDICAL WASTE

BMW is specified as waste that has been generated because of medical care activities in humans or animals; it can be generated by any research, therapeutic, diagnostic, and immunization purpose (Rajan et al., 2019). In 2004, the World Health Organization (WHO) reported that improper management of BWM (e.g., using hypodermic needles) caused 21 million recent cases of hepatitis B infection, 2 million recent cases of hepatitis C infection, and 260,000 cases of deadly HIV infection in 2000. In 2018, WHO reported that only 15% of the total quantity of BWM is hazardous in terms of infectious agent, radioactive element, toxic compound, even deadly multidrug-resistant microorganisms, while the remaining 85% of waste is referred to as non-hazardous or general BWM (WHO, 2018). Different BMW and their sources are shown in Figures 16.1 and 16.2.

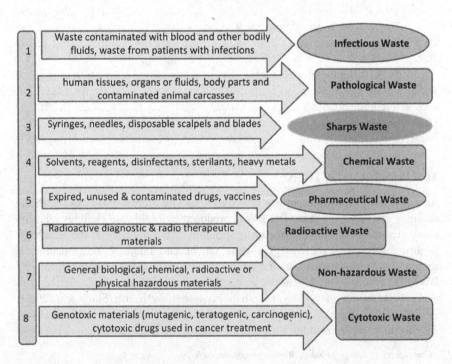

FIGURE 16.1 Types of biomedical waste.

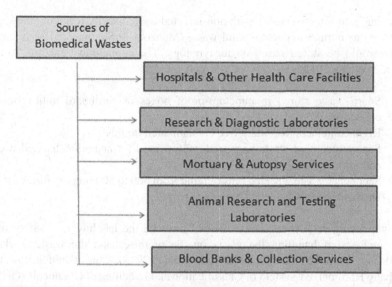

FIGURE 16.2   Different sources of biomedical waste.

16.3   BIOMEDICAL WASTES: TREATMENT AND DISPOSAL

BMW must always adhere to international and national regulatory requirements, as the unsafe management of BWM could lead to severe public health consequences such as the spread of infectious disease or dangerous pathogens. This section will highlight the steps to follow for healthcare waste management (HCWM) in low- and middle-income countries. The first step in efficient HCWM at facility level is the development of a Healthcare Waste Management Plan (HCWMP), which provides a comprehensive guide that includes a clear organizational chart for the healthcare facility, including the contracted collection service, a complete list of potential sources of healthcare waste alongside the anticipated generation rate and the method of internal waste collection and containment until external collection (Kreith & Tchobanoglous, 2002). At a more senior level, either at municipal or national level, it must include a full mapping of waste streams from the healthcare facility to the transfer station (if any) and to final disposal in the form of an incinerator or a sanitary landfill after treatment.

16.3.1   CONTAINMENT

The mapping of all potential sources of BWM in the HCWMP would be utilized to manage waste appropriately within the healthcare facility (Kreith & Tchobanoglous, 2002). First, different waste streams are developed based on the BWM typologies generated in the healthcare facility and a segregation system is implemented that follows the national respective ministry of health requirements. This segregation system would be based on a labeling and color-coding system, which the healthcare facility staff must be trained in. The two main waste streams are infected waste and non-infected waste, with non-infected waste usually receiving the same treatment as normal municipal solid waste (Manzoor & Sharma, 2019). Infected waste would be stored based on its typology. The containment method would include (WHO, 2014):

- Sharp waste stored in puncture-proof boxes or cardboard until external collection
- Rigid containers to contain free contaminated liquids
- Separate colored waste bags (red, yellow etc.) for anatomical/soiled waste and plastics
- Secondary waste wheeled bins ranging from 500 to 800 liters to further store and isolate the waste from humans.

Accompanying each containment method must be the labeling as a safety precaution for staff handling the waste on the premises and the waste workers collecting the BWM (Dehghani & Rahmatinia, 2018). This would follow the Globally Harmonized System of Classification and Labelling of Chemicals (GHS), developed by the United Nations (UN, 2017). The labeling and packaging must be either implemented by the external collection service and staff should be trained on handling it, or vice versa.

Containment in the facility also includes safely transporting the waste from the medical cubicle to the storage secondary waste bin within the premises of the healthcare facility. The HCWMP must be designed to ensure that there is an absolute minimal handling of BWM involved in the internal collection of waste (Singh et al., 2001). This should be done via the use of medical waste transport trolleys, which are designed to be convenient for healthcare staff (WHO, 2014). The containers used to store the waste until its collection must be separate for hazardous and non-hazardous BWM. This would include the utilization of plastic barrels for hazardous waste and secondary wheeled bins for infectious and non-hazardous BWM (Rajan et al., 2019).

16.3.2 COLLECTION AND TRANSPORTATION

The BWM generated in the facility must be safely collected regularly. A designated vehicle cargo area must be established in the facility (Kreith & Tchobanoglous, 2002). Collection via appropriate trucks is the only sustainable method to transport the generated BWM to disposal facilities. The collection vehicle must be a specialized truck that is well maintained, appropriately labeled to show the load it is carrying, regularly cleaned, with a well-trained driver or crew handling it, and be equipped with waste-handling equipment (WHO, 2014). The contractor responsible for transporting the waste must have a monitoring plan, to ensure vehicle operations are safe and the vehicle is always in a suitable condition. Vehicles must not refuel during a transportation trip; rather the vehicle should be fully prepared to send the BWM to the disposal facilities without the need to make unnecessary stops. Similarly, a vehicle cargo area must be established in the treatment or disposal facility to receive safely the waste from the transport truck (Kreith & Tchobanoglous, 2002).

16.3.3 TREATMENT

BWM is directly sent to an incinerator or to a treatment facility followed by a sanitary landfill. The purpose of BWM treatment is to eliminate all the pathogens and microorganisms that pose a risk to the environment and public health before sending the BWM to a landfill (Dehghani & Rahmatinia, 2018). The selection of a treatment method depends on several elements that include the characteristics and generation rate of the BWM alongside the technological availability of equipment and expertise. Other elements are location of healthcare facility, transportation costs, and environmental considerations (Raj, 2009). There are different methods to treat BWM, including:

- Autoclaving: This is a treatment process that uses steam sterilizer units usually alongside shredding machinery to treat the BWM and remove most harmful microorganisms. The process combines mechanical and thermal technologies to disinfect the medical waste. This process does not involve any combustion, making it more environmentally friendly than incineration, and does not disinfect many BWMs.
- Microwaving: Similarly to autoclaving, the BWM is shredded and intensely heated to reduce massively the volume of the waste while also killing the microorganisms present. This process also does not involve any combustion.
- Chemical disinfection: This is a process that uses chemicals to inactivate or destroy microorganisms and pathogens in the BWM. It is more suitable for treating liquid medical waste (WHO, 2014). It usually requires a shredder.

The treated waste is then transported to a suitable landfill, or with chemical disinfection to a sewer system if pollutants are under the required national limits (Rao et al., 2017).

16.3.4 DISPOSAL

The two primary options for final waste disposal are landfilling and incineration (Kreith & Tchobanoglous, 2002). Treated BWM will be transported to a licensed landfill suitable for receiving it. Direct disposal of BWM into a landfill is not advisable by WHO standards, and the BWM must be treated prior to burial (WHO, 2014). For BWM containing heavy metals, burial must be avoided unless they are encapsulated in a block then buried (WHO, 2005). For sharp BWM, if they are to be disposed directly into landfill, they must also be encapsulated in a safe container before burial. Animal carcasses, alongside anatomical, go through either deep burial or special incinerators. Incineration is usually the preferred method of BWM disposal, as it is cheaper, faster, and much easier to manage compared to landfill (Dehghani & Rahmatinia, 2018). However, they release serious combustion gaseous byproducts and pollutants that could affect human health if not treated appropriately before leaving the incineration system. They also generate residual ash that must be disposed of. The different incineration systems include (WHO, 2014):

- Dual-chamber incinerators (starved-air incinerators)
- Multiple-chamber incinerators
- Rotary kilns.

The choice of an incineration system depends on the volume of waste that requires incineration, the composition of the waste, and the financial feasibility regarding energy and transportation (Kreith & Tchobanoglous, 2002). Each system has a different design, and combustion or gasification occurs at different temperatures ranging from 800 to 1600°C.

In low- and low-middle-income countries, these disposal facilities may not exist and healthcare facilities will be faced with the impossible task of sustainable BWM disposal (Dieng et al., 2020). In such cases, the waste should ideally be sent to a municipal landfill, since this would be the best option to protect public health. If landfills are not available, healthcare facilities can explore a controlled dumpsite and upgrade a portion to be a minimal version of a sanitary landfill, to bury the BWM safely away from public health (Liao & Ho, 2014). Figure 16.3 summarizes HCWM by highlighting the flow of BWM from source to disposal.

16.4 BIOMEDICAL WASTE MANAGEMENT IN LOW-INCOME COUNTRIES

The management of BWM in low-income countries and low-middle-income countries in the Global South has been much less of a priority, especially since there

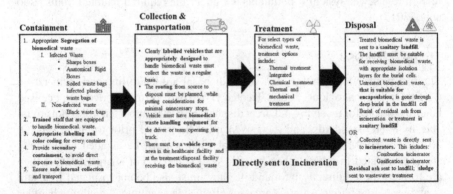

FIGURE 16.3 The flow of biomedical waste from source to disposal.

is a lack of regulative measures and resources (Khan et al., 2019). In countries such as Nigeria and Ethiopia, consistent open burning of BWM has been noted (Yazie et al., 2019); this is a massive threat to public health. This is usually due to the lack of any overarching BWM management system in the country or locality, and because there are no better means of disposal. With low-income countries, the efficient management of BWM requires special commitment from healthcare facilities, to ensure that they are disposed of in a manner that is safe for the environment and the people. To achieve that, they must go above and beyond financially and technically. There are no suitable disposal facilities for the BWM, and thus the only workable option is usually to dispose of the waste via dumping or open burning (Yazie et al., 2019).

To appropriately and sustainability manage BWM in low-income countries requires a special focus on reduction of waste at source and the segregation of waste during containment (Sowande et al., 2014). To achieve that, healthcare workers and staff handling healthcare waste must be trained in how to handle BWM. At the other end of the spectrum, there must be campaigns and interventions to raise awareness of BWM collectors and waste pickers, who must be informed about the serious health risks associated with direct exposure to BWM without appropriate personal protective equipment (PPE) and waste containment (Raj, 2009). This includes diseases such as hepatitis B and C, and HIV. These workers must be provided with better alternatives to dispose of the collected BWM, such as nearby sanitary landfills and temporary transfer stations for storing the waste for up to 48 hours.

16.5 REGULATIONS

The improper disposal and management of BWMs from unique sources such as clinics, hospitals, and other medical facilities lead to public and occupational health hazards affecting health workers, patients, waste handlers, haulers, and the public. Air, water, and soil also become contaminated, affecting all forms of life and the natural ecosystem. The management and regulation of BWM are more challenging in developing countries as compared to developed countries. This may be because of the lack of research on HCWM, disposal methods, lack of infrastructure, awareness, participation, shortage of resources, weak implementation of laws, financial constraints, and technological limitations (Zafar, 2019).

Most African countries like Ghana, Eritrea, and Lesotho lack legislation for medical waste management, lack of sanitary landfills, lack of disposal methods, and have financial issues, while the Gambia, Nigeria, and Kenya are participants in the Stockholm Convention with few significant laws. There is increased use of crudely designed incinerators for the absence of sanitary landfills. There is a lack of landfills in the Gambia, Ghana, Lesotho, Nigeria, Senegal, and Tanzania, while Zambia and Kenya only have crude dumpsites. There are approximately more than 1,000 incinerators in Africa, but many of them are inoperative or operating below standards (Zafar, 2019).

In developed countries like the USA and the UK, the BWM is properly managed and regulated following legislation. In the UK, the Environmental Protection Act 1990 (Part II), Waste Management Licensing Regulations 1994, and the Hazardous Waste Regulations (England and Wales) 2005, and the Special Waste Regulations in Scotland are applicable legislation. In the USA, BWM is regulated by The Medical Waste Tracking Act, which allowed the Environmental Protection Agency to establish rules for the management of medical waste in states. In California, the Medical Waste Management Act is used to regulate and manage BWMs. The Medical Waste Management Program regulates the generation, handling, storage, treatment, and disposal of medical waste.

From the above discussions it can be seen that, compared to developed countries, developing countries suffer more as they are resource-constrained and inadequate in management of hospital waste, causing environmental and occupational health risks. Also, the legislation and implementation of rules vary between different places and countries, so there is no uniformity in method and regulations. Developing countries are also deprived of infrastructure, excellent research, technology, and finance. Thus, conditions of BWM management in developing countries are poor because of poor waste segregation, collection, storage, transportation, and disposal practices (Ali et al., 2017). Lack of training for hospital staff and less knowledge regarding proper waste management lead to less awareness and risks. The health hazard risks increase as most of the hospital sanitary workers, and scavengers, operate without the provision of safety equipment or immunization. The risk increases when unsegregated waste is illegally recycled. Thus, it can be concluded that overall, developing countries face more challenges in waste management, leading to several health hazards, as compared to developed countries.

16.6 CHALLENGES

Perhaps the greatest test the administration of medical clinics and small health care facilities will confront, during the execution of BMW 2016 standards (MoE, 2016) will be the absence of resources. To eliminate chlorinated plastic packs, gloves, and blood sacks and to build up a standardized identification framework for sacks/compartments, the cost will be high. The time range for doing this, for example, two years, is excessively short (MoE, 2016). There is an extraordinary need for fast improvement to satisfy requirements for treatment and removal of all BMW produced. Incinerators transmit harmful air toxins, and incinerator debris is unsafe.

16.6.1 INCINERATOR HAZARDS

The main solution for removing BMW was to consume the waste. The last decade witnessed a substantial increase in the quantity of incinerators being introduced. The incinerators depend on the high temperature that kills microorganisms and in the process demolishes the material in which those microorganisms live (Mattiello et al., 2013). However, during incinerator activity several poisons are delivered, for example, as a result of inadequate ignition. During cremation and post-ignition cooling, waste particles separate and recombine, framing new particles, which are harmful. Metals are not yet demolished and are scattered into nature, generating genuine medical problems. Dioxins are an unexpected byproduct of waste ignition created during incinerator activity. These are a gathering of 75 synthetic substances which exist together alongside furans, another gathering of poisons. These poisons have the propensity to aggregate in greasy tissues and travel up the food chain. Clinical gadgets made of polyvinyl chloride (PVC) which is the biggest dioxin maker in the environment (Vilavert et al., 2015) are used. Furthermore, metals present in the clinical waste are an impetus for dioxin arrangement. These are very harmful: they are known to cause cancer, and cause harm to the human endocrine system. In 2007, Subramanian et al. discovered an elevated level of dioxin in human milk gathered from New Delhi, Mumbai, and Kolkata (Subramanian et al., 2007). In addition, incinerator debris is hazardous and should be checked for poison before being sent to landfill. In this manner, keeping these focuses in mind, most nations are moving towards elective natural well-disposed strategies for BMW removal. The Philippines has restricted the use of incinerators, and Denmark has restricted their development.

16.7   FUTURE INSIGHTS

Even general hospital waste should be sterilized before disposal and the PPE of healthcare staff to reduce the risk for both health workers and rag pickers. Strict hygiene and sanitation practices are an integral part of infection control measures and disease prevention. As far as treatment is concerned, other technologies such as autoclave, gas, other than incineration, known as high-temperature combustion technology, irradiation from microwave processing and thermal inactivation may be viewed as safe treatment methods for BWM.

The following are several policy guidelines for policy makers that will help build a framework to cope better with BMW management. Waste management should be included in the disaster recovery strategies, which are currently solely focused on waste. Response steps and recommendations should be tabled to handle and adjust the waste dynamics created. Such a charter and disaster waste management guideline must be implemented in uniting centers and countries. While solid waste is included in disaster waste provision, the management plan must ensure that participants are qualified to manage hazardous BWM by setting up a common international forum to share information. An effective and reliable waste management system is the foundation for a national policy framework with legislation and technical guidance.

Based on the legal structure, most countries have developed color-coded BMW segregation. Comprehensive coding standardization based on the form and nature of waste and health training would avoid excessive waste production in the treatment of infectious waste. Systems need to be updated to accommodate waste management intricacies. Technology-based solutions such as automatic waste recovery processes, including pyrolysis, gasification, and hydrothermal carbonization, should be sponsored. These offer high-quality byproducts and guarantee full workplace safety and protection for the workers concerned. In addition, the promotion of research and investment should be ensured in these new technologies. Social viability, besides environmental and economic feasibility, should also be integrated into their design.

Innovative technologies are required to recycle mixed and other complex plastic forms. A modern technique known as hydrothermal carbonization (mostly non-infectious plastic fraction) was recently applied to medical waste using high-pressure carbonization and autoclaving methods (Shen et al., 2017). Integrating machine learning for sorting and processing into recycled components ensures higher recyclability rates. Broad, economically impossible recycling plastic packaging and goods should be tracked. Strategies should be put in place to efficiently create and incorporate homogeneous plastics, environmentally friendly bioplastics, and circular technology.

16.8 RECOMMENDATIONS

- Allocate a special budget in each healthcare facility to supply tools to handle and manage BWM.
- Provide all healthcare facilities with special tools for BMW such as PPE and safety boxes.
- Train healthcare staff on adequately handling BWM.
- Instruct cleaners to wear PPE such as gowns, gloves, and facial masks while performing their daily duties in handling BWM.
- Segregate BWM at their source of origin by hazard degree in differently colored collecting bags.
- Prohibit disposal of BWM with other domestic waste.
- Allocate special trucks to collect BWM from both public and private healthcare facilities.
- Create a committee for BMW in each town.
- Enforce BMW regulations in both public and private healthcare facilities.
- Provide legal powers to the BMW committee to enforce penalties such as fines where the environment has been contaminated.

16.9 CONCLUSION

Recently, for the growing population, there has been a swift proliferation in both public and private healthcare facilities, and therefore, the amount and hazard of BWM have been greater than expected. BWM should be sorted by type, source, and hazard degree in relation to treatment, housing, and finally disposal. Separating BWM at the source of origin is a vital step while accounting for reducing, reusing, or recycling as deemed appropriate. Novel measures to raise state and healthcare facilities' civil attention towards adopting at least essential regulations after waste production, and particularly BMW, raises both direct and indirect expenses for the community. Systematically controlling increasing amounts of BWM is challenging, hence both healthcare authorities and the public should be held accountable for safeguarding public health and the ecosystem. Ultimately, to improve the world and our own well-being, it is important to sensitize ourselves. That is why understanding waste control, waste minimization at source, waste segregation, proper waste transport, and proper care is of great concern not only to society but also for relevant personnel. This helps ensure the preservation of biodiversity and ecological stability and global population well-being.

REFERENCES

Ali, M., Wang, W., Chaudhry, N., & Geng, Y. (2017). Hospital waste management in developing countries: A mini review. *Waste Management & Research: The Journal of the International Solid Wastes and Public Cleansing Association, ISWA, 35*(6), 581–592. https://doi.org/10.1177/0734242X17691344.

Dehghani, M. H., & Rahmatinia, M. (2018). Dataset on the knowledge, attitude, and practices of biomedical waste management among Tehran hospital's healthcare personnel. *Data in Brief, 20,* 219–225. https://doi.org/10.1016/j.dib.2018.08.002.

Dieng, C., Mberu, B., Dimbuene, Z. T., Faye, C., Amugsi, D., & Aboderin, I. (2020). Biomedical waste management in Dakar, Senegal: Legal framework, health and environment issues; policy and program options. *Cities & Health, 1,* 1–15. https://doi.org/10.1080/23748834.2020.1786228.

Khan, B. A., Cheng, L., Khan, A. A., & Ahmed, H. (2019). Healthcare waste management in Asian developing countries: A mini review. *Waste Management & Research, 37*(9), 863–875. https://doi.org/10.1177/0734242X19857470.

Kreith, F., & Tchobanoglous, G. (2002). *Handbook of Solid Waste Management* (2nd edition). USA: McGraw-Hill Education.

Liao, C.-J., & Ho, C. C. (2014). Risk management for outsourcing biomedical waste disposal – Using the failure mode and effects analysis. *Waste Management, 34*(7), 1324–1329. https://doi.org/10.1016/j.wasman.2014.03.007.

Manzoor, J., & Sharma, M. (2019). Impact of biomedical waste on environment and human health. *Environmental Claims Journal, 31*(4), 311–334. https://doi.org/10.1080/10406026.2019.1619265.

Mattiello, A., Chiodini, P., Bianco, E., Forgione, N., Flammia, I., Gallo, C., Pizzuti, R., & Panico, S. (2013). Health effects associated with the disposal of solid waste in landfills and incinerators in populations living in surrounding areas: A systematic review. *International Journal of Public Health, 58*(5), 725–735. https://doi.org/10.1007/s00038-013-0496-8.

MoE. (2016). *Bio-Medical Waste Management Rules 2016.* https://vikaspedia.in/energy/environment/waste-management/bio-medical-waste-management/bio-medical-waste-management-rules.

Pasupathi, D. P. (2011). Biomedical waste management for health care industry: A review. *International Journal of Biological Medicine Research.* www.academia.edu/1327770/Biomedical_waste_management_for_health_care_industry_A_review.

Raj, M. R. R. (2009). Biomedical waste management: An overview. *Journal of Indian Academy of Oral Medicine and Radiology, 21*(3), 139. https://doi.org/10.4103/0972-1363.58757.

Rajan, R., Robin, D. T., & Vandarani, M. (2019). Biomedical waste management in Ayurveda hospitals – current practices and future perspectives. *Journal of Ayurveda and Integrative Medicine, 10*(3), 214–221. https://doi.org/10.1016/j.jaim.2017.07.011.

Rao, M. N., Sultana, R., & Kota, S. H. (2017). Chapter 4 – Biomedical waste. In M. N. Rao, R. Sultana, & S. H. Kota (Eds.), *Solid and Hazardous Waste Management* (pp. 127–157). India: Butterworth-Heinemann. https://doi.org/10.1016/B978-0-12-809734-2.00004-3.

Shen, Y., Yu, S., Ge, S., Chen, X., Ge, X., & Chen, M. (2017). Hydrothermal carbonization of medical wastes and lignocellulosic biomass for solid fuel production from lab-scale to pilot-scale. *Energy, 118*(C), 312–323. https://ideas.repec.org/a/eee/energy/v118y2017icp312-323.html.

Singh, V. P., Biswas, G., & Sharma, J. J. (2007). Biomedical waste management – an emerging concern in Indian hospitals. *Indian Journal of Forensic Medicine & Toxicology, 1*(1), 39–44. www.i-scholar.in/index.php/ijfmt/article/view/45850.

Singh, Z., Bhalwar, R., Jayaram, J., & Tilak, V. (2001). An introduction to essentials of bio-medical waste management. *Medical Journal, Armed Forces India, 57*(2), 144–147. https://doi.org/10.1016/S0377-1237(01)80136-2.

Sowande, A. O., Amaefule, K. E., Pearson, J., & Iyortim, I. (2014). Healthcare waste management in low resource countries – Nigerian experience. *International Journal of Infection Control*. www.ijic.info/article/view/12542.

Subramanian, A., Ohtake, M., Kunisue, T., & Tanabe, S. (2007). High levels of organochlorines in mothers' milk from Chennai (Madras) city, India. *Chemosphere, 68*(5), 928–939. https://doi.org/10.1016/j.chemosphere.2007.01.041.

UN. (2017). *Globally Harmonized System of Classification and Labelling of Chemicals (GHS) (7th ed.)*. www.un-ilibrary.org/environment-and-climate-change/globally-harmonized-system-of-classification-and-labelling-of-chemicals-ghs_e9e7b6dc-en.

Vilavert, L., Nadal, M., Schuhmacher, M., & Domingo, J. L. (2015). Two decades of environmental surveillance in the vicinity of a waste incinerator: Human health risks associated with metals and PCDD/Fs. *Archives of Environmental Contamination and Toxicology, 69*(2), 241–253. https://doi.org/10.1007/s00244-015-0168-1.

WHO. (2004). Health-Care Waste Management, Rapid Assessment Tool. Geneva: WHO.

WHO. (2005). *Preparation of National Health-Care Waste Management Plans in Sub-Saharan Countries: Guidance Manual*. Geneva: World Health Organization. https://apps.who.int/iris/handle/10665/43118.

WHO. (2014). *Safe Management of Wastes from Health-Care Activities*. Geneva: World Health Organization. www.who.int/water_sanitation_health/publications/wastemanag/en/.

WHO. (2018, February 8). *Health-Care Waste*. www.who.int/news-room/fact-sheets/detail/health-care-waste.

Windfeld, E. S., & Brooks, M. S.-L. (2015). Medical waste management – A review. *Journal of Environmental Management, 163*, 98–108. https://doi.org/10.1016/j.jenvman.2015.08.013.

Yazie, T. D., Tebeje, M. G., & Chufa, K. A. (2019). Healthcare waste management current status and potential challenges in Ethiopia: A systematic review. *BMC Research Notes, 12*(1), 285. https://doi.org/10.1186/s13104-019-4316-y.

Zafar, S. (2019, September 29). *Medical Waste Management in Developing Countries. BioEnergy Consult*. www.bioenergyconsult.com/medical-waste-management/.

Unit VII

Pandemics
Challenges and Way Forward

17 Environment-Friendly Plant-Based Edible Vaccines – A Novel Technique to Fight SARS-CoV-2 and Other Pandemics

A Review

*Anurag Chanda**

CONTENTS

* Corresponding author: Anurag Chanda. anurag.chanda01@gmail.com

DOI: 10.1201/9781003095422-17

17.1 INTRODUCTION

Biological preparations capable of eliciting an immune response in the human body, especially in the event of invasion by a foreign pathogen, are called vaccines or conventional vaccines.

With the help of medical advances in genetic engineering and molecular biology, vaccines have been primed in such a way that they activate the innate defenses of our body. In the vaccinated individual, the T and B cells specific for the particular pathogen, proliferate faster and clamp down on the invader, providing abstract immunity to that disease, in comparison to an unvaccinated person who would be susceptible to the disease. The immunological response generated varies with different strains with respect to pathogen, antigenic shift, and drift and also with various other unrevealed mechanisms, directly hampering its construction. These factors lead to complexity in the adoption process of the specific peptide sequence to which the antigen-specific immune response is to be primed, as individual strains are naturally bound to be different. But conventional vaccines also incorporate the danger of acquiring the disease, since at times during vaccine design live attenuation of the pathogenic microorganism is required, leading to destruction rather than protection (Langridge, 2000).

Polynucleotide immunization involves utilization of sophistically designed DNA vaccines to slow progression of the disease. DNA inoculated into the body undergoes transcription and translation to yield protein which then stimulates specific T and B cells to grow and differentiate. These processes make the immunological system ready to quickly combat any invading pathogens attacking the body before they can hamper the existing equilibrium inside. Though conventional and DNA vaccines have time and again proven their mettle in the domain of medical science, with the advent of oral vaccines, everything began to change.

Firstly, oral vaccines eased the process of host inoculation as formerly professional medical expertise had been needed to administer conventional vaccines. These newly developed oral vaccines not only offer the advantage of painless oral administration, increasing patient complience, but as they do not involve needle insertion, this reduces the perils of cross-contamination and the spread of deadly diseases, especially in many third-world developing countries. In some countries there have been numerous reports of reuse of injection needles in multiple hosts; this practice can lead to the uncontrolled proliferation of many life-threatening and lethal diseases. In addition, oral vaccines have been proved to be more cost-effective than to conventional vaccines.

Edible vaccines are similar to subunit vaccines which use genetic engineering technology incorporating pathogen-derived proteins or glycoproteins as antigens. This gives an added advantage over conventional vaccines as the risks associated with handling pathogenic microorganisms are reduced. However, as edible vaccines do not contain any genes, the formation of a whole pathogen does not take place. Their mechanism of action is very similar to that of DNA vaccines, where a peptide sequence similar to the infectious pathogen synthesizes and triggers the formation of humoral (B-cell) and cell-mediated (T-cell) immunity. The only difference is that these are stored in plant tissues which can be consumed by eating. In edible vaccines the plant genome is encoded by genetic engineering with specific protein sequences which then result in genesis of desired proteins. These are then consumed as fruit or vegetables.

In the first instance, successful antigen expression in plants was achieved for rabies virus (G-protein) in tomato plants. Tobacco and potato plants have been also used as vectors to express Norwalk capsid proteins as well as hepatitis B surface antigen (HB$_s$Ag). While numerous plants have been studied: the main ones are potato, tomato, rice, soybean, banana, wheat, corn, and legumes.

17.2   PRODUCTION OF EDIBLE VACCINES

Genetic encoding (Mishra et al., 2008) of the antigens from already characterized pathogenic microorganisms (virus, bacteria, or parasites) and for which antibodies are available are managed in two ways. First, the whole structural genetic material is inserted into the plant genome for transformation, specifically between the 5' and 3' of the regulatory elements, which ultimately allows transcription of the entire coding sequence into the plant genome (Figure 17.1).

Second, the epitopes containing the antigen to be planted are identified. Subsequently, employed the genes of the DNA fragments are constructed by fusion, encoding them along with a coat of the protein gene from the plant virus, e.g., cytomegalovirus or tobacco mosaic virus. Then, the recombinant virus thus formed is directed to infect stabilized plants and through these methods edible vaccines are formed.

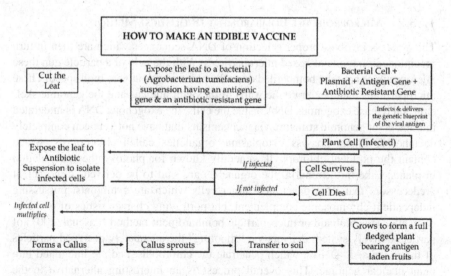

FIGURE 17.1   How an edible vaccine is made (adapted from Langridge, 2000).

17.3   METHODS FOR TRANSFORMATION OF GENES/DNA INTO PLANTS

These methods can be broadly classified into two main types: plasmid/vector carrier system and microprojectile bombardment (biolistics) method.

17.3.1   PLASMID/VECTOR CARRIER SYSTEM

This method harnesses *Agrobacterium tumefaciens,* a common soil bacteria. *A. tumefaciens* can be used to transfer small segments of DNA into the plant genome using the technique of transformation. With this technique, the entire plant is reproduced into an individual plant cell. Studies reveal that, thanks to this methodology, genes have successfully expressed themselves when they have been administered via the oral route to animals (Kurup and Thomas, 2020). Studies also reveal that *A. tumefaciens* is one the most stable vectors that can be utilized to transport the antigen into the plant genome, and thus it can be widely exploited in the preparation of plant-based edible vaccines. *A. tumefaciens* have this unique property to integrate DNA (T-DNA) with infected cells in the genomic skeleton. The entry of the exogenous genes into adequately modified T-DNA of the *Agrobacterium* cells and on consequent infection of a vegetable tissue led to stable integration of the gene into the plant genome. Initially this methodology was limited to a few species such as tobacco but later it was extended to other plant species to investigate its versatility, especially to plants belonging to the Graminae and Leguminosae family, opening new avenues for research and development on edible vaccines as a better alternative to conventional vaccines.

17.3.2   MICROPROJECTILE BOMBARDMENT (BIOLISTICS) METHOD

This process involves proper selection of DNA sequences which are then in turn precipitated on to metal-based microparticles. With the help of a particle gun these microparticles are then bombarded on to the plant tissues at very high speed. These microparticles then penetrate the walls of the plant nucleus and the genomic skeleton and release exogenous DNA inside the cells; the exogenous DNA is integrated into the plant genomic structure via mechanisms that have not yet been completely deciphered. Plants possess cytoplasmic organelles called chloroplasts, which contain the pigment chlorophyll, generally known for photosynthesis regulation in plants. Like mitochondria, the organelles are said to be derived from ancient predecessors that have penetrated larger cells which are symbionts, possessing independent chromosome complement, but portraying characteristics of prokaryotic cells. This biolistic or microparticle bombardment method (Pascual, 2007) of particle delivery system delivers via "shooting" the adequately designed particles of the processed "DNA", which penetrate the chloroplast and are integrated into plant nuclear genome. This overall process is an interesting alternative to the nuclear transformation process.

17.4   MECHANISM OF ACTION

Edible vaccines are capable of activating the mucosal immune system (MIS). This is advantageous in comparison with conventional vaccines. Mucosal immunity has an edge over others since it possesses both innate and adaptive arms (T and B cells) of the immune system. Also, most pathogenic agents on invading the host body come into contact with the first line of defense, i.e., the mucosal linings forming the surface of the digestive, respiratory, and uroreproductive tracts, collectively known as the largest immunologically active tissues in our body. The MIS predominantly acts in the first line to defend the body by fighting viral antigens entering our body through opening inlets like nose and mouth. MIS activation strengthens our fight against these infectious agents, making it one of the most effective ways of immunization. Edible vaccines are developed with the aim of activating both sentinels, MIS and humoral immune system, against harmful foreign pathogens.

Consumption of edible plant tissue via the oral route leads to mastication of the products consumed. On reaching the stomach and then the intestine the digestive and bacterial enzymes come into play and further act to disintegrate and degrade plant cells into respective simpler products (Figure 17.2). Peyer's patches (PP) carry out the function of immunosurveillance, are highly enriching sources of immunoglobulin A (IgA), produced by plasma cells in the lamina propria, populate mucosal tissue, and serve as mucosal effector sites.

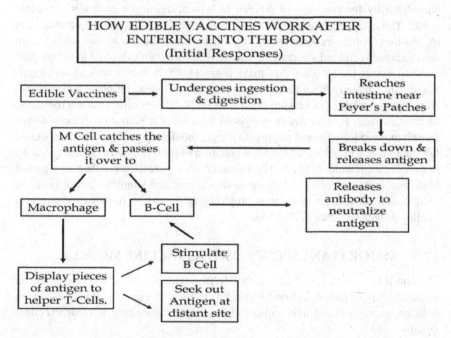

FIGURE 17.2   How an edible vaccine works after entering the body (initial responses) (adapted from Langridge, 2000).

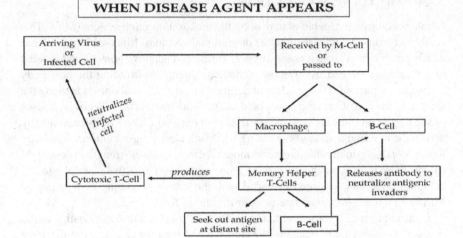

FIGURE 17.3   When a disease agent appears (adapted from Langridge, 2000).

Edible vaccine breakdown occurs near the PP, which reside in the mucous membrane. PP carry out a sampling function as 30–40 lymphoid nodules at the exterior surface, mainly in the ileum of the intestine. PP also contain follicles which, when stimulated by the presence of antigen in lumen, develop a protruding geminal center. The antigens penetrate through this follicle site in intestinal epithelial cells or, in other words, are sampled through these sites, and are accumulated within an organized lymphoid structure. These antigens are then subjected to the M cells residing next to the PP. They then make contact with the lumen with a broad membrane which already has a deep invagination in its basolateral plasma membrane. Now, these available pockets are filled with the T cells, B cells, and macrophages. M cells activate B cells within lymphoid follicles. On activation B cells depart from lymphoid follicles and migrate to trigger the diffusion of mucosal-associated lymphoid tissue (MALT), where differentiation of plasma cells secreting IgA antibodies occurs (Daniel et al., 2004). The antibodies generated are then transported back into lumen secretions, leading to interaction and simultaneous disposal of antigens on subsequent entry, thus providing immunity to further exposure to a similar antigen (Figures 17.3–17.5).

17.5   MAJOR PLANT SPECIES USED AS VACCINE MODELS

The aim is to create a search engine that derives evidence-based knowledge and an understanding of factors influencing health. The search engine will help us design policies, strategies, and interventions that can steer humanity towards excellent health.

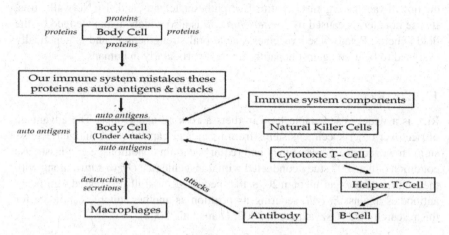

FIGURE 17.4 How an edible vaccine helps to stop autoimmunity (before treatment) (adapted from Langridge, 2000).

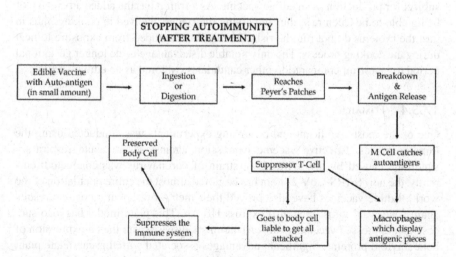

FIGURE 17.5 How an edible vaccine helps to stop autoimmunity (after treatment) (adapted from Langridge, 2000).

17.5.1 POTATO

Potato has proven to be an appropriate model when used as a vehicle for the production of vaccines against hepatitis B, diphtheria, tetanus, and also Norwalk virus. Its use in enteritis caused by *Escherichia coli* is also widely acknowledged by the field experts. Potato-based vaccines enable oral strengthening, and is genetically designed to be used against hepatitis B virus, particularly in humans.

17.5.2 RICE

Rice is a widely used staple food in diets across all age groups. The advantage of rice over other specimens stems from its greater capability for antigen expression. However, rice grows slowly and requires certain conditions, e.g., glasshouse conditions. In a 2007 study conducted with transgenic rice *Orzya sativa* along with the confirmatory experiment in 2008, the species successfully expressed significant antibodies against *E. coli*, securing its position as another suitable candidate for this research field (Oszvald et al., 2007; Qian et al., 2008).

17.5.3 BANANA

Banana is found abundantly throughout the Indian subcontinent and is an excellent subject for production as an edible vaccine. As a fruit it has the added advantage of being able to be eaten raw, thus bypassing the stages involved in cooking, thus in turn the proteins do not run the risk of becoming degraded from exposure to heat during the cooking process. The only notable disadvantage is the longer gestational period to bear fruit compared to other candidates explored as an edible vaccine.

17.5.4 TOMATO

One of the most significant and promising experiments was conducted using the tomato species. Effective vaccine expression against severe acute respiratory syndrome caused by the SARS-CoV strain of coronavirus was conducted; currently, the new SARS-CoV-2 strain has engulfed almost the entire population of the world. Edible vaccines have also proved their mettle by showing positive results against Norwalk virus; they also express HB_sAg. This plant model has also successfully expressed vaccine against Alzheimer's disease, with the co-expression of beta-amyloid proteins. Significant advantages associated with this candidate plant include low gestational and growth period, it can be grown in the backyard as a garden plant, and it is rich in vitamin A and carotenoids which act as an immunological booster.

17.6 APPLICATIONS OF EDIBLE VACCINES

Science is a tool we use to try to understand how nature functions. We can achieve this understanding by either a reductionistic or a holistic approach.

The WHO (1958) definition of health says, "Health is a state of physical, mental and social well-being in which disease and infirmity are absent."

17.6.1 MALARIA

Malaria remains a major cause of human morbidity worldwide. There are 300–500 million new cases every year, leading to nearly 1.5–2.7 million deaths every year, and this has only grown worse over the decades. Many studies carried out to explore and establish the advantage of mass reach have shown new hope in mass immunization processes, thanks to easy availability and accessibility. Although there are little data on exact dosage, effective studies have reported that edible vaccines can surely minimize deaths due to mishandling in many third-world countries.

17.6.2 HEPATITIS B

Data reveal that more than 400 million people are affected by hepatitis B worldwide. It is one of the most common pathogens known to affect human life adversely. As immunization is known to be the only pre-emptive step to fight this virus, any possible effort to reduce the numbers worldwide would require huge quantities of vaccine HB_sAg (Tripurani et al., 2003), successfully expressed in plant-based vaccines.

17.6.3 MEASLES

Measles causes 800,000 deaths every year globally. In addition individuals who are affected and survive have been reported to develop conditions like deafness and also encephalitis. As a major life-threatening disease, mass immunization is the only remedy in such cases. Studies have suggested that using edible vaccines effectively can help us fight the war against measles, on a global platform (Arntzen, 1997).

17.6.4 DIABETES

Diabetes is a very common disease worldwide; it affects more than 100 million people each year. Type 1 or juvenile-onset diabetes has a history of affecting children and the young adults. It is categorized as an autoimmune disorder of pancreatic beta cells, leading to destruction of insulin produced by the body (Sharma et al., 1999). Plants expressing antigenic proteins have demonstrated considerable responses to this disease, providing positive results in minimizing the devastating effects of diabetes.

17.7 CONCLUSION

Edible vaccines can be a one-stop solution to fight pandemics globally. Their positive effects help to curtail and, if possible, eliminate the hazards inherent to conventional parenteral vaccines with toxic or allergic compounds. Edible vaccines provide an excellent opportunity to deliver vaccines orally, along with elimination of the need for cold-chain maintenance (where parenteral ampoules must be maintained at refrigeration temperatures – i.e., less than 8°C – to protect vaccines from degradation), and they are also economical in terms of cost-effective transportation. They are effective against chemical warfare and bio-weapons (Meloen et al., 1998). Edible vaccines are a milestone in the creation of cost-effective vaccine subunits. The future is bright if these novel techniques can be utilized in every country, whether developed or developing, especially in such times when the world is fighting against one of the deadliest virus outbreaks.

REFERENCES

Arntzen, Charles J. Edible vaccines. *Public Health Reports*, volume 112, May–Jun 1997.

Daniel, Henry, Carmona-Sanchez, Olga, Burns, Britany E. *Chloroplast Derived Antibodies, Biopharmaceuticals and Edible Vaccines.* Molecular Farming: Plant-Made Pharmaceuticals & Technical Proteins. Weinheim: Wiley-Vch Verlag, 2004.

Kurup, Vrinda M., Thomas, Jaya. *Edible Vaccines: Promises and Challenges.* Molecular Biotechnology, volume 62(2), pages 79–90, 2020.

Langridge, William H.R. *Edible Vaccines.* Scientific America, volume 283(3), pages 48–53, 2000.

Meloen, R.H., Hamilton, W.D.O., Casal J.I., Dalsgaard, K., Langeveld, J.P.L. Edible Vaccines. Veterinary Quarterly, volume 20(Supp. 3), 1998.

Mishra, Neeraj, Gupta, Prem N., Khatri, Kapil, Goyal, Amit K., Vyas, Suresh P. *Edible vaccines: A new approach to oral immunization,* Indian Journal of Biotechnology, volume 7, July 2008.

Oszvald, M., Kang, T.J., Tomoskozi, S., Tamas, C., Tamas, L., Kim, T.G., Yang, M.S. Expression of a synthetic neutralizing epitope of porcine epidemic diarrhea virus fused with synthetic B subunit of *Escherichia coli* heat labile enterotoxin in rice endosperm. *Molecular Biotechnology,* volume 35, pages 215–222, 2007.

Pascual, David W. Vaccines are for dinner, *Proceedings of the National Academy of Sciences of the United States of America*, June 2007.

Qian, B., Shen, H., Liang, W., Guo, X., Zhang, C., Wang, Y., Li, G., Wu, A., Cao, K., Zhang, D. Immunogenicity of recombinant hepatitis B virus surface antigen fused with preS1 epitopes expressed in rice seeds. *Transgenic Research*, volume 17, 2008.

Sharma, Arun K., Mohanty, Amitabh, Singh, Yogendra, Tyagi, Akhilesh K. Transgenic plants for the production of edible vaccines and immunotherapy, Current Science, volume 77, August 1999.

Tripurani, Swami Krishna, Reddy N.S., Rao, Sambasiva K.R.S. Green revolution vaccines, edible vaccines, African Journal of Biotechnology, volume 2, December 2003.

World Health Organization. The First Ten Years of the World Health Organization. Geneva: WHO, 1958.

18 Exploring the Relationship between the Emergence of Zoonotic Diseases and the Inhuman Touch of Habitat Loss and Wildlife Trade

Nawin Kumar Tiwary, Govind Singh and Asani Bhaduri*

CONTENTS

18.1 INTRODUCTION

A large number of wild animals inhabit every landscape and create their own ecological niche in the world. The enormous diversity of vertebrate and invertebrate species harbors an equally imposing assemblage of pathogens with potential negative impact on the health of human beings. Destruction of wildlife habitat and anthropogenic intrusion into wild spaces are primarily responsible for increased interactions between humans and wildlife. Such interactions very often lead to an unpleasant discourse where the wildlife is physically threatened, forced to retreat, harmed or captured.

* Corresponding author: Asani Bhaduri. asanii.bhaduri@gmail.com

DOI: 10.1201/9781003095422-18

Alteration of the physical environment is also responsible for ecological and behavioral changes in wildlife which, combined with other factors such as loss of habitat and demand for animal products, often brings wildlife in close proximity to humans. This has increased the risk of emerging zoonotic diseases in human populations. Legal wildlife trade and illegal trafficking of wildlife products are documented all over the world, and are often cited as primary reasons for pathogen spillover to human hosts. Movement of animals and animal products across countries and several agricultural practices which bring wild and domesticated animals together facilitate transmission of pathogens from wild populations to humans. Consumption of non-domesticated waterfowl and other wild birds has also been proved to be a medium of zoonotic disease transmission (Burgos & Burgos, 2007). Proximity of humans with non-human populations in practices like rearing of livestock, captive rearing of wild animals and contact-based research on free-ranging wild animals also pose the threat of reverse zoonosis (Brondízio & Moran, 2013).

The upsurge of zoonotic diseases worldwide has the potential to turn into a pandemic ravaging human lives and destroying global resources. The country of origin of the pandemic often faces a global backlash leading to an economic and political spurning. Increasing human population and frequent local and international travel have speeded up the rate of human-to-human transmission of pathogens. Once the pathogen enters and adapts into the human population, human-to-human transmission spreads the disease on a much larger scale that is sustained until the transmission chain is broken. Diseases like acquired immune deficiency syndrome (AIDS), influenza A, severe acute respiratory syndrome (SARS), Ebola and the current COVID-19 pandemic are a few examples where humans transmit the disease to each other through various levels and forms of contact (Bengis et al., 2004).

Another pattern of pathogen transmission is vector-mediated where the main pathogen reservoir is the wild population which is the direct source of infection into humans. Pathogens like hantavirus, Nipah virus, rabies and plague are a few examples where such transmission occurs (Bengis et al., 2004). Increased instances of such diseases have now made people more aware of exploring links between wildlife and disease transmission.

Increasing awareness and involving local communities can help to bring a positive attitude towards wildlife and will reduce hunting and poaching. Effective implementation of dedicated wildlife and environmental legislation is paramount to ensure wildlife hunting is reduced. Transboundary laws like the Convention on International Trade in Endangered Species of Wild Fauna and Flora (CITES), which bans the commercial trade of wildlife between signatory countries, are important to curb the illegal trade of wildlife. However, merely enforcing regulatory measures without understanding the economic and social actuality of the wildlife trade is probably a reason why CITES has been less productive on many fronts (Challender et al., 2015; Dongol & Heinen, 2012). It is very important to work on human behavioral change to reduce consumption of wildlife and wildlife-based products. Improving the existing regulatory framework to ensure maximum trade bans will minimize the possibility of future pandemics.

The exceptional increase in global epidemics in recent decades necessitates implementation of preventive measures rather than spending resources on containing outbreaks. Incorporating scientific approach and understanding the travel pathways of various pathogens will help us to devise standard protocols and a unified solution to regulate trade in wildlife and reduce such epidemics. Adopting the One Health approach, which included environmental, ecological and anthropogenic factors, will create a greater chance for success in dealing with infectious diseases (Cunningham et al., 2017).

18.2 HABITAT LOSS AND IMPACT ON BIODIVERSITY

The decade of 2011–2020 was earmarked by the United Nations (UN) as the UN Decade on Biodiversity (UN, 2011). The objective behind this declaration was to promote the implementation of conservation of biodiversity strategic schemes and the overall vision of human beings living in harmony with nature. Despite this and several other measures taken by the UN in the preceding decade, the 2019 global assessment report of the Intergovernmental Science-Policy Platform on Biodiversity and Ecosystem Services (IPBES) presented a grim picture. At the outset it has become clear that no substantial reason exists to celebrate the closing year of the UN Decade on Biodiversity. This report by the IPBES, an intergovernmental body comprising more than 130 member governments, estimates that around 1 million animal and plant species are now threatened with extinction (IPBES, 2019). What is even more concerning is that, in many projections, we will begin to witness the majority of these extinctions in the next few decades.

It is now widely accepted and understood that loss of habitat is the leading reason for this drastic decline in global biodiversity (Chase et al., 2020). Increasing human population is exerting tremendous pressure on land resources, engendering large-scale changes in land use patterns around the world. Rising population and resource demand along with the constraints of changing climate are pressing challenges faced by governments around the world. As a response to this challenge, the first concern of most – if not all – governments is to do whatever is necessary to meet the requirements of the burgeoning human population (Figure 18.1). Concerns about wildlife survival and biodiversity conservation take a back seat, as can be seen from a decline in biodiversity, human–wildlife conflicts and a consequent reduction in the biodiversity and ecosystem services obtained from nature.

Recent research is now indicating, and has largely established, the relationship between ongoing land use changes and declining ecosystem services in several countries (Hasan et al., 2020). The Millennium Ecosystem Assessment Report (Reid et al., 2005) had elaborated the direct link between ecosystem services and human well-being. We have therefore known for more than a decade that any loss of habitat or biodiversity can have deleterious impacts on our own health and survival on the planet. The cascading effect on the entire food chain and web due to even one species loss has been known for decades. Despite the availability of this

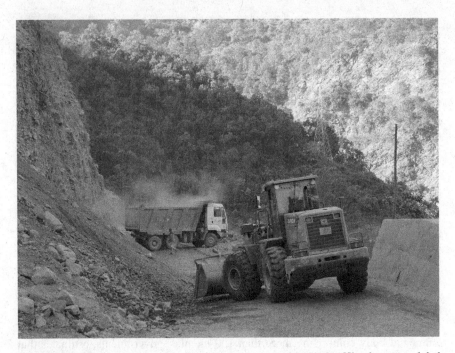

FIGURE 18.1 Rampant construction and road expansion in the Himalayas, a global biodiversity hotspot, continue to threaten its fragile ecosystem.

knowledge and information, there has been a lack of concrete action which is significant for biodiversity conservation. On the contrary, poaching and illegal sale of animals through wildlife markets, habitat fragmentation and continual use of pesticides have become the norm. These activities have put us in harm's way and the first and most prominent indicator of this are the greatly reduced ecosystem services today in comparison to a few decades ago. As a result, we are now beginning to explore and understand the link between loss of biodiversity and the emergence of infectious diseases (Wilkinson et al., 2018). This is clearly going to continue and become the focus of most biodiversity-related research in the post-COVID-19 pandemic world.

18.3 HUMAN INTERFERENCE AND ANIMALS

Human beings and fellow animal species on earth are heterotrophs – dependent on food from different sources. This inevitably brings about an innate inter/intra-specific competition for food and resources. With availability of shelter and food, the population increases manifold until it reaches a carrying capacity. In this Anthropocene era with lunatic growth and simultaneous conquering of nature and natural riches, human beings have overpowered all the other animal species. We are unrelenting in annihilating the environment of which we are an inextricable part (Otto, 2018). The devastation that humans are causing worldwide is glaringly obvious. It ranges from forest encroachment and deforestation; draining out water from all available freshwater resources; creating unnecessary and unplanned dams in every river; burning fossil fuel at an alarming rate, and thus releasing more stored carbon; creating a plastic garbage dump in oceans; to hunting and poaching for animals and animal parts (wildlife trade) – not sparing any part of nature through our anthropogenic activity. The freshwater sources of the planet are becoming scarcer every decade, thanks to wasteful usage by a plethora of human beings. Rivers and wetlands, not only rich water sources but also rich in bioresources, are the worst hit. Most river dams are without a fish ladder, thus restricting upward breeding of fishes in the rivers and creating fragmented freshwater habitats (Barbarossa et al., 2020). Add to this sudden hydropeakings by dam authorities which are often detrimental for reproductive success downstream (Kennedy et al., 2016). Similarly, systemic draining of water for irrigation and daily usage from wetlands and subsequent filling in with earth depleting wetlands in every continent is an alarming practice. In the 'Great Acceleration', everything in the planet is human-controlled and it is thus pertinent that we take care of the planet's biodiversity and resources before wiping everything out.

Not everything is lost to 'human touch' though. Despite being targeted by poachers, developers and anti-environment lobbies worldwide, dedicated groups of people are working diligently in every country to preserve the minuscule yet pristine environment that is still left. Equivalently, there are many ongoing projects for restoration of mines and degraded forests. Environmentalists are keen to plant native plants with the aim of slowly reclaiming a natural space. For endangered species, designated protected areas are created. In the recent past cryopreserving genetic materials has been initiated; this could be utilized for *in vitro* fertilization or even cloning critically endangered or extinct species in the near future.

However, the continued illegal trade of animals and animal parts remains an alarming trend. The market exists for exotic pets, which encourages poachers to capture animals alive (Wyler & Sheikh, 2013). Death is more often the result, thereby substantially depleting flora and fauna in a certain nature reserve. The other form of hunting is for animal parts, including horns, tusks, leather, caviar, shells and even bushmeat (Wyler & Sheikh, 2013).

18.4   WILDLIFE TRADE, ILLEGAL TRAFFICKING AND ZOONOTIC DISEASES

Hunting is considered to be a grave threat to wildlife across the world, and is largely carried out for food, trade and leisure. In some parts of India and the world many endangered, vulnerable and near-threatened species are killed in ritualistic hunting by tribes and forest-dwelling communities (Aiyadurai et al., 2010). The growing human population, increased access to remote forest areas and use of modern technology and weapons have upscaled the entire process. Hunting pressure on the wildlife population of several species is intense, and this has led to a reduced and scattered population. There have been several reports from TRAFFIC on the vast numbers of animal parts being traded and transported illegally (Rosen & Smith, 2010). The fact that known or estimated figures of wildlife trade are just the tip of the iceberg is even more alarming. An analysis of the CITES data has shown that over 11 million live individuals of 1316 wild species were traded among 189 countries of the world in a span of just four years, from 2012 to 2016 (Can et al., 2019). Some of the countries exporting large numbers of wild animals in the above-mentioned period were China (mammals), Nicaragua (amphibians), South Africa (birds) and Peru (reptiles). Several wild species like wild boar, masked palm civets, barking deer, hedgehogs, squirrels, bamboo rats and snake species, domestic dogs, cats and rabbits have been reported to be sold in the wet market at Guangzhou, China (Cook & Karesh, 2008). In Indonesia, up to 90,000 mammals are sold every year in a market in North Sulawesi (Milner-Gulland & Clayton, 2002). The local consumption of bushmeat in central Africa is reported to be over 1 billion kg/year (Wilkie & Carpenter, 1999). International trade of wildlife products and wild animals is a huge market with an upside valuation of around US$ 20 billion (Barber-Meyer, 2010).

Zoonoses is a generic term used for diseases that are transmitted from animals to human beings. The reason why zoonotic pathogens are entering the human population is the increased contact of humans with wildlife. Wildlife trade and consumption of wildlife products is one way in which such interactions are escalated. Domestication and rearing of formerly wild species and interactions of wildlife with domesticated livestock in agricultural systems can also be responsible for bringing wildlife-harbored pathogens into human populations.

Wildlife trade and intensified poaching are documented in more than 120 countries and are considered to be a source of at least 75% of all zoonotic diseases (Daszak et al., 2007). Such trade, which is largely fueled by an unquenchable appetite for wildlife products (Figure 18.2), food, medicine and decoration, has not only led to the reckless destruction of biodiversity but has presented itself as an incubator for transboundary disease movement and also the risk of reverse zoonosis. Many frequently traded and sold wild animals have proved to have an epidemiologically significant role in disease transmission. Shrinking habitat and reckless interference have resulted in pathogens jumping from one host to another. Expansion of agriculture, livestock rearing and the increased rate of global travel and migrations are some of the proximate factors which can escalate contact rates between humans and wildlife, providing a bridge for pathogen transfer.

18.5 ZOONOSIS – EMERGENCE AND RE-EMERGENCE

Zoonotic diseases are effectuated by an alteration in a pathogen's host target: human beings are infected directly from the customary host (animal) or through a vector. Subsequent human-to-human transmission often results in local spread which, if not contained, can lead to an epidemic or even a pandemic (Dhiman and Tiwari, 2018). Although fungi, nematodes, protists and even prions have been shown to

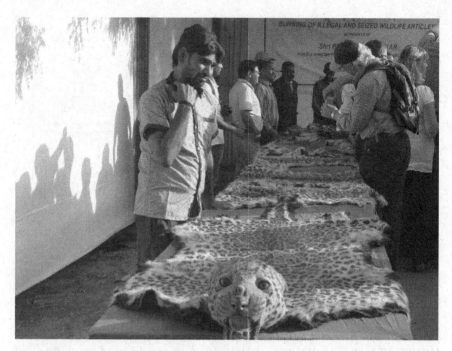

FIGURE 18.2 Image showing seized wildlife articles displayed during the 69th World Association of Zoos and Aquariums (WAZA) annual conference and Conservation Breeding Specialist Group (CBSG) annual meeting held on November 2, 2014 (Nawin K. Tiwary).

possess zoonotic characters, it is the diseases caused by bacteria and viruses which are often most pestilential. Viruses and bacteria are generally well-established pathogens in the natural world with their ability to mutate and adapt in the hostile environment of the host immune system. Zoonotic pathogens become special in that they can stay hidden in other animal hosts and re-emerge later with a modified structure thereby, avoiding a successful vaccination program. Several other factors instigate such zoonotic spillover becoming epidemic (Figure 18.3) – these include animal hosts containing the pathogen, pathogen transmission, pathogen load, population movement and population density in humans, timely and successful detection and extermination of the pathogen, to name a few (Dhiman, 2014). However, morbidity is often high in zoonotic diseases, albeit locally, due to the suddenness of the outbreak, which is generally caused by a tweak in pathogen eco-physiology or a variation in the environment in the asymptomatic natural/reservoir host.

Outbreaks often happen in a densely populated area and the world increasingly has such urban/rurban pockets with densely populated human inhabitants. To check such outbreaks numerous precautions have to be taken; first and foremost is identifying potential zoonotic pathogens. This is a herculean task as different

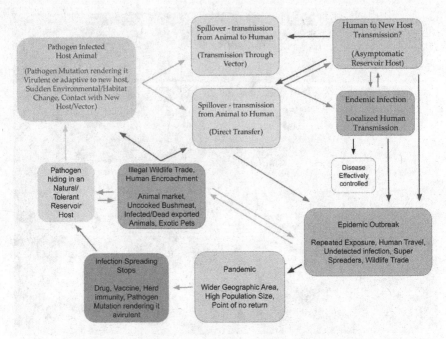

FIGURE 18.3 A schematic diagram highlighting the complexity of transmission and emergence of zoonosis. Human interference, from habitat destruction and illegal wildlife trade to superspreading, enormously affects the extent of spread.

pathogens have different hosts and, for a virus or bacteria, mutation in selected genes and reassortment of surface proteins and macromolecules give way to high evolvability through modularity.

The next task is to check human–animal interactions on a regular basis. This involves controlling illegal wildlife trade as well as enforcing firmly regulations for animal farming and import/export of wild species (Beltran-Alcrudo et al., 2019). This is easier said than done. For example, bird flu in poultry farms is often associated with an infection which starts with a migratory bird that came into contact with the domestic ones (Bengis et al., 2004). It is observed that a human outbreak often appears following another outbreak in a certain animal host. A prompt and proper extermination of such infected animals is warranted, which again is not successful in most cases as infected animals are often transported from farms or wildlife markets to other cities or even countries before being checked for infection. For scientific investigation, the most decisive step is identification and subsequent isolation of the pathogen. Although genomic sequencing is a potent tool for identification, it often takes time as the animal host may not always be identified in the initial period of an outbreak. Moreover, sequencing may reveal the identity and classification details but creating a biotherapeutic particle or a potent drug or suitable vaccine may take decades and involves many insurmountable challenges (Moleirinho et al., 2020). Often in certain cases of viral infection like influenza it may be an impossible task. The next step in an outbreak becoming an epidemic or pandemic also depends on human behavior. The COVID-19 epidemic has shown our inability to curb our innate desire not to follow rules and our callousness, resulting in superspreader groups worldwide.

Given that human beings are indulging in habitat loss of many animal species in such an alarming way, more and more zoonotic cases are going to come out in the open. Adding to this is the uncertainty of how global climate change can affect the planet in the near and distant future. Recent findings suggest that several archaic glacial viruses are lurking within icy glacier cores in the Tibetan plateau (Zhong et al., 2020). With anthropogenic global warming melting glaciers all over the world, pathogens unknown to modern humans and animals can reemerge, spread and establish in new hosts.

The illegal trade of animals, whether for bushmeat, as imported pets or for aesthetically desired animal parts or even for traditional medicine, is another instigator for zoonosis outbreaks. Often the illegal trade involves export to different countries, bypassing existing quarantine rules (Beltran-Alcrudo et al., 2019). In recent years, it has become evident that collaboration between forest officials, quarantine regulators and border security forces of different countries is extremely important in containing possible zoonotic spread.

18.6 MEASURES TO TACKLE FUTURE PANDEMICS AND WAYS OF SUSTAINABILITY

The year 2020 witnessed the rapid spread of coronavirus in almost every country in the world, almost like a proverbial forest fire. The resulting COVID-19 pandemic directly affected many people and many lost their lives. The indirect impacts of COVID-19 pandemic have proven to be as sinister as the direct impacts and a plenitude of human livelihoods has been threatened by it. COVID-19 is definitely the worst pandemic in recent times. It is certainly not the last one and should be taken as a warning sign by us and prompt us to be prepared with action plans and pandemic handbooks for similar threats in the near future. The origin of the COVID-19 pandemic remains under question and it may never be substantially established due to initial delays in the reporting and investigation of this pandemic. That is Learning 101 and all nations, irrespective of governance structure, must work with full transparency in their healthcare and disease control departments. This must become a necessity for any nation to exist as a sovereign state, and be regarded as the responsibility of every nation state.

The need to strengthen existing strategies and plans for the conservation of biodiversity, especially wildlife, is of paramount importance today. This can begin with steady support to all the biodiversity hotspots of the world with resources needed to ensure natural resources and wildlife conservation. Habitat encroachment by humans and illegal trading of animals are the main reasons behind the prevalence of zoonotic diseases. There should be greater impetus in the implementation of strategies stopping poaching, hunting and trading of wild animals from protected areas and this should be supervised by the highest monitoring agencies of the respective nations. A simultaneous campaign both to generate awareness in the masses about the need to conserve wildlife and biodiversity and the risk associated with zoonotic diseases should be initiated. Each nation must work on a war footing in order to understand host–pathogen relationships in the wild, finding the reservoir hosts of hitherto unknown pathogens to mankind. The awareness and identification process should continue alongside ensuring endangered species conservation and preservation of most vulnerable habitats and ecosystems. This will require harsh decisions that may seem adverse to human society in the short term but will certainly have long-term benefits in ensuring the sustained survival of human beings on the planet.

REFERENCES

Aiyadurai, A., Singh, N. J., & Milner-Gulland, E. J. (2010). Wildlife hunting by indigenous tribes: A case study from Arunachal Pradesh, north-east India. *Oryx*, *44*(4), 564–572. https://doi.org/10.1017/S0030605309990937.

Barbarossa, V., Schmitt, R. J., Huijbregts, M. A., Zarfl, C., King, H., & Schipper, A. M. (2020). Impacts of current and future large dams on the geographic range connectivity of freshwater fish worldwide. *Proceedings of the National Academy of Sciences*, *117*(7), 3648–3655. https://doi.org/10.1073/pnas.1912776117.

Barber-Meyer, S. M. (2010). Dealing with the clandestine nature of wildlife – trade market surveys. *Conservation Biology*, *24*(4), 918–923. https://doi.org/10.1111/j.1523-1739.2010.01500.x.

Beltran-Alcrudo, D., Falco, J. R., Raizman, E., & Dietze, K. (2019). Transboundary spread of pig diseases: the role of international trade and travel. *BMC Veterinary Research*, *15*, 64. https://doi.org/10.1186/s12917-019-1800-5.

Bengis, R. G., Leighton, F. A., Fischer, J. R., Artois, M., Mörner, T., & Tate, C. M. (2004). The role of wildlife in emerging and re-emerging zoonoses. *Revue Scientifique et Technique*, *23*(2), 497–511. https://doi.org/10.20506/rst.23.2.1498.

Brondízio, E. S., & Moran, E. F. (2013). Human–environment interactions: current and future directions. *Human-Environment Interactions: Current and Future Directions*, 1–404. https://doi.org/10.1007/978-94-007-4780-7

Burgos, S., & Burgos, S. A. (2007). Influence of exotic bird and wildlife trade on avian influenza transmission dynamics: animal–human interface. *International Journal of Poultry Science*, *6*(7), 535–538. https://doi.org/10.3923/ijps.2007.535.538.

Can, Ö. E., D'Cruze, N., & Macdonald, D. W. (2019). Dealing in deadly pathogens: taking stock of the legal trade in live wildlife and potential risks to human health. *Global Ecology and Conservation*, *17*. https://doi.org/10.1016/j.gecco.2018.e00515.

Challender, D. W. S., Harrop, S. R., & MacMillan, D. C. (2015). Understanding markets to conserve trade-threatened species in CITES. *Biological Conservation*, *187*, 249–259. https://doi.org/10.1016/j.biocon.2015.04.015.

Chase, J. M., Blowes, S. A., Knight, T. M., Gerstner, K., & May, F. (2020). Ecosystem decay exacerbates biodiversity loss with habitat loss. *Nature*, *584*(7820), 238–243.

Cook, R. A., & Karesh, W. B. (2008). Emerging diseases at the interface of people, domestic animals, and wildlife. In *Zoo and Wild Animal Medicine* (Issue 1, pp. 136–146). St. Louis: Elsevier.

Cunningham, A. A., Daszak, P., & Wood, J. L. N. (2017). One health, emerging infectious diseases and wildlife: two decades of progress? *Philosophical Transactions of the Royal Society B: Biological Sciences, 372*(1725). https://doi.org/10.1098/rstb.2016.0167.

Daszak, P., Epstein, J. H., Kilpatrick, A. M., Aguirre, A. A., Karesh, W. B., & Cunningham, A. A. (2007). Collaborative research approaches to the role of wildlife in zoonotic disease emergence. *Current Topics in Microbiology and Immunology, 315*, 463–475. https://doi.org/10.1007/978-3-540-70962-6_18.

Dhiman, R. C. (2014). Emerging vector-borne zoonoses: eco-epidemiology and public health implications in India. *Frontiers in Public Health, 2*, 168. doi: 10.3389/fpubh.2014.00168.

Dhiman, R. C., & Tiwari, A. (2018). Emergence of zoonotic diseases in India: a systematic review. *Medical Reports and Case Studies 3*, 163. doi: 10.4172/2572-5130.1000163.

Dongol, Y., & Heinen, J. T. (2012). Pitfalls of CITES implementation in Nepal: a policy gap analysis. *Environmental Management, 50*(2), 181–190. https://doi.org/10.1007/s00267-012-9896-4.

Hasan, S. S., Zhen, L., Miah, M. G., Ahamed, T., & Samie, A. (2020). Impact of land use change on ecosystem services: a review. *Environmental Development, 34*, 100527.

Intergovernmental Science-Policy Platform on Biodiversity and Ecosystem Services (IPBES). (2019). UN Report: Nature's Dangerous Decline 'Unprecedented'; Species Extinction Rates 'Accelerating'. URL: www.un.org/sustainabledevelopment/blog/2019/05/nature-decline-unprecedented-report/ (accessed on 23 October 2020).

Kennedy, T. A., Muehlbauer, J. D., Yackulic, C. B., Lytle, D. A., Miller, S. W., Dibble, K. L., Kortenhoeven, E. W., Metcalfe, A. N., & Baxter, C. V. (2016). Flow management for hydropower extirpates aquatic insects, undermining river food webs. *Bioscience, 66*(7), 561–575. doi:10.1093/Biosci/Biw059.

Milner-Gulland, E. J., & Clayton, L. (2002). The trade in babirusas and wild pigs in North Sulawesi, Indonesia. *Ecological Economics, 42*(1–2), 165–183. https://doi.org/10.1016/S0921-8009(02)00047-2.

Moleirinho, M. G., Silva, R. J. S., Alves, P. M., Carrondo, M. J. T., & Peixoto, C. (2020). Current challenges in biotherapeutic particles manufacturing. *Expert Opinion on Biological Therapy, 20*(5), 451–465. doi: 10.1080/14712598.2020.1693541.

Otto, S. P. (2018). Adaptation, speciation and extinction in the Anthropocene. *Proceedings. Biological Sciences, 285*(1891), 20182047. https://doi.org/10.1098/rspb.2018.2047.

Reid, W. V., Mooney, H. A., Cropper, A., Capistrano, D., Carpenter, S. R., Chopra, K., & Kasperson, R. (2005). *Ecosystems and Human Well-Being: Synthesis: A Report of the Millennium Ecosystem Assessment*. Washington, DC: Island Press.

Rosen, G. E., & Smith, K. F., (2010). Summarizing the evidence on the international trade in illegal wildlife. *Ecohealth, 7*, 24–32. https://doi.org/10.1007/s10393-010-0317-y.

United Nations (UN). (2011). Resolution adopted by the General Assembly on 20 December 2010. A/RES/65/161. www.un.org/en/ga/search/view_doc.asp?symbol=A/RES/65/161 (accessed on 23 October 2020).

Wilkie, D., & Carpenter, J. (1999). Bushmeat hunting in the Congo Basin. *Biodiversity, 8*, 927–955. https://link.springer.com/content/pdf/10.1023%2FA%3A1008877309871.pdf.

Wilkinson, D. A., Marshall, J. C., French, N. P., & Hayman, D. T. (2018). Habitat fragmentation, biodiversity loss and the risk of novel infectious disease emergence. *Journal of the Royal Society Interface, 15*(149), 20180403.

Wyler, L., & Sheikh, P. (2013). International Illegal Trade in Wildlife: Threats and U.S. Policy Congressional Research Services. Retrieved from: https://fas.org/sgp/crs/misc/RL34395.pdf (accessed on 23 October 2020).

Zhong, Z. P., Solonenko, N. E., Li, Y. F., Gazitúa, M. C., Roux, S., Davis, M. E., Van Etten, J. L., Mosley-Thompson, E., Rich, V. I., Sullivan, M. B., & Thompson, L. G. (2020). Glacier ice archives fifteen-thousand-year-old viruses. BioRxiv. doi:10.1101/2020.01.03.894675.

Unit VIII

Perspectives on Environmental and Human Health Management

19 Contribution Towards a Greener Environment by Using Specific MAP Species

A Case Study Among the Tribes of Tripura, India

Sujit K. Dutta* and Ratul Arya Baishya

CONTENTS

19.1 INTRODUCTION

The tiny little state of Tripura is located in the far corner of North-East India. The state has an enormous repository of diverse medicinal plant resources with great potential for alleviating poverty by enhancing the rural economy. A large number

* Corresponding author: Sujit K. Dutta. sujitk1953@gmail.com

DOI: 10.1201/9781003095422-19

of the poorest indigenous people of India use herbal plants collected from forest areas. Thus, the tribes of Tripura, like other tribes of India, use their traditional ecological knowledge (TEK) from their ancestors, inculcate it and transmit it further to contemporary society for primary healthcare requirements. Further, TEK of a tribal community is closely linked to geography as well as ecological and cultural factors (Gesler, 1992; Wiley, 2002).

19.1.1 Climate Change and MAP Species

Earth's climate is warming and changing at an exponential rate, as is explicitly clear. The increasing levels of greenhouse gases (GHGs), higher temperatures, frequent droughts and floods and rising sea levels are gradually having an impact on MAP species growth, yield and production, resulting in increased vulnerability, especially to resource-poor farmers (Harish et al., 2012; Marshall et al., 2015; Das et al., 2016). Biodiversity may be at risk of mass extinction as the planet Earth warms and the rate at which the global climate is changing creates problems of adaptation issues to the plant communities (Das, 2010; Hatfield and Prueger, 2015; Das et al., 2016).

There has been a worldwide change in environmental factors, e.g. erratic temperature and rainfall patterns, climate change, global warming, ultraviolet irradiation, intense sunlight and shade, ozone, GHG concentrations in the atmosphere, drought, salinity, nutrient deficiency, agro-chemicals, waste, heavy metals, nano materials, weeds, pests and pathogen infections that can be attributed to global climate change (Das et al., 2016). There is no doubt that Climate change will affect lifecycles and distributions of the Earth's vegetation, including wild MAP species across the globe (Hatfield and Prueger, 2015). Such challenges are the major cause of concern as regards the survival and genetic integrity of some highly valued MAP species that are the subject of discussion in various academic/scientific platforms and forums.

Furthermore, the challenge of finding an appropriate solution to adapt to climate change will unquestionably pose a greater or more immediate threat to the existence of these MAP species. Moreover, scientists are uncertain whether climate change has the potential to increase pressure on MAP species and/or their population. It is certain that the impact of climate change may have an effect on the distribution and existence of MAP species around the globe, as these MAP species are economically viable plant species and have enormous medicinal properties.

Traditional systems of medicine together with the practice of folklore continue to serve a large section of the rural population, particularly in the tribal inhabitant areas of the state, even with the existence of modern medicine. The traditional practices of medicine in developing countries based on plants are considered important for the primary healthcare system (Sheldon et al., 1997; Gautam and Richhariya, 2015; Murmu and Pramanik, 2018). The World Health Organization (WHO) has estimated that about 80% of the world's population still mostly relies on conventional medicine for their primary healthcare necessities (Azaizeh et al., 2003).

The consequences of the impact of environmental factors on MAP species would lead to their secondary metabolism activities (Yang et al., 2018; Mohiuddin, 2019; Yanqun et al., 2020). In recent years, it has been noticed that the use of bio-active compounds from natural resources has gained momentum. The presence of vital chemical compounds (secondary metabolites) in MAP species – alkaloids, glycosides, essential oils and other miscellaneous active substances – enabled these plant species to cope with any kind of environmental and/or external stimuli in a rapid, reversible and ecologically meaningful manner. In addition, environmental factors play an important function in regulating the metabolic production of biologically active molecules in MAP species. Understanding how MAP species counteract these environmental degradation and climate changes could open up new avenues in MAP species production in cultivable and wild nature, where succeeding innovation is urgently needed to meet the threatening challenges of climate change and global food security issues.

19.1.2 HERBAL REMEDIES – AN EFFECTIVE MEANS OF TREATMENT

Herbal remedies used by ethnic groups were generally effective, although they contained many inert compounds in addition to the bioactive compound(s) (Kamboj, 2000; Sannomiya et al., 2007; Verma and Singh, 2008). The studies made by Katewa et al. (2004) highlight that indigenous medicines which are harmless, effective and inexpensive are gaining recognition in both rural and urban areas in countries like India. Many Indian tribes and rural communities still continue to practice TEK to heal a number of diseases and ailments (Jain and Dam, 1979; Katewa et al., 2001; Kshirsagar and Singh, 2001; Jagtap et al., 2006; Sajem and Gosai, 2006; Kala and Sajwan, 2007; Sajem et al., 2008; Katewa, 2009; Gautam and Richhariya, 2015; Murmu and Pramanik, 2018). Among the world's 12 bio-diversity centers, India is one such important biodiversity hotspot, having over 49,441 different plant species (Mao and Dash, 2018). The forest is the principal storehouse of MAP species in large quantities in India; there is estimated to be over 20,000 plants which have good medicinal values, of which only 7,000–7,500 species are used by traditional communities (Matthews, 2005; Mao et al., 2009).

19.1.3 BACKDROP TO THE STUDY

Tripura is the richest reservoir of MAP species, especially in hilly and forest areas. Out of the total geographic area of the state of 10,492 km², 59.98% is forest (34.2% reserve forest, 4.85% proposed reserve forest and 20.93% unclassified forest). The tribes in this region have been living in close proximity to nature and maintaining close links with the environment. In India, from 18,864 species of higher plants (Mao and Dash, 2018), over 2,000 species are documented and 1,100 species have medicinal usage in different systems of medicine. About 95% of MAP species are obtained from wild sources, of which only 150 species have commercial use. In India, Tripura has a maximum plant diversity index of 5.23 (Kshirsagar and Upadhvyay, 2009). The state also borders part of both Himalayan and Indo-Burman biodiversity regions that have a large number of flora and fauna, making this region a 'biodiversity hotspot' (Dutta and Dutta, 2005).

At present, there are 19 different tribes of Tripura. The Tripuri, Reang, Noatia, Jamatia, Halam, Kuki, Chaimal and Uchai were historically immigrants from outside the state but they are now regarded as the original settlers of the state. Each tribe with its unique ethnic criteria has distinctive ethnic features with its respective socio-cultural heritage, language and food habits, among others. Each tribe has its own dialect but *Kokborok* is customary as standard lingua franca for the purpose of communication among the tribes.

The diversity of culture, people and plant species is an added advantage for developing each tribe's own traditional knowledge, but with the passage of time, these diversifications have gradually diminished due to negligence about knowledge management. The tribal/rural ethnic communities in the state have been engaged in subsistence agriculture, *jhum*, piggery, fishery and hunting. Moreover, in due course, these tribes/rural ethnic communities have achieve immense knowledge on the usage of fundamental plant products in the therapeutic treatment of various ailments/diseases (Maheswari et al., 1986, Gautam and Richhariya, 2015; Murmu and Pramanik, 2018). They have developed a profound belief in their indigenous folk medicine for remedial purposes; their ancestral knowledge about native remedial techniques treating various diseases was transmitted orally from one generation to another. Further, the era of modernization has rapidly taken root in the society; traditional knowledge has day by day become mislaid and very few studies have been carried out in the field of state ethno-medico-botany. Scholars have reported several medicinal plants and their utilization as proposed by indigenous tribes, yet the state listing of highly valued MAP species is still deficient. According to a study conducted by Dutta et al. (2013) on Meghalaya and a study by Rai and Lalramnghinglova (2010) on Mizoram, the trading of highly valued MAP species in all North-East India is somewhat limited. Thus, the authors have attempted to explore the herbal practices of tribes in Tripura that are contributing livelihood options in a greener environment.

19.2 MATERIALS AND METHODS

19.2.1 STUDY AREA

The study focuses mainly on the contribution towards a greener environment made by the usage of specific MAP species by tribal communities with their distinctive culture. The study continued for about two years to generate time series data. Tripura is located in the bio-geographic zone of 9B-North East Hills between 22°56' N and 24°32' N latitude and 90°09' E and 92°20' E longitude. The length of the international boundary between Tripura and Bangladesh is 839 km in the north, west and south-east peripheries, while the boundaries with the states of Assam and Mizoram were 53 km and 109 km respectively (Majumdar et al., 2006).

The total geographic area of Tripura is about 10,486 km² or 0.32% of the total area of the country. The forest coverage of Tripura is about 7977 km² (FSI, 2019). The temperature ranges between 10°C and 36°C and average annual rainfall is about 247.9 cm.

19.2.2   MAP SAMPLE COLLECTION AND METHODOLOGY

For collecting, documenting and assessing the impact of climate change on highly valued ethno-botanical MAP species, the entire state forest was included in the study based on the accessibility and similarity in physical habitat (Figure 19.1).

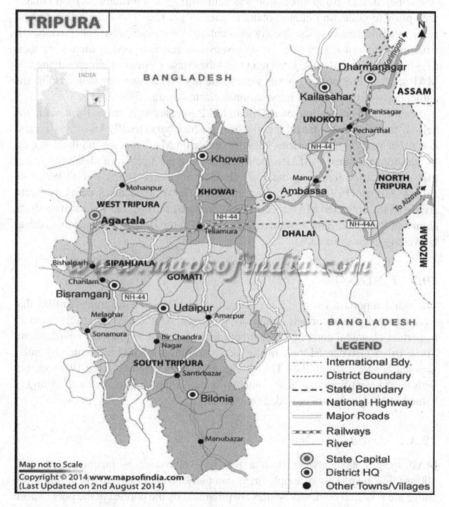

FIGURE 19.1   Map showing the entire state of Tripura, India.

The locations of the sampling sites were documented by global positioning system (GPS) receiver.

During the ethno-botanical survey in the sample study area, the authors purposively identified several herbalists, local healers of a tribal community who are more sensitive to local conditions. The authors accompanied them on several study visits conducted regarding medicinal plant usage to evaluate the impact of climate change on these MAP species. After collecting relevant materials on the subjects, an interface discussion was conducted with government officials, such as the Chief Executive Officer, National Medicinal Plant Board (NMPB), Tripura; Principal Chief Conservator of Forests, Tripura; and local healers (both men and women) on the data already collected.

Further, a brief group discussion was held with local informants at each village/area prior to collecting ethno-botanical data to get their consent; in this discussion, valuable data on these locally available MAP species were collected. Semi-structured interview schedule, group discussion and field observation were used to generate information on knowledge and the consequences of climate change on MAP species. Frequent site visits were made in different seasons to determine the authenticity of the data and information collected during field survey.

Scientific identification of different MAP species was carried out with the help of forest officials, traditional medical practitioners (locally known as *auchai*, *kabiraj* or *vaidyas*) and persons knowledgeable on MAP species and their usages. In addition, samples of MAP species collected were further validated for scientific identification following the research of Anonymous (1985), Deb (1989), Jain and De-Filipps (1991) and Kritikar and Basu (2005). Voucher specimens (herbarium) of the collected MAP species were prepared through conventional methods (Jain and Rao, 1977); these were then deposited at the Botanical Museum, Gauhati University, Assam, India.

19.3 FINDINGS

The study reports a list of 15 highly valued MAPs in 12 different families that were ethnically used for self-healthcare purposes. All these MAP species contain important chemical compounds that help them to adapt to the local environment. These tribes also earned their livelihood by trading the same in the nearby international border zone market. The species have been listed in Table 19.1 together with their scientific name, and ailments treated. Photographs of these 15 highly valued MAP species are provided in Appendix I.

19.3.1 LIVELIHOOD OPTIONS

MAP species have always been a prospective avenue of income, generating 100 million man days of employment annually (Negi et al., 2010). Further, the fringe areas of rich biodiversity sites are inhabited by the poorest of the poor, whose incomes can be augmented by a comprehensive strategy aimed at capacity building

TABLE 19.1
List of 15 highly valued traditional medicinal and aromatic plant (MAP) species used by the tribal communities of Tripura

Serial no.	Scientific name [family]; exsiccate	Local name	Plant parts used	Ailments treated
1.	*Aegle marmelos* (Linn.) Correa ex Roxb. [Rutaceae]	Bel/Shirphal	Roots, leaves and fruit	Diarrhea, dysentery, dyspepsia, vomiting, intermittent fever, gastric irritability, etc.
2.	*Andrographis paniculata* (Burm.f.) Wall. ex Nees [Acanthaceae]	Kalmegh	Whole plants, mainly leaves	Viral fevers like chikungunya, swine flu, typhoid, etc.
3.	*Asparagus racemosus* Willd. [Liliaceae]	Shatavar/ Satamuli	Roots, leaves	Diabetes, stomach disorders, blood pressure, etc.
4.	*Emblica officinalis* Gaertn. [Euphorbiaceae]	Amla	Fruit	Ulcers, treatment of jaundice, dyspepsia, blood pressure, hyperacidity, etc.
5.	*Gmelina arborea* Roxb. [Verbinaceae]	Gamhar/ Gambhari/ white teak	Roots, barks, flowers and fruit	Stomachic, galactagogue, laxative and anthelmintic; improves appetite, piles, pains, burning sensations, fevers and urinary discharge
6.	*Moringa oleifera* Lam. [Moringaceae]	Sajna	Roots, barks, flowers and leaves	Dyspepsia, anorexia, verminosis, diarrhea, colic, flatulence, paralysis, inflammation, amenorrhea, dysmenorrhea, fever, etc.
7.	*Mucona pruriens* (L) DC. [Fabaceae]	Gonca/ Koncha	Seeds and flowers	Male sexual dysfunction and snakebites
8.	*Piper nigrum* L. [Piperaceae]	Gulmirch/ Kalimirch	Fruit	Stomachic, stimulant, aphrodisiac and carminative properties

(continued)

TABLE 19.1 Continued
List of 15 highly valued traditional medicinal and aromatic plant (MAP) species used by the tribal communities of Tripura

Serial no.	Scientific name [family]; exsiccate	Local name	Plant parts used	Ailments treated
9.	*Rauvolfia serpentina* Bentham ex Kurz. [Apocynaceae]	Sarpagandha/ Chota Chand	Roots	Malaria, chickenpox, tuberculosis, high blood pressure, snake poison, stomach pain, fever, etc.
10.	*Saraca asoca* (Roxb.) de Wildeman [Caesalpiniaceae]	Asoca/Sita Asoca	Flowers, seeds and bark	Hemorrhagic dysentery, urinary trouble, menstruation, etc.
11.	*Terminalia arjuna* (Roxb. ex DC.) Wight & Arn. [Combretaceae]	Arjun	Bark	Hearing diseases, contusions, fractures and ulcers
12.	*Terminalia bellerica* Roxb. [Combretaceae]	Bahera	Fruit	Cough, tuberculosis, eye diseases, anti-HIV-1, dyspepsia, diarrhea, dysentery, etc.
13.	*Terminalia chebula* (Gaertner) Retz. [Combretaceae]	Haritaki/ Harar	Fruit	Digestive diseases, urinary diseases, diabetes, skin disease, parasitic infections, heart disease, irregular fevers, flatulence, constipation, ulcers, etc.
14.	*Tinospora cordifolia* (Willd.) Miers [Menispermaceae]	Gulancha/ Giloe	Stems	Anthelmintic, anti-arthritic, antiperiodic, anti-pyretic, aphrodisiac, blood purifier, cardiac, carminative, digestive, diuretic and expectorant
15.	*Wedelia chinensis* (Osbeck) Merr. [Compositae]	Bhingaraj	Leaves	Jaundice, helminthiasis, hair growth stimulant, hair dying, rheumatic fever and headache

and value addition facilities with several interfaces between the representatives of industrial institutions and the local community. NMPB has always played a supportive role in executing projects to provide value added infrastructure and capacity building for rural peoples. These specific projects are implemented by Joint Forest Management Committees (JFMCs), Biodiversity Management Committees (BMCs) and Self Help Groups (SHGs). In this process, about 1,052 JFMCs, 592 Panchayats, 456 BMCs and 600 SHGs have been developed up to March 2019 as project-implementing agents in Tripura. This is a boon for the marginalized producers of medicinal plant-based raw materials towards income augmentation. NMPB has also collaborated with the National Rural Livelihood Mission (NRLM) of the Ministry of Rural Development to forge synergy between NMPB and NRLM initiatives.

Panchakarma therapy has been practiced to treat ailments by the people of Tripura from ancient times. This system is being practiced at (1) *Panchakarma* Research and Training Centre, and (2) Sepahijala for basic healthcare necessities under the administration of expert Ayurvedic practitioners. From 2009, this system, which is beneficial for diseased individuals, has been executed under the supervision of the Medicinal Plant Board, Tripura (MPBT). Thus, this becomes an important livelihood option for the ethnic communities of the region.

19.3.2 SOCIAL ENTREPRENEURS

Social entrepreneurs may also be involved as social actors with an ideology to organize, create and manage such ventures to make social changes. These types of entrepreneurs develop self-driven social agents devoted to achieve a social purpose focusing mainly on marginalized sections of society. Further, they use innovative and systematic approaches towards the marginalized, the disadvantaged and the disenfranchised in society, such as the one we have taken as a sample, and expect that these would help in several ways. It is the prerogative of the social entrepreneur who tries to solve community-based issues in a professional manner (Roy, 2011).

19.3.3 INTELLECTUAL PROPERTIES

The tribes of Tripura have been utilizing MAP species for their health problems, viz. diarrhea, viral fevers, stomach disorders, jaundice, malaria, chickenpox. At times there is an instant cure or sometimes they look for alternative MAP species or modern medical treatment. It has largely been found that their knowledge of plant identification was tremendous, but they lack proper endorsement and established rights over MAP resources. It is highly recommended that under Intellectual Property Rights (IPRs), the Geographical Indication (GI) should be established as a trademark to protect the rights of these local indigenous people. The other option would be to share royalties and proceeds of sales of these MAP species with local tribes.

19.4   DISCUSSION

At the very outset of the investigation, the authors documented 15 highly valued MAP species, mostly used by the tribal communities of Tripura, containing important chemical compounds that help these plant species to survive in local environmental conditions. The documented 15 MAP species are categorized as herbs (one species), shrubs (three species), climbers (two species) and woody trees (nine species) respectively. Among these 15 MAP species, only five are cultivated in homestead lands and the *jhum* lands of the tribes, while the rest are grown naturally in wild form in the forest adapted to local climatic conditions. The investigation data further reveal that roots and leaves are mostly used in the treatment of many major ailments, whereas fruit, barks and seeds are used for general minor ailments. Maximum formulations are a mixture of two or more plant parts, whereas mixtures with preservatives like honey, sugar, ajwain, asafoetida, ghee, and so forth, have also been found to be utilized in several ailments. It was also learned during this research that similar formulations are being used to treat different types of ailments/diseases due to the presence of vital chemical constituents in these MAP species. A few of the demonstrated MAP species in this present study had already been reported but their purposes and usage methods were different; for example, *Andrographis paniculata* (Burm.f.) Wall. ex Nees is used for viral fevers like chikungunya, swine flu, typhoid, etc., that are prevalent in this part of the country; *Asparagus racemosus* Willd. is used in frigidity and sexual weakness; *Mucona pruriens* (L.) DC is used in male sexual dysfunction and snakebites; and *Wedelia chinensis* (Osbeck) Merr. is used in jaundice, helminthiasis, as a hair growth stimulant, in hair dying, rheumatic fever and headache. From this exploration, it was assessed that the Tripura has enormous TEK on the ethno-medicinal usage of MAP species in curing various ailments/diseases.

The present research also depicts that the tribes of Tripura have acquired substantial knowledge about the traditional usage of MAP species that are grown locally in the region which are well adapted to local climatic conditions. Different parts of these valuable MAP species, such as leaf, stem, bark, fruit, seed and root, were used in different forms like crude, power, juice, decoction, infusion and paste for curing various ailments/diseases. It was also learnt that these different tribal communities of Tripura inhabiting the hilly and forested area still have faith in traditional/ethnic herbal drugs.

The need of the hour is to assess climate change and the global warming effect (elevated CO_2) on these MAP species with a focused approach, especially on the accumulation of secondary metabolites (Courtney, 2009; Harish et al., 2012). The feasible climatic effects on these MAP species are significant due to their immense traditional medicinal valuation with reasonable cost. The loss of some MAP species in the region may hamper livelihood opportunities of large sections of tribes that depend on the trade of such MAP species. Sudden warming of temperature disrupting seasonal events cannot be understood easily, while appropriate human interference can always thwart biodiversity. Hence, a detailed focused research approach must be carried out, especially on the accumulation of secondary metabolites of significance for health (Harish et al., 2012). Scientific research studies on MAP species with respect to climate change are very sporadic and insignificant in comparison with other commercial crops.

Given the undisputed role of MAP species in today's healthcare requirements, prioritization must be made so that these MAP species are cultivated and propagated on a large scale. Besides their beneficial medicinal attributes, these MAP species have trade properties and market potentiality. This in turn will provide a livelihood opportunity for cultivators and entrepreneurs dealing with it within the region and, thus, would reduce pressure on natural resources, as forests still contribute the greatest share towards the pharmaceutical industry. This is regardless of the fact that, though the wealth of available MAP resources in the region is abundant, the trade sector is still marginalized because of the absence of standardized market institution and low product values.

19.5 CONCLUSIONS AND RECOMMENDATIONS

The tribal communities living in the forested area of Tripura are largely dependent upon traditional herbal practices. Although disorganized management, non-scientific and non-sustainable harvesting, shifting cultivation and other developmental projects had gradually reduced the usage of MAP species by rural/local communities, the laxity of the state government's authority and cost of allopathic medicines had deepened their faith in old treaties and tradition. Yet, in addition to all these, there is concern as improper market regulations and global warming effects are making a number of MAP species vulnerable in their natural habitat.

Knowledge about various MAP species being used as medicine by these tribal communities following ancient practices has been receding for generations. The passage of this indigenous/ethnic knowledge from an older generation to the present generation has been stopped as the present generation is not at all interested in establishing themselves as traditional medicinal practitioners by profession. The younger generation has been following the trend of leaving their villages due to economic changes and instability. Thus, indigenous/ethnic practices and knowledge regarding the sustainable harvest and proper utilization of MAP species resources as medicine need to be documented and preserved before they disappear unrecorded.

It is therefore, recommended that the state government and scientific research organizations together with non-government organizations should take an active part in research and development activities of the MAP sector and their conservation.

APPENDIX I

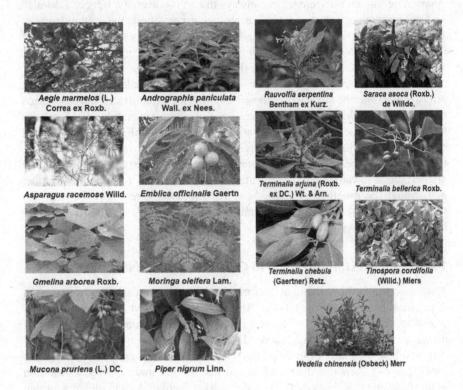

Aegle marmelos (L.) Correa ex Roxb.

Andrographis paniculata Wall. ex Nees.

Rauvolfia serpentina Bentham ex Kurz.

Saraca asoca (Roxb.) de Willde.

Asparagus racemose Willd.

Emblica officinalis Gaertn

Terminalia arjuna (Roxb. ex DC.) Wt. & Arn.

Terminalia bellerica Roxb.

Gmelina arborea Roxb.

Moringa oleifera Lam.

Terminalia chebula (Gaertner) Retz.

Tinospora cordifolia (Willd.) Miers

Mucona pruriens (L.) DC.

Piper nigrum Linn.

Wedelia chinensis (Osbeck) Merr

ACKNOWLEDGMENT

The authors are obliged to the tribal and non-tribal people of the study area for their cooperation during the study. The authors are grateful to the Ministry of Ayurvedic, Yoga and Naturopathy, Unani, Siddha and Homeopathy (AYUSH), Tripura, for sharing information on MAP species. The authors are much indebted to Mr. Jatindra Sarma (IFS), CF of Northern Assam Circle for his valuable comments, critical review and support on MAP species.

REFERENCES

Anonymous. (1985). *The Wealth of India: A Dictionary of Raw Materials and Industrial Product Raw Materials* (Vol. I). New Delhi: Publications and Information Directorate, p. 10.

Azaizeh, H., Fulder, S., Khalil, K. and Said, O. (2003). Ethnomedicinal knowledge of local Arab practitioners in the Middle East region. *Fitoterapia, 74*, 98–108.

Courtney, C. (2009). The effects of climate change on medicinal and aromatic plants. *HerbalGram (American Botanical Council), 81*, 44–57.

Das, M. (2010). Performance of Asalio (*Lepidium sativum* L.) genotypes under semi-arid condition of middle Gujarat. *Indian Journal of Plant Physiology, 15*(1), 85–89.

Das, M., Jain, V. and Malhotra, S.K. (2016). Impact of climate change on medicinal and aromatic plants: Review. *Indian Journal of Agricultural Sciences, 86*(11), 1375–1382.

Deb, D.B. (1989). *The Flora of Tripura State.* New Delhi: Today and Tomorrows Printers and Publishers, p. 5.

Dutta, B.K. and Dutta, P.K. (2005). Potential of ethnobotanical studies in North East India: An overview. *Indian Journal of Traditional Knowledge, 4,* 7–14.

Dutta, S.K., Baishya, R.A. and Singh, B. (2013). Potential tradable medicinal and aromatic plants of Meghalaya, India. *Indian Forester, 139*(5), 467–468.

FSI. (2019). *India State of Forest Report.* Dehradun, India: Forest Survey of India, p. 26.

Gautam, P. and Richhariya, G.P. (2015). Ethnoveterinary medicinal plants used by tribals and rural communities of Chitrakoot, Distt.-Satna (M.P.). *International Journal of Pharmacy & Life Science, 6*(4), 4427–4430.

Gesler, W.M. (1992). Therapeutic landscapes: Medical issues in light of the new cultural geography. *Social Science & Medicine, 34,* 735.

Harish, B.S., Dandin, S.B., Umesha, K. and Sasanur, A. (2012). Impact of climate change on medicinal plants – A review. *Ancient Science of Life, 32 (Suppl. 1),* S32.

Hatfield, J.L. and Prueger, J.H. (2015). Temperature extremes: Effect on plant growth and development. *Weather and Climate Extremes, 10,* 4–10.

Jagtap, S.D., Deokule, S.S. and Bhosle, S.V. (2006). Some unique ethnomedicinal uses of plants used by the Korku tribe of Amravati district of Maharashtra, India. *Journal of Ethnopharmacology, 107,* 463–469.

Jain, S.K. and Dam, N. (1979). Some ethnobotanical notes from Northeastern India. *Economic Botany, 33*(1), 52–56.

Jain, S.K. and De-Filipps, R.A. (1991). *Medicinal Plant of India.* Algonac, MI: Reference Publications.

Jain, S.K. and Rao, R.R. (1977). *A Handbook of Field and Herbarium Methods* (Vol. XVI). New Delhi: Today and Tomorrow's Printers and Publishers, p. 157.

Kala, C.P. and Sajwan, B.S. (2007). Revitalizing Indian systems of herbal medicine by the National Medicinal Plants Board through institutional networking and capacity building. *Current Science, 93*(6), 797–806.

Kamboj, V.P. (2000). Herbal medicine. *Current Sciences, 78,* 35–39.

Katewa, S.S. (2009). Indigenous people and forests: Perspectives of an ethnobotanical study from Rajasthan (India). In K.G. Ramawat (Ed.), *Herbal Drugs: Ethnomedicine to Modern Medicine* (p. 33). Berlin: Springer-Verlag.

Katewa, S.S., Chaudhary, B.L. and Jain, A. (2004). Folk herbal medicines from tribal area of Rajasthan, India. *Journal of Ethnopharmacology, 92,* 41–46.

Katewa, S.S., Guria, B.D. and Jain, A. (2001). Ethnomedicinal and obnoxious grasses of Rajasthan, India. *Journal of Ethnopharmacology, 76,* 293–297.

Kritikar, K.R. and Basu, B.D. (2005). *Indian Medicinal Plants.* Dehradun: International Book Distributors, p. 23.Kshirsagar, R.D. and Singh, N.P. (2001). Some less known ethnomedicinal uses from Mysore and Kodagu districts, Karnataka State, India. *Journal of Ethnopharmacology, 75,* 231–238.

Kshirsagar, R. and Upadhyay, S. (2009). Free radical scavenging activity screening of medicinal plants from Tripura, Northeast India. *Natural Product Radiance, 8,* 117–122.

Maheswari, J.K., Kalakoti, B.S. and Brijlal. (1986). Ethnomedicine of Bhil tribes of Jhabua district, Madhya Pradesh. *Ancient Science Life, 5,* 255–261.

Majumdar, K., Saha, R., Datta, B.K. and Bhakta, T. (2006). Medicinal plants prescribed by different tribal and non-tribal medicine men of Tripura State. *Indian Journal of Traditional Knowledge, 5,* 559–562.

Mao, A.A. and Dash, S.S. (2018). *Plant Discoveries 2018 – New Genera, Species and New Records*. Salt Lake City: CGO Complex, Botanical Survey of India, p. 182.

Mao, A.A., Hynniewta, T.M. and Sanjappa, M. (2009). Plant wealth of Northeast India with reference to ethnobotany. *Indian Journal of Traditional Knowledge, 8*, 96–103.

Marshall, E., Aillery, M., Malcolm, S. and Williams, R. (2015). Agricultural production under climate change: The potential impacts of shifting regional water balances in the United States. *American Journal of Agricultural Economics, 97*(2), 568–588.

Matthews, S. (2005). Ayurveda. In T. Robson (Ed.), *An Introduction to Complementary Medicine* (pp. 15–32). Crows Nest, NSW: Allen & Unwin.

Mohiuddin, A.K. (2019). Impact of various environmental factors on secondary metabolism of medicinal plants. *Journal of Pharmacology & Clinical Research, 7*(1), 555704. DOI: 10.19080/ JPCR. 2019. 07. 555704.

Murmu, S.C. and Pramanik, R. (2018). Medicinal plants in primary health care: A traditional knowledge. *Asian Resonance, 7*(3), 84–92.

Negi, V.S., Maikhuri, R.K., Phondani, P.C. and Rawat, L.S. (2010). An inventory of indigenous knowledge and cultivation practices of medicinal plants in Govind Pashu Vihar Wildlife Sanctuary, Central Himalaya, India. *International Journal of Biodiversity Science, Ecosystem Services and Management, 1*, 1–10.

Rai, P.K. and Lalramnghinglova, H. (2010). Ethnomedicinal plant resources of Mizoram, India: Implication of traditional knowledge in health care system. *Ethnobotanical Leaflets, 14*, 274–305.

Roy, R. (2011). *Entrepreneurship* (2nd ed.). New Delhi: Oxford University Press, p. 461.

Sajem, A.L. and Gosai, K. (2006). Traditional use of medicinal plants by the Jaintia Tribes in North Cachar Hills district of Assam, Northeast India. *Journal of Ethnobiology and Ethnomedicine, 2*, 33.

Sajem, A.L., Rout, J. and Nath, M. (2008). Traditional tribal knowledge and status of some rare and endemic medicinal plants of North Cachar Hills District of Assam, Northeast India. *Ethnobotanical Leaflets, 12*, 261–275.

Sannomiya, M., Cardoso, C.R.P., Figueiredo, M.E., Rodrigues, C.M., dos Santos, L.C., dos Santos, F.V., Serpeloni, J.M., Colus, I.M.S., Vilegas, W. and Varanda, E.A. (2007). Mutagenic evaluation and chemical investigation of *Byrsonima intermedia* A. Juss. leaf extracts. *Journal of Ethnopharmacology, 112*, 319–326.

Sheldon, J.W., Balick, M.J. and Laird, S.A. (1997). Medicinal plants: Can utilization and conservation coexist? *Economic Botany, 12*, 1–104.

Verma, S. and Singh, S.P. (2008). Current and future status of herbal medicines. *Veterinary World, 1*, 347–350.

Wiley, A. (2002). Increasing use of prenatal care in Ladakh (India): The roles of ecological and cultural factors. *Social Science & Medicine, 55*(7), 1089–1102.

Yang, L., Wen, K.S., Ruan, X., Zhao, Y.X., Wei, F. and Wang, Q. (2018). Response of plant secondary metabolites to environmental factors. *Molecules, 23*(4), 762–787.

Yanqun, L., Kong, D., Fu, Y., Sussman, M.R. and Wu, H. (2020). The effect of developmental and environmental factors on secondary metabolites in medicinal plants. *Plant Physiology and Biochemistry, 148*, 80–89.

20 Creating a Search Engine for a Multidimensional and Personalized Healthcare Solution

*C. R. Desai**

CONTENTS

* Corresponding author: C. R. Desai. satayushi@gmail.com

DOI: 10.1201/9781003095422-20

20.1   INTRODUCTION

The World Health Organization (WHO) definition of health says, "Health is a state of physical, mental and social well-being in which disease and infirmity are absent".[1] This is a definition of ideal health, a state of health that we can work towards. It does not, however, define actual health. The journey to ideal health has to begin from the actual health of the individual. It is imperative, therefore, to understand what actual health is. Health of an individual is studied at multiple levels – physical, mental and social levels. Each human being is born with a unique genetic profile or DNA. The DNA carries the blueprint of the life cycle of the human species from conception to birth, maturing, ageing and death. The internal changes in health as age advances are dictated by this blueprint. These are genetic or intrinsic influencing factors. The genetic profile of the individual translates into the unique constitution that the individual is born with. The DNA or constitution of an individual is a given and does not change through life. As the child grows, its health is shaped by external influencing factors like geo-climatic conditions, parents and their education, socio-economic status, the country, culture and religion that it is born in, the events and geo-political changes that take place in its life, and so on. Besides, there are other influencing factors like diet, lifestyle, education, vocation, hobbies, entertainment, marriage, children, and so forth. These are known as epigenetic or extrinsic influencing factors. They are factors that do not change the genetic profile of a person but definitely influence the manifestation and expression of the genes and have an impact on the health of the individual. Thus, there are multiple factors that impact the health of a human being. Further, each of these influencing factors has multiple variations or options. That is why each person is a unique individual; no two individuals are the same. Nevertheless, individuals can be grouped together according to their similarities in age, gender, race, constitution, and so on. Identifying the similarities among unique individuals or unity in diversity can help create a roadmap of what happens to normal individuals in their normal life span.

20.1.1 THE ROADMAP OF HEALTH

To generate a roadmap of health, we zoom out and look at the human race as a species, follow the human race as we would any other species and view their health journey from birth to death. Observation shows us that individuals with a similar constitution tend to follow a certain pattern of changes in health with age. They seem to have similar characteristics as they become adults. As they age, the group shows a predilection towards particular diseases. These can be understood as the impact of intrinsic or genetic influencing factors. The difference between this group and the other groups becomes obvious as age advances. We can see these as the different highways of the roadmap of health taken by various types of genetic profiles. Closer observation of each group shows us that in each group there are forks at which one section of the group separates from the rest. This happens because of the impact of some major extrinsic influencing factors. Tracing back shows us which extrinsic influencing factors could have made the group split. We are now discovering the main streets of the roadmap. As data start accumulating, minor influencing factors are revealed. These are the byways, dead ends and the roads less travelled on the roadmap of human health. Individuals are clustered together according to their similarities and the history of their health is traced back to their childhood in a retrospective study. Analysing the data reveals emerging patterns of sequential changes in health.

Though each individual is unique, the changes in the health of the human race fall into a few patterns. Each influencing factor subtly steers an individual towards a particular pattern of changes in health. What emerges is the roadmap of what happens to normal human beings in their normal life span (Desai, 2018a). On this roadmap, each influencing factor is seen as a fork that diverts a particular group of individuals. As the map gets populated, the roadmap gives us insights into the impact of intrinsic and extrinsic influencing factors.

20.1.2 TIME

Health is not a static entity; it is a continuous series of changes due to intrinsic and extrinsic influencing factors. The roadmap of health unfolds as time progresses. Time or t-axis plays a significant role in the study of human health. The sequence in which the influencing factors appear, the age at which they were introduced into the life of the individual and the duration for which they were part of his or her life definitely matter in shaping the life and health of the individual. For example, loss of parents is a common event in everyone's life. At what age the person lost his or her parents has a big impact on life. To give another example, we all know that yoga is good for health but at what age one begins and for how many years one practises it will matter in the impact that yoga asanas have on the health of the individual. In short, the potatoes being mashed before boiling or boiled before being mashed and how long they were boiled have a definite impact on the final dish. Thus, studying the impact of environmental factors on human health is a scientific feat.

Each individual starts from a unique initial state or genetic profile. As time passes, health is influenced by multiple influencing factors – genetic (intrinsic) and epigenetic (extrinsic). Matters get even more complicated because each influencing factor, such as diet, lifestyle, seasons, geo-climatic conditions, education, job profile, etc., has multiple options and only a few of them can be quantified or graded. In effect, we are dealing with multiple, multi-optional, qualitative and quantitative influencing factors. The time factor, sequence and duration of each influencing factor should be considered when designing a predictive module of human health.

The final and most challenging influencing factor to include in a design is the free-will choices that each individual makes. And free will is the most important and only factor that we can control.

> Human health is a canvas of infinite possibilities governed by the laws that steer an individual towards a particular health destination as time progresses. The aim of scientific research is to derive the laws that govern the probability of changes in human health.

Classical research methodology is designed to establish deterministic laws and represent them as an equation. Reality, however, is not deterministic; it is probabilistic. Added to this is the unpredictability of human free will. It becomes clear that human health cannot be studied with a deterministic approach. Besides, many of the influencing factors are qualitative; they cannot be quantified or graded. Influencing factors cannot be ignored just because they cannot be quantified. Hence, classical science and mathematics cannot be applied to the study of the impact of changing environmental factors on human health. There is another form of science which has the capacity to deal with multiple influencing factors that have multiple options and are not quantifiable. It is the Science of Classification.

20.1.3 SCIENCE OF CLASSIFICATION

Scientists in modern medicine are not too familiar with the Science of Classification but it is extensively used in computer science and information technology, retrospective studies and evidence-based scientific research. Pattern recognition, machine learning and artificial intelligence also use the Science of Classification quite extensively. These techniques are used to derive the laws that increase or decrease the probability of particular health destinations. Influencing factors that cannot be quantified can be classified and dealt with scientifically with Science of Classification. The form of mathematics that applies to the Science of Classification is the Set Theory. In fact, Set Theory forms the basis of computer science and information technology. For centuries, Indian philosophy and the science of Ayurveda have been using the Science of Classification. There is a lot that we can learn by understanding the worldview of the East.

20.2 AIMS AND OBJECTIVES

The aim is to create a search engine that derives evidence-based knowledge and an understanding about factors influencing health. The search engine will help us design policies, strategies and interventions that can steer humanity towards excellent health.

Evidence-based learning that emerges from data analysis improves understanding of predilection and susceptibility to disease, facilitating early diagnosis and intervention. Influencing factors are defined and separated from non-influencing factors. Knowing the influencing factors and their incubation period makes it possible to navigate the individual towards excellence in health. Hypotheses generated by the search engine will guide us towards the changes that need to be made at the social level.

Finally, government agencies can be guided in designing more effective, efficient and economical healthcare policies and strategies. Strategies for proactive healthcare and health enhancement can be defined at individual, social and government levels.

The need of the hour is a comprehensive, multidimensional and personalized health solution. The search engine, using the Science of Classification, will make this possible with the help of machine learning. Health for all will become a scientific possibility.

20.3 HEALTH AND ITS DIMENSIONS

Science is a tool we use to try to understand how nature functions. We can achieve this understanding either by a reductionistic approach or by holistic approach.

The human being is much more than just the physical body. Each individual is blessed with an emotive mind, a sharp intellect, fertile imagination, dreams and aspirations. The human being is a social animal that has to find his or her place in society and learn to live in co-operation and harmony with society. At the personal or spiritual level, an individual strives to live a happy, contented and meaningful life. Good health means balance at every level of existence. Health is not a static phenomenon. Life itself is a continuous interaction of the individual with his or her environment; the environment is constantly changing and the individual is changing, evolving and growing at every moment of life. At the physical level, with each breath we inhale oxygen and give out carbon dioxide; we take in food, absorb nutrition, convert it to body cells and the energy that drives us and we give out waste. At the emotional level, we are constantly dealing with the stress and demands of survival, protection, provision, procreation and bringing up the young ones. At the intellectual level, we are learning from experience and from our peers, priests and teachers. At the spiritual level, we are trying to understand the meaning of life and to give meaning to our life.

The human being is a constantly changing, growing and evolving entity. The life of a normal human being can be divided into four stages: childhood, youth, adulthood and old age. Each stage is marked by certain pre-programmed physical changes like primary dentition, secondary dentition and age-related secondary sexual characters like body hair, development of breasts and commencement of menses in women. As age advances, signs of ageing appear: greying hair, loss of muscle mass and slowing down of internal functions. Eventually, a person gets old, falls ill and dies.

This is normal.

Birth, growth, maturity, ageing, disease and death – this is the normal life cycle of a normal human being.

Objective evaluation of health assesses a person at all levels. At the physical level, the main parameters to be assessed are strength, stamina and flexibility. These parameters assess the potential of the individual. At the physiological level, the efficiency of the organs and the systems is assessed – cardio-pulmonary, musculoskeletal, digestive, metabolic and endocrine systems. Mental health deals with what the person feels about his/her life, about him-/herself, his/her relationships and so on. It also considers the worldview of the person, his/her beliefs, values and principles. Spiritual health deals with desires, aspiration, ideals and idols of the individual. Psychometric evaluation is done to assess health on these parameters. These parameters together help us assess the actual health of an individual.

In addition, assessment of imbalances, discomforts and disease is a necessary part of health assessment. Discomforts and diseases are assessed on their intensity, duration, frequency and resultant loss of activity. Health is a process of change due to intrinsic and extrinsic influencing factors, driven by desires and fears. It is unfair to represent health by a static health score since health is dynamic and changes as age advances. On a lighter note, you know a person is healthy when you see a glint in the eyes, a smile on the face, a song on the lips, a spring in the step, enthusiasm in welcoming each day, appreciation of nature, the desire to learn, compassion for others and dreams in the eyes. This, of course, is a poetic definition of health. Nevertheless, it is realistic and applies to all ages and stages of life.

This understanding of health gives us the chance to design a strategy for proactive healthcare. We can enhance the health of an individual at each level. At the physical level one can improve strength, stamina and flexibility. At the mental level one can improve awareness, empathy and compassion. At the intellectual level there is ample scope for improvement through education, experimentation and experience. At the social level one can improve the art of collaboration and co-operation. At the spiritual level one can rearrange priorities towards personal evolution and the common good of society. Health needs to be enhanced at all levels; hence a multidimensional approach is needed. Recognizing your strengths, honing your skills and using them to give meaning to life and making yourself and the people around you happy are indicators of good health.

20.4 CURRENT HEALTH

The health of an individual at any stage is the sum total of the impact of intrinsic and extrinsic influencing factors. These factors can be categorized into three groups: nature, nurture and the free-will choices that an individual makes (Figure 20.1).

20.4.1 INTRINSIC INFLUENCING FACTORS

Nature: genetic profile, constitution or Prakruti and gender remain unchanged through life.

20.4.1.1 Nature (Intrinsic Influencing Factor)

The genetic profile or DNA of an individual defines the unique initial state or constitution that a child is born with. In Ayurveda, the traditional Indian medical system, the unique constitution of an individual is called his or her Prakruti. The genetic profile, constitution or Prakruti of an individual defines his or her inherent unique physical, physiological and psychological characteristics. The significant point in the health profile of an individual is that the DNA or Prakruti and gender do not change through life.

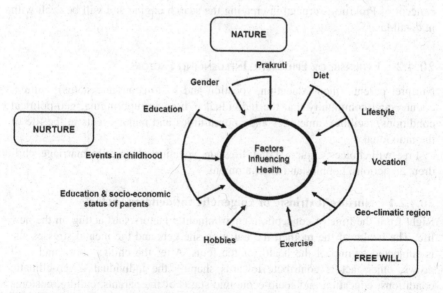

FIGURE 20.1 Factors influencing health.

The genetic profile or Prakruti of an individual plays a major role in defining how the individual reacts or responds to extrinsic influencing factors. The Prakruti of the individual influences his/her predilection and susceptibility to certain diseases. It leaves its mark on the psychological profile, behaviour pattern, learning style and coping skills, and his/her strengths and weaknesses.

We know that some people are naturally tall and lanky, and do not put on weight in spite of having a healthy appetite. They are generally restless and move with short jerky movements. Another type of normal people have naturally an enviable build; they are forceful personalities, generally leaders. People with the third type of constitution or Prakruti are stocky in build, have a slow languid style of moving and tend to put on weight quite easily. These three types of constitution are all normal but definitely different from each other, as dictated by their Prakruti.

Every individual starts life from a different initial state which is similar to other individuals, though never the same. The similarities in the Prakruti of individuals are used as a basis to classify them into clusters in which the initial state of two individuals in a cluster resembles each other more than it resembles the initial state of any other individual from any other cluster. *Individuals can be classified into clusters of different types of normal individuals according to their Prakruti and gender.*

Over centuries of observation and research, Ayurveda has established a system to diagnose the Prakruti of an individual from observable physical, physiological and psychological characteristics, to establish the cluster that he/she belongs to. People belonging to one Prakruti react differently to changes in extrinsic influencing factors from people belonging to any other Prakruti (Desai, 2018b). The concept of Prakruti is crucial in creating the search engine and will be dealt with in detail later.

20.4.2   EXTRINSIC OR EPIGENETIC INFLUENCING FACTORS

Nurture: parents (their education, vocation and socio-economic status), culture, country and community that the individual is born in, upbringing, geo-political conditions, facilities, amenities and opportunities and major events in the life of the individual.

Free-will choices: choice of diet, lifestyle, vocation, job profile, marriage, children, addictions, hobbies and entertainment.

20.4.2.1   Nurture (Extrinsic or Epigenetic Influencing Factor)

Right from the time of conception, environmental factors start acting on the new life. The health of the mother, the nutrition she gets and the mental stresses she is subjected to impact the health of the fetus. After the child is born and as it grows, other factors contribute towards shaping the individual – geo-climatic conditions, education and socio-economic status of the parents, culture, customs and traditions, facilities, amenities and opportunities, to name a few. Besides, there are other factors like drought, famine and other natural calamities, up-bringing, peers, priests and events in the life of the individual, such as the death of a parent, right up to this moment.

20.4.2.2 Free-Will Choices (Extrinsic or Epigenetic Influencing Factor)

The third set of influencing factors is the choices that an individual makes throughout life. Ayurved has classified the free-will influencing factors as *Ahar* (diet), *Vihar* (vocation), *Achar* (habits/addictions, hobbies), *Vichar* (values, principles, attitude), *Nidra* (sleep pattern), *Maithun* (sex life), *Dinacharya* (lifestyle), *Rutucharya* (changes in lifestyle with seasons), *Desh* (infrastructure, facilities, amenities) and *Kaal* (geo-political conditions, religious practices) (Ranade et al., 2004). In addition, choices in marriage, number of children, forms of entertainment, passions, desires, ambitions and activities like social service impact health. These factors, along with those described under nurture, are known as extrinsic or epigenetic influencing factors.

20.4.2.3 Mechanism of Action of Extrinsic or Epigenetic Influencing Factors

Prakruti and gender are known as intrinsic or genetic influencing factors. All other factors are known as extrinsic or epigenetic influencing factors. Epigenetics (beyond genetics) is a budding science but it gives us some insights that are worth understanding. Epigenetic factors do not change the structure of inherited genes but they definitely impact the function. Scientists have identified two chemical reactions through which epigenetic factors act on the function of the genes. *The two reactions are methylation and acetylation.*

There are thousands of genes in the gene bank of an individual but not all are constantly active. Some genes from the gene bank are switched on and some are switched off during the process of cell differentiation. This process may also be responsible for age-related changes like dentition, secondary sexual characteristics and ageing. The process that switches off certain genes is methylation. The second process is acetylation. Acetylation defines the extent or magnitude of the function of the gene. Acetylation explains the impact of habits, practice, addictions and attitude; the more an action is repeated, the stronger its impact. In short, methylation is the on–off switch and acetylation is the volume control of the impact of epigenetic influencing factors. Further research will surely throw more light on the mechanism of action of epigenetic factors.

20.4.3 DEALING WITH THE IMPACT OF INFLUENCING FACTORS

The most important point to be remembered while dealing with the impact of factors influencing health is that the past cannot be changed. The genetic profile or Prakruti of the individual does not change throughout life. Factors like nurture and all the choices made up to the present moment have already had their impact; their effect cannot be erased. The influencing factors that can be modified are the free-will choices that the individual makes in every present moment. Here too, the

> ## Concepts at a Glance 1
>
> - Each individual begins life from a unique initial state, gender and prakruti.
>
> - The individual lives at multiple levels — physical, mental, social and spiritual.
>
> - Health is a dynamic entity constantly responding to intrinsic and extrinsic influencing factors.
>
> - There are innumerable qualitative and quantitative genetic and epigenetic influencing factors that impact the health of an individual.
>
> - Identifying the influencing factors that can be changed, designing a strategy to change them and empowering the individual, community and country to make the changes is the foundation of the multidimensional approach to dealing with the impact of changing environmental factors.

FIGURE 20.2   Concepts at a glance 1.

consistency, duration and frequency with which any good habit is followed play a major role in the impact on health. The foundation of multidimensional healthcare is cultivating good habits and practising them with sincerity, perseverance and consistency. There is no short cut to remaining healthy.

The good news is that a surprisingly large number of epigenetic influencing factors are under the direct control of the individual. The individual deserves to be empowered to actively participate in his/her health enhancement. Certain influencing factors need correction at the family, community or national level.

The strategy involves identifying influencing factors that can be modified, defining their relative and cumulative impact and identifying the corrective measures to be implemented. These scientific insights help to guide the individual, community or government to proactively make the necessary changes (Figure 20.2).

20.5   SCIENTIFIC APPROACH TO HEALTH ENHANCEMENT

The approach to health enhancement has to be a seamless blend of modern science, traditional wisdom and the latest technology backed with consistent logic and reason.

20.5.1   MODERN MEDICAL SYSTEM

In the late 19th century, Louis Pasteur put forth his 'germ theory', stating that infections are caused by germs. About three decades later, Alexander Fleming discovered penicillin; it triggered a revolution in medicine, and the era of antibiotics started. Up until then, average life expectancy was about 40 years or less. Whole generations were lost to bacterial infections. Infant deaths were more than 350 per thousand births.

Antibiotics changed the face of medicine. Modern medicine surged ahead of all other medical systems. The approach to medical research was quite simple – isolate the causative agent, identify its weakness, create a molecule that kills the bacteria and develop a mode of administration (oral/injectable). The world is witness to the magical impact of this simple approach.

The second surge in modern medicine was the invention of vaccines; they largely control diseases like smallpox, polio, measles, mumps, rubella, typhoid and even tuberculosis. The approach was 'one disease–one cause–one standardized treatment'. Thanks to advances in modern medicine, average life expectancy today is between 65 and 70 years. People do not easily succumb to infections.

The third surge that put modern medicine on a pedestal was computerization, advances in cell biology, laboratory investigations, advanced imaging techniques, laser, ultrasound, magnetic resonance imaging (MRI), positron emission tomography (PET) scans, genetic engineering, advanced surgical techniques and robotics. The approach was still one disease–one cause–one standardized treatment. Clinicians became more dependent on investigations to establish diagnosis. Identification of the one cause and standardized treatment became the pillars of modern medicine. We could treat rare diseases and congenital deformities. Genetic engineering became possible.

All the sophistication did not have as dramatic an effect on life expectancy as antibiotics and vaccines had had. The reason was that 90% of hospitals and super-specialists are now working on 10% of diseases. Diseases are getting more attention than health. The fact remains that, at any given time, about 5% of people need medical attention; 95% are the 'not-yet-ill' people. Hardly anything is being done for the not-yet-ill. We are doing more and more for less and less. We can't see the forest for the trees.

Early detection, early intervention, new drugs, advanced surgical techniques, rehabilitation, group therapies and insurance are all a reactive approach to disease. It is a strategy of playing not to lose but we all lose eventually; everyone who is born eventually dies. There is no strategy for playing to win. Winning is being healthy, happy, productive and enthusiastic all through life. The answer lies in proactive healthcare and a strategy for health enhancement in the physical, mental and social dimensions. These are receiving scant attention today.

In the past three decades, the patient pattern has changed. Today, 70% of deaths are due to non-communicable disease (NCD), diabetes, hypertension, autoimmune diseases, psychosomatic diseases, psychological and psychiatric disorders, suicides and, of course, cancer. A problem that has been brought out in the open by the COVID-19 pandemic is that antibiotics are ineffective against viruses. The infection spreads rapidly and it takes more than a year to produce a vaccine against it. Doctors, hospitals, super-specialists and intensive care units step in after the event and have a limited role to play. It is now amply clear that:

> The first and last line of defence is robust health and the strong immune system of the individual.

It became obvious that studying health as a concept independent of disease is mandatory. The cracks in the current system started showing.

20.5.1.1 The Issue

- Health is not a static entity that can be represented by an equation.
- Health is a dynamic algorithm that is constantly evolving and unfolding with age.
- There are many types of normal individuals and they be can classified into groups that have a similar response to influencing factors.
- The health of an individual has multiple dimensions – physical, physiological, mental, social and spiritual. A healthcare strategy has to address each of these dimensions.
- Changes in health status are an effect of intrinsic and extrinsic influencing factors.
- Most influencing factors are qualitative and cannot be quantified or graded.
- The chronology, duration and frequency of influencing factors play a major role in the impact that they have on health.
- The aetiology of NCDs is multi-factorial and NCDs develop over long periods of time.
- Susceptibility to communicable disease is a function of the efficiency of the immune system of the individual, history of previous exposure, age, constitution and other influencing factors.
- The health of an individual is a unique combination of nature, nurture and choices made through life; a standardized solution cannot be applied across the board (Desai, 2020).
- The current approach to healthcare of decreasing deficiencies has to be replaced by a proactive approach of increasing efficiency.
- Empowering the individual, the society and the government to make informed, proactive and scientific free-will choices is the key to healthcare.

The healthcare solution that we seek has to be (Desai, 2019) (Figure 20.3):

- Multidimensional
- Comprehensive
- Personalized
- Proactive.

20.5.1.2 The Problem

Problems with the current approach to healthcare are as follows:

- We do not know the different types of normal individuals in a region.
- We do not know the actual health status of normal people.
- We do not know enough about the influencing and non-influencing factors that impact health.
- We do not know the relative or cumulative impact of the influencing factors.

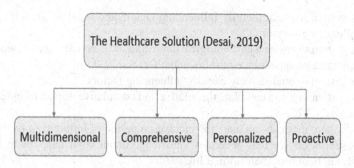

FIGURE 20.3 The ideal healthcare solution (Desai, 2019).

- We do not have a strategy to enhance the health of normal individuals since our focus has been on treatment of diseases.
- Our current research methodology is prospective, experimental and works on the principle of 'one disease–one cause–one standardized treatment'.
- Data analytics is not equipped to deal with multiple, multi-optional influencing factors.
- Data analytics cannot deal with qualitative influencing factors unless they are graded. Many influencing factors cannot be quantified or graded.
- The current method of data analytics is not equipped to deal with multiple, multi-optional, qualitative and quantitative influencing factors that are continuously changing as time progresses.
- There is no database of individuals in whom all parameters are the same.
- There is no comprehensive knowledge bank of best practices for health enhancement.
- Standardization is the main pillar of modern medicine; hence, personalization is difficult.
- Doctors are trained in curative medicine and not in health enhancement.
- The individual is not conditioned or empowered to proactively participate in healthcare.

20.5.1.3 The Solution
The solution should have certain features that help to create a multidimensional, comprehensive, personalized and proactive healthcare system (Desai, 2019).

- A method and system to identify and classify normal human beings in clusters in which the members in each cluster resemble each other more than they resemble any member from any other cluster
- A system that captures influencing factors in the sequence that they appear in the life of an individual
- A method and system to classify human beings into groups according to similarities in all parameters

- A system that can identify influencing factors and separate them from non-influencing factors
- A system to create a chronological algorithm of each individual based on the sequence of appearance of influencing factors
- A system to qualitatively classify influencing factors
- A system that can calculate the relative and cumulative impact of influencing factors
- A system that can calculate the incubation period of influencing factors
- A search engine that generates knowledge about what happens to normal human beings in their normal life span
- An intelligent search engine that uses the latest techniques of pattern recognition, machine learning and artificial intelligence and comes closer to real time each time it is used
- A concurrent and iterative system of health assessment, personalization, knowledge dissemination, real-time monitoring of compliance and reassessment.

Harnessing the free will of the individual is a crucial part of healthcare. The paradox is that, though all the progress in science originates from the free will, passion, determination, perseverance, innovativeness and creativity of scientists, science itself is not equipped to deal with free will or any of the other human qualities. Free will and determinism cannot co-exist and the other qualities cannot be measured. The science of quantification cannot deal with desire, passion, fear, greed, altruism, creativity, values, principles and love, though these are exactly the qualities that drive human behaviour. It cannot deal with reality because reality is not deterministic; like the quantum world, reality is a world of infinite possibilities governed by the laws of probability. We can avoid facing reality but we cannot avoid facing the consequences of avoiding reality.

> No problem can be solved from the same level of consciousness that created it.
>
> **(Albert Einstein)**

The current problem was created from the current level of consciousness or paradigm; hence the need to explore a different level of consciousness or paradigm. It is time to see the world from a different set of eyes. For thousands of years, the East has been following a philosophy and medical system that was born from a different worldview. Let us invest time in seeing the world differently.

20.5.2 THE PARADIGM SHIFT

- Western science believes that the universe is a continuous process of matter changing into energy and energy changing into matter according to fixed predetermined laws of nature. The East perceives the world as a hologram of algorithm within algorithm within algorithm – a continuous process of qualities (guna) changing according to inherent properties (dharma).

- To Western scientists, the universe is a relentless process of mindless change dictated by deterministic laws. The East believes that the universe is an ever-evolving algorithm; each moment manifests as hitherto unseen, new, emerging qualities and properties.
- Scientists believe that if we can measure the mass and velocity of a particle we can derive the ultimate set of deterministic laws and scientifically reconstruct the past and predict the future. Eastern scientists understand that human beings perceive change as constantly changing qualities (gunas); each moment the world is similar but never the same as the moment before (Desai, 2018a). Observation makes us aware of a pattern that change follows. Scientists believe that if we can understand the pattern and design of change we can derive the laws that drive change. We can then proactively align ourselves, our desires, thoughts and actions to synchronize with the grand design.

We need to invest time in understanding the thought process of Eastern scientists.

20.6 EASTERN SCIENCE

Ancient seers of India were well aware that the universe is a continuous on-going process of change; the only constant in the universe is change. The universe and everything in it is momentary; it is constantly changing its qualities and properties. Studying the pattern of change is the way to understand how the universe functions. We are not very familiar with this method of scientific enquiry but it is worthy of our attention because it directly opens the doors to our current enquiry. The aim of this chapter is to understand the impact of changing environmental factors on the health of a human being and further to design a multidimensional approach to deal with it. Ayurveda is the key because it directly deals with interactions of individuals with the ever-changing environmental factors and its impact on health. Therefore, we need to dig a bit deeper into Eastern science, especially Ayurveda. *Ayur* means life and *veda* means science; Ayurveda is the science of life.

Eastern philosophy and science are based on experience, observation and *Chintan/Manan* (deep thought in an effort to fit the observed phenomenon into the grand picture or jigsaw puzzle of reality). The aim is to perceive the pattern of change and the role that each participant plays in the interaction. It begins with the way the human being experiences reality. We experience qualities or gunas through our senses – size, shape, colour, texture, smell, sound and taste. We observe that over time these qualities change. For instance, we see a bud in the morning; by afternoon it has blossomed into a beautiful flower. We think over the phenomenon, compare it with other similar observations and perceive a pattern; within a few hours a bud blossoms into a lovely flower. Though the size, shape and fragrance have changed, the basic character of the flower persists. This we understand as the dharma, the inherent property or character of the flower.

Gunas are experienced through our senses as qualities; dharma is an inference made through observation of changes in gunas over time. Dharma can be understood as properties.

With experience, we infer the pattern of change and learn that day follows night, summer follows winter and that an animal gives birth to an offspring of the same species or that like begets like. This is dharma, the inherent character of reality.

The unique set of qualities and properties, gunadharma, is the identity or unique character of a substance, mountain, river, plant, animal or person.

Gunadharma of the human race shows the normal progression of changes in form or gunas of the individual as age advances, from birth, childhood, adolescence, youth and maturity to old age. We can thus understand dharma as the *intrinsic influencing factor*. Dharma dictates the sequential changes in health of an individual as age advances.

The second step is to recognize the association between gunas and dharma, so that one can understand the character of a substance from the qualities that one perceives. Over centuries of observation and experimentation, scientists have raised this ability to the state of the art. Diagnosing the character or Prakruti of an individual from observable gunas forms the basis of *Prakruti Nidan* or diagnosing the basic constitution of an individual. Prakruti of an individual can be diagnosed from his/her observable physical, physiological and psychological characteristics.

20.6.1 DOSHA OR TENDENCY

We have seen that:

- Qualities like touch, smell, taste, sound and shape of any substance are its gunas.
- The intrinsic changes over time form the property of the substance; it is its dharma.

There is, however, a third aspect of reality that needs to be understood – dosha. Scientists found that each substance brings its inherent character (gunadharma) to an interaction. The gunadharma of each participant in an interaction influences the gunadharma of the end product.

This phenomenon can be best seen in the process of cooking. Each ingredient brings its gunadharma to the table. The taste of the final product is a combination of the gunadharma of each of the ingredients. The end product is not a mere addition of the tastes of all the ingredients. It is a new substance that has its own gunadharma. Though the gunadharma of all the ingredients has changed, there is something of each substance that persists all through the changes and that is its tendency or dosha.

We need to invest a little more effort in understanding the Ayurvedic concept of dosha because it is slightly tricky to understand. Let us begin from the basics. According to Ayurved, the universe and everything in it is made of five elements known as *pancha mahabhuta*. The five elements are: Prithvi (earth), Aap (water), Tej (light/heat), Vayu (air) and Akash (space).

Each element has its signature gunadharma (qualities and properties). Prithvi represents solidity and strength. Aap characterizes fluidity and interaction. Tej represents conversion, heat and power. Vayu represents movement and dynamism and Akash represents the space required for change and growth.

Scientists clearly understood that qualities and properties (gunadharma) constantly change. Yet there is something of the substance that persists all through the changes in gunadharma as its signature identity. They call this signature character dosha. Dosha is the natural tendency of a substance that is carried forward through all changes in form.

The five principal elements combine to create three basic tendencies: Vata dosha, Pitta dosha and Kapha dosha. Prithvi (earth) and Aap (water) combine to create Kapha dosha, Tej (light/heat) creates Pitta dosha and Vayu (air) and Akash (space) together create Vata dosha. The gunadharma of the five principal elements are reflected in the dosha they create. In Ayurved, everything in the universe is classified under the three doshas; hence, Ayurved is known as the Tridosha system of medicine.

The dosha of a substance also dictates the direction in which the substance tends to steer an interaction.

Earth, water, sun, wind and space change with every season yet each element retains its inherent character. Earth retains its solidity, water its fluidity, sun its heat, wind its movement and space its capacity to envelop the world. The principal element Aap or water is seen in nature in different forms – water vapour, clouds and flowing water or ice, yet it does not lose its wateriness.

Here is another example. Sugar can be identified by its white colour, granular structure, sweet smell and taste; these are its gunas. We know that it becomes sticky when it interacts with moisture, melts when heated and becomes caramelized when burnt. This is its dharma. In any interaction, sugar lends its sweetness and stickiness to the end product. This tendency is its dosha. The chemical structure of water in any form retains its H_2O-ness and sugar in any form remains a hydrocarbon; this could be understood as its dosha; a signature identity that persists through all change.

On the same grounds, the Prakruti of an individual can be understood as his/her genetic profile. The form of the individual changes as age advances but his/her Prakruti, his/her individuality, remains the same throughout life. It is very important to be able to diagnose the Prakruti of an individual to understand how the intrinsic and extrinsic influencing factors impact him/her.

The analogy brings forth another point of difference. Western science is analytical and structure-oriented, looking for mass, chemical formula, active ingredient and structure of the cell and the gene. Eastern science has always been holistic and function-oriented. The universe changes as a whole, simultaneously. How a substance interacts with other substances is more important than what the substance is. How you live, evolve and interact with the world is more important than what you are or what you have. The structure of the chromosome is the genome of the individual; the functional manifestation of the genome is his/her Prakruti.

20.6.2 PRAKRUTI

Ayurved, also known as the Tridosha system of medicine, has defined the three basic doshas or tendencies: Vata (V), Pitta (P) and Kapha (K). Each individual is born with a unique Prakruti or combination of the three doshas. We can understand it as the basic constitution of a person. Since there are three doshas, mathematically there are ten possible combinations of Vata, Pitta and Kapha:

- Three single-dosha Prakrutis: Pure Vata (V), pure Pitta (P) and pure Kapha (K) are known as single-dosha Prakruti.
- Six combination Prakrutis: One dosha is dominant, the second dosha less so and the last dosha is very low or recessive. For instance, the Prakruti of a person with dominant Kapha dosha, secondary Vata dosha and weak Pitta dosha is read as Kapha Pradhan Vata or Kapha/Vata (K/V) Prakruti. In this way, there are six possible combinations, namely, K/V, K/P, P/V, P/K, V/K and V/P.
- One equal dosha Prakruti: Here all three doshas, V/P/K, are equal. In practice, however, pure V, P or K and equal V/P/K are rarely seen. Most individuals fall within the six basic Prakruti combinations K/V, K/P, P/V, P/K and V/P, V/K.

We have seen that the character of a substance can be diagnosed by observing its gunas or qualities. Over centuries, Ayurvedic physicians have drawn a ready reckoner of physical, physiological and psychological gunas or characteristics that are used to diagnose the Prakruti or basic constitution of an individual. Some physicians may use pulse diagnosis (*Nadi Parikshan*) to confirm the diagnosis.

A person with Kapha pradhan (Kapha-dominant) Prakruti is typically stocky, sedate, humble, trustworthy, persevering and tending towards obesity. He/she reflects the tendency of Prithvi (earth) and Aap (water) mahabhutas.

A person with Pitta pradhan Prakruti is muscular, sharp, analytical, short-tempered and tends towards acidity and high blood pressure. He/she reflects the tendencies of Tej (light/heat) mahabhuta.

A person with Vata pradhan Prakruti is lean, flitting from one topic to another, open to new ideas and has disturbed digestion and cracking joints. He/she reflects tendencies of Vayu (air/wind) and Akash (space) mahabhutas.

These attributes remain with the person all through life. We see these people every day. They are so different from each other and yet all of them are normal. Each Prakruti has its strengths and weaknesses and every Prakruti is susceptible to and has a predilection for certain diseases.

20.6.3 TRIDOSHA SYSTEM OF CLASSIFICATION

In Ayurved, not only the Prakruti of the human being but also all the influencing factors have been classified under the Tridosha system of classification. Therein lies its brilliance. Thousands of dietary items, various wines, cooking styles, food-processing techniques, vocations, lifestyle, sleep patterns, sex life, emotions, thoughts, activities, geo-climatic conditions and even seasons have been classified into Vata, Pitta and Kapha. Diagnosis in Ayurved is more about pattern recognition. It takes into consideration not only the Prakruti of the person but also the doshas of the influencing factors that he/she interacts with. A typical Ayurvedic observation will be: if a Pitta Prakruti person has spicy (pitta) food, in summer (pitta season), in the afternoon (pitta time) his/her pitta (acidity) will increase and he/she will start sweating, become irritable and his/her blood pressure will increase. Interacting with other pitta influencing factors increases the overall pitta tendency.

The most important significance of classifying all influencing factors and the individual under one system of classification is that it helps us understand why a particular individual responds strongly to a particular factor while another person does not. The fact that the individual has been classified under the same method of classification as all influencing factors makes Ayurved a complete Science of Classification. It can deal with multiple, multi-optional, qualitative and quantitative influencing factors. We shall see how it does so as we proceed.

20.6.4 AYURVEDA AND HEALTH

Health according to Ayurved is maintaining the balance of doshas as close to the proportion (of doshas) that one was born with.

Balance is health; imbalance is disease; rebalancing of doshas is treatment.

The aim of an Ayurvedic physician is to guide a person in all practices that will help him/her to maintain the balance of Prakruti. Since all influencing factors have been classified as Vata, Pitta or Kapha, the physician can advise a person on judicious choice of the extrinsic influencing factors that are most suited to his/her Prakruti, age, gender, vocation, and so forth. This is the pinnacle of personalized proactive healthcare. A person belonging to Pitta Prakruti is advised to avoid excessive exposure to pitta influencing factors such as spicy food, hot sun in the afternoon, late nights, heavy physical work in summer, and so on. All these factors increase Pitta dosha and cause imbalance. A whole section in Ayurved, known as Swasthavrutta, deals with the science of maintaining balance and staying healthy.

There is a system in Ayurved to diagnose imbalance or Vikruti and a system to make subtle corrections at all levels to re-establish balance. Only if all above strategies fail is a person put on medication. Ayurved is truly a scientific, rule-based, multidimensional and proactive healthcare system; it deserves the name Ayurved – the science of life.

This is just a simplistic overview of Eastern philosophy, science and Ayurved (Figure 20.4).

Concepts at a Glance 2

- Eastern philosophy and science have been studying the world as a continuous process of changing and evolving qualities and properties.
- A system has been established to recognise the pattern of change.
- The Science of Classification followed by Eastern philosophy is capable of dealing with multiple, multi-optional, qualitative and quantitative influencing factors that impact human health.
- The influencing factors have been identified and classified under the same system of classification used to classify types of normal human beings.
- The system of classification helps us understand why different types of people react differently to the same influencing factors.
- There is a system of rule-based advice that can help an individual to proactively maintain the balance of health.
- The Science of Classification has the capacity to deal with the sequence, duration and frequency of influencing factors.
- Personalising healthcare to the Prakruti, age, gender, current health status, diet, lifestyle, current diseases and discomforts is possible with the Science of Classification

FIGURE 20.4   Concepts at a glance 2.

The paradigm shift in our worldview from matter/energy to qualities/properties (gunadharma) and from determinism to probability enables us to create a system that can derive the laws that govern the changes in health of human beings. The aim is to harness free will of the individual to build habits that will steadily increase the probability of leading a healthy life at physical, mental and social levels up to a ripe old age. The system can guide the individual, community and country to deal with the impact of changing environmental factors on health.

We need to create an evidence-based search engine of health that can navigate a person from illness to wellness and further to excellence in health.

20.7 CREATING A SEARCH ENGINE

The foundation of a search engine is Data. The most important tool for creating the search engine is the questionnaire that is designed to capture relevant data. The questionnaire has to capture the following:

- The physical, physiological and psychological characteristics of an individual to diagnose his/her Prakruti
- Information about intrinsic and extrinsic influencing factors in the life of the individual
- The age at which the influencing factors appeared and the duration for which it was active
- The current health status at physical, physiological and psychological levels
- The current diseases and discomforts that the person is suffering from

- The intensity, duration, frequency and loss of activity due to the current diseases/discomfort
- The medical history of the person and family history of diseases (Figure 20.5).

Each individual in the search engine is represented by a story or an algorithm that is held together by Prakruti, as a string holds together a necklace. The story begins with the current health status and traces its way backwards to the initial state. This is known as a retrospective study. It helps us to create a roadmap of health of the human species. It is a virtual map of what happens to normal human beings in their normal life span. The data collected define the Prakruti of each individual. The picture becomes clearer as individuals are grouped according to their initial state or Prakruti. Individuals from each group resemble each other more than they resemble any other person from any other cluster. It becomes easier to trace the history of people belonging to each Prakruti (cluster) and compare their health with people belonging to other Prakrutis and the general population.

Analysis of the resulting data gives us scientifically significant insights. These insights are validated because they are evidence-based.

The normal method of scientific enquiry is to define a hypothesis, define research methodology and define the sample of the study. Relevant data are then collected and subjected to analysis in order to validate the hypothesis. In a retrospective study, the process is reversed. The data are already available; the event has already taken place. These individuals have already been subjected to multiple influencing factors. The resultant health status has been recorded. The data are analysed to establish statistically significant associations between any two parameters in a group in whom all other parameters are the same.

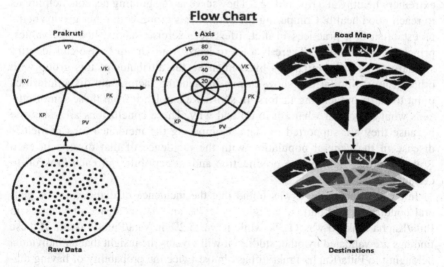

Flow Chart

FIGURE 20.5 A flowchart of data analysis.

When we see the health data of senior citizens who have lived a full life, we see the path that brought them to their current health destination. The data show us that most human beings in the age group 60 and above have complaints involving one or two systems. Many suffer from one or more diseases like arthritis, cardiac problems, diabetes, autoimmune diseases or even cancer. The data contain sequential information about influencing factors and their duration and frequency. It tells us when the diseases were detected and the early signs that were noticed.

20.7.1 INSIGHTS

Initial analysis of the data gives us the following pointers:

- The types of normal individuals in the region
- Prakruti distribution among the general population; percentage incidence of each Prakruti
- Gender distribution of Prakruti
- The normal health status of individuals belonging to a particular age, gender and Prakruti in the region
- The various diseases and discomforts that the population under study is suffering from
- Prakruti distribution of diseases and discomforts
- Age at which the early signs of a disease appear
- The questionnaire is the tool that has established the co-ordinates of an individual on the roadmap of health.

Study of this data shows us that individuals from Group E in Figure 20.6 are extremely healthy at a ripe old age. They serve as the guiding beacon, helping us to reach good health. Comparing the data of this group with other groups helps us establish best practices in diet, lifestyle, exercise, habits, hobbies, values, principles and attitude. There is a lot to learn from Group E. We can identify similarities and dissimilarities by comparing the attributes of this group with other groups. Similarities show us non-influencing factors and dis-similarities point towards influencing factors. In short, we can learn from these senior citizens what to do and what not to do and why. These conclusions are scientific because they are supported by data. Comparing the incidence of a particular disease in the general population with the incidence of that disease in each Prakruti throws light on the predilection and susceptibility of each Prakruti to certain diseases.

In an ongoing study, it was found that the incidence of diabetes in the general population in a particular region was 7% and the incidence of diabetes in Pitta/Kapha Prakruti was 11.3% while it was 5.2% in Vata/Pitta Prakruti. If these findings are validated by other studies, it will give us the insight that an individual belonging to Pitta/Kapha Prakruti has almost twice the probability of having diabetes as compared to people belonging to Vata/Pitta Prakruti.

Flow Chart

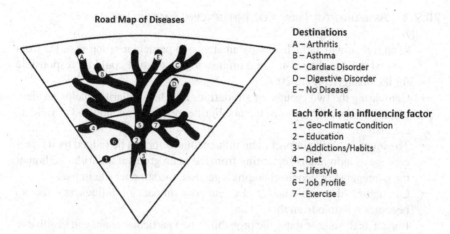

Road Map of Diseases

Destinations
A – Arthritis
B – Asthma
C – Cardiac Disorder
D – Digestive Disorder
E – No Disease

Each fork is an influencing factor
1 – Geo-climatic Condition
2 – Education
3 – Addictions/Habits
4 – Diet
5 – Lifestyle
6 – Job Profile
7 – Exercise

FIGURE 20.6 The roadmap.

Another study has shown that Pitta Prakruti has a predilection for hypertension, cardiac disease, acid-peptic disease and acne. Vata Prakruti people show a higher incidence of arthritis and digestive disorders and Kapha Prakruti people tend towards obesity. This is just the beginning; a lot more research needs to be done. One thing is sure; these findings give a direction to research.

20.7.2 *t*-Axis – Time

Human health is not a fixed, deterministic entity that can be represented by an equation. Like reality, health is an ever-changing and evolving algorithm. In the case of an individual, the common thread that retains its identity through that person's life is his/her Prakruti. It does not change through life. This thread sequentially strings together the beads of all the changes and events that have taken place in the life of a person. The algorithm thus created represents the unique story of the individual. Each individual is a unique story or algorithm that unfolds over about 70 years of change and evolution. Hence the *t*-axis – time – cannot be eliminated from the picture.

As data of individuals belonging to younger age groups 40–60 years and 20–40 years accumulate, the system comes alive; it becomes dynamic because the *t*-axis – time is added to the roadmap. It is like watching a movie in reverse. The data show younger people steadily walking towards the destination reached by the elders in their Prakruti. The roadmap traces the journey of individuals belonging to a particular Prakruti from the initial state through childhood, youth, adulthood and ageing; the data come alive and narrate the life story of individuals belonging to a particular Prakruti.

20.7.3 ASSESSING THE IMPACT OF INFLUENCING FACTORS

- Each fork at which the health parameters of a particular group separate from the rest points a finger at some influencing factor that could be responsible for the change (Figure 20.7).
- Comparing the two groups for similarities and dis-similarities helps us identify the influencing factor or factors. Further research is conducted to validate the insight.
- The intensity of the impact of an influencing factor can be judged by the percentage of individuals separating from the main group at the fork; the higher the percentage of people changing direction, the stronger the impact.
- Calculating the individual and cumulative impact of influencing factors becomes possible from these data.
- Impact analysis calculates the probability of a particular change in health due to the impact of an influencing factor.
- As data start accumulating, the predictive capacity of the search engine improves through pattern recognition and machine learning.
- The more the search engine is used, the better it gets at predicting pattern of change and the closer it gets to real time.

This is reverse engineering. Machine learning and artificial intelligence also work on the same principle of pattern recognition as used by Ayurved.

Flow Chart

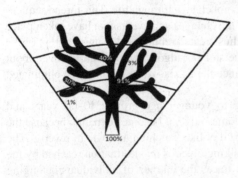

Each fork is an influencing factor
The % deviation is the impact of each factor

FIGURE 20.7   Impact analysis.

The search engine tells us what happens to a normal human being, why it happens and how much time it takes for the changes to manifest. The machine generates knowledge about the health of human beings. It validates existing hypotheses and generates data-based new hypotheses. The insights can prove to be extremely useful to the individual to design a health enhancement programme. The learning from the search engine can guide the government in designing health policies and laying down efficient, economical and effective strategies, thus saving time, effort and money.

20.7.4 How the Search Engine Works

The search engine has a system that is capable of incorporating innumerable, qualitative and quantitative influencing factors, each with its multiple options. It is also capable of incorporating the t-axis – time along with the sequence, duration and frequency of events, interventions and influencing factors. This system of data storage is known as Active Directory.

Each individual is an algorithm, which is a record of all the events and parameters in his/her life, in the sequence in which they appear. One can choose any of the variables like age, gender, Prakruti, disease and exercise. The data in an amorphous form arranges itself to define a group of people with similar algorithms. It creates a group in whom all parameters asked for are the same. Comparing the algorithm of this group with the algorithm of other groups shows similarities and dis-similarities. Similarities between two groups are non-influencing factors; they have *not* contributed to the change. The dis-similarities point a finger at the influencing factors.

20.7.5 Mathematics of the Science of Classification

The form of mathematics used in the Science of Classification is the Set Theory, which also forms the foundation of computer science.

In computer science, the formula of an algorithm is:

Data + program = changed data

The search engine has captured data (initial state) and changed data (current health status). It also has a record of major influencing factors; they represent the program that was responsible for the change. Since we have (data) and (changed data) we can derive the program responsible for the change. The answer comes in the form of an algorithm and not as an equation.

The structure of an algorithm is: If (this) and (this) and (this) but not (this) nor (this) … then (this) happens (action). In this algorithm, each bracket represents a set, subset or superset. The brackets are connected with syntax and the algorithm ends with an action or a conclusion. The structure of shlokas in Ayurved is identical to that of an algorithm. It always ends with a verb, which indicates action. A typical shloka from Ayurved will read as follows: If a Pitta Prakruti person has spicy (pitta) food, in summer (pitta season), in the afternoon (pitta time), his pitta (acidity) will increase, he will start sweating, become irritable and his blood pressure will increase.

Classifying the influencing factors under the same system of classification as the individual tells us why a group of similar individuals responds to an influencing factor in a particular way while another group responds in a different way. Including the *t*-axis – time makes it possible to calculate the incubation period of influencing factors and interventions.

20.7.6 ACTIVATING THE SEARCH ENGINE

The search engine is a concurrent, iterative cycle that creates a continuous cycle from customization to standardization back to customization and further standardization (Figure 20.8). It is a seamless blend of traditional knowledge, modern science and latest technology. Today, the best way to reach each individual is to present the solution in the form of an application on smart phones. A large percentage of the population today owns a smart phone.

The search engine has:

- A knowledge bank of best practices in diet, lifestyle, exercise, yoga, pranayama and meditation
- A tool for health assessment and Prakruti diagnosis
- An algorithm to personalize rule-based advice to the age, gender, Prakruti, current health status and current disease status of an individual

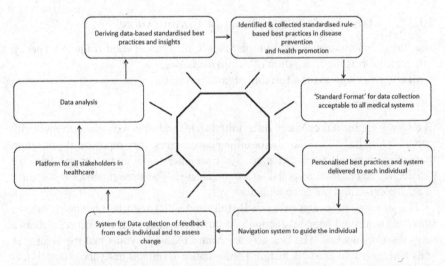

FIGURE 20.8 The concurrent and iterative cycle of customization to standardization and back.

- An app that can collect data and disseminate knowledge using the latest technology of a smart phone
- A feature that can record follow-up, compliance and re-assessment
- A system for real-time data collection of initial state, intervention, compliance and reassessment
- Research tools for data analysis, pattern recognition and machine learning
- A system that continuously converts the knowledge bank from rule-based to data-based knowledge of best practices.

As the search engine is populated with actively participating users, its predictive capacity will improve and the advice given will steadily approach real time.

20.8 SCOPE AND SIGNIFICANCE

The search engine has the potential to benefit the individual, the society and science.

20.8.1 BENEFITS TO AN INDIVIDUAL

- Understanding his/her Prakruti, its characteristics and the impact on physical, physiological and mental aspects of health, as well as on his/her diet and lifestyle choices
- Understanding his/her current health status based on age, gender, diseases, discomforts, lifestyle, habits and daily routine as compared to his/her peer group
- Advice on diet, lifestyle, exercises and yoga personalized to his/her age, gender, body mass index, current health status and Prakruti
- A personalized plan to enhance health and immunity
- A sustainable diet plan to suit his/her geo-climatic conditions and his/her Prakruti, taking care of macro- and micro-nutrient needs
- Home-based therapies to take care of imbalances as soon as they appear
- Better chance of fighting communicable diseases and avoiding NCD.

The significance of *Sanskar* or upbringing as an influencing factor will be scientifically established. This will be a guide for every parent, leading to informed parenting.

20.8.2 BENEFITS TO SCIENCE

- For the first time, we will know what a normal human being is.
- We will also know the types of normal people in a given region.
- For the first time, we will know the actual and average health of human beings belonging to a particular age group, gender, Prakruti and geo-climatic and socio-economic conditions.

- Medical research will have a data bank of groups of individuals in whom all parameters are the same. This is important for selecting a scientifically valid sample for a research project. At present, no such database is available.
- The search engine will make it possible to separate influencing from non-influencing factors.
- We will know the impact of intrinsic and extrinsic influencing factors – the roles that nature, nurture and free will play in the health of an individual.
- We will know what happens to a normal individual in his/her normal life span – the roadmap of health.
- We will have a tool to establish the co-ordinates of a person, a group or a community on the roadmap of health.
- We will know the improvements that need to be made to remain in excellent health (active healthcare) and can steer an individual towards health enhancement (proactive healthcare).
- We can identify the Prakrutis that respond well to a drug and the Prakrutis that suffer the adverse effects.
- We can guide pharmaceuticals to create Prakruti-specific drugs for each disease and thus reduce incidences of adverse effects.
- Healthcare systems can be made proactive, efficient, effective and economical.
- We will know the inherent predilection of each type of individual towards particular diseases.
- We will get insights on ways to reduce the possibility of contracting the disease.
- We will know when (the age at which) the early signs appear and how the disease progresses.
- Early detection and early intervention drives will be made more efficient and economical.
- Prakruti, age, gender and socio-economic distribution of any disease will be established.
- Prakruti, age, gender and socio-economic distribution of addictive and criminal tendencies will be established.
- We will validate existing hypotheses of modern and traditional medical systems.
- We will create a common language of communication between the various medical systems and make integration of various medical systems possible.
- We will generate new hypotheses for further research, using the research tools in the search engine; we will also have the database to validate these hypotheses.

20.8.3   BENEFITS TO SOCIETY

- The inferences drawn can guide the government to design health strategies customized to region, gender, geo-climatic conditions, communities, age groups, socio-economic class and vocation.

- Seamless communication between central government agencies, district hospitals, private hospitals, pharmaceutical industries, research organizations, non-government organizations, insurance agencies, primary health centres and Accredited Social Health Activist (ASHA) workers can be established.
- The search engine will offer a common platform of communication between all stakeholders in healthcare.
- Secondary data from these organisations will contribute to centralized data analysis.
- The search engine has global significance and the potential to make India the world leader in healthcare.
- Health for all will become a scientific possibility.

NOTE

1   https://www.hsl.gov.uk/media/202146/5_kim_who.pdf.

REFERENCES

Desai, C. (2018a, September). Transdisciplinary Education. Talk delivered at University of Trans-Disciplinary Health Sciences and Technology, Bangalore.

Desai, C. R. (2018b, December 14–17). Empowering the Individual: The need of the Hour. Paper presented at the World Ayurved Congress, Ahmedabad.

Desai, C. (2019, July). IMA Plus Monthly Newsletter, Pune Branch, Vol XIII, Issue No. 12.

Desai, C. R. (2020, March 8). Presentation at IMA, Pune.

Ranade, S., Paranjpe, G. R., Sathye, B. V. (2004). Swasthavrutta, Anmol Prakashan.

21 Health Sector Resilience to Climate-Related Disasters

India's Experience of National Health Adaptation Planning

Anil Kumar Gupta, Atisha Sood* and Anjali Barwal

CONTENTS

21.1 CLIMATE CHANGE RISK AND RESILIENCE

Among the major riveting rationales for studying the consequences of climate change is its impact on human health. Health is the finest tool to see the combined effect of climate change on the ecosystem, physical environment, economy and society. Climate change, in the long haul, can shake the basic stipulations of good health like adequate safe drinking water, secure housing and sufficient nutritious food. Any delay in action on climate change is bound to only increase the risks and its impact on human health. It is further a direct infraction of the global commitment to achieve health for all, a basic human right (United Nations General Assembly, 1949).

* Corresponding author: Atisha Sood. soodatisha@gmail.com

DOI: 10.1201/9781003095422-21

In the past few years, interest in climate change and health research has grown substantially among the public health community, resulting in a better understanding of the overlapping domains of climate change and health, sensitization on specific health risks and finding sustainable solutions keeping in mind the mitigation costs. Many organizations are working together to meet the commitments made for climate change negotiation at the World Health Assembly, including United Nations agencies, government and non-governmental bodies (World Health Organization, 2016).

The Intergovernmental Panel on Climate Change (IPCC) in its recent report unveiled the urgent need for decision makers to make sure global warming is maintained under 1.5°C before this narrow window of opportunity shuts (IPCC, 2018). To ensure maximum benefits for climate as well as health a greater coordination between different sectors like health, transport, agriculture and urban planning is of utmost importance. The health sector specifically can support nations by providing evidence-based analysis that can benefit both human health and global climate change. When supported by unified governance and policy frameworks the effects can be amplified to another level (World Health Organization, 2018).

21.2   NEED FOR ADAPTATION PLANNING

Climate change and variability are now visible all across the globe. The adverse effects of climate change are being felt all round and are at the top of global issues. If we are not in a position to deal with climate change and its adverse effects in an integrated and cooperative manner, it might ruin the social, environmental, economic and political achievements gained so far. Initiatives of Climate Resilient Green Economy (CRGE) and many other studies have revealed that the health sector is one of the top three vulnerable sectors to climate change and to build a green economy (National Health Adaptation Plan to Climate Change, 2018).

A 'one size fits all' set of criteria is not appropriate for adaptation. Countries with smaller populations (e.g. Ireland, Luxembourg, New Zealand) have reported fewer health adaptation initiatives than countries with larger populations (Austin et al., 2016).

Adaptation basically involves taking all the initiatives necessary to lower the negative effects of climate change. Such measures may range from technological options, early-warning or surveillance systems, to behavioral interventions.

The main aim of developing the National Health Adaptation Plan (NHAP) is to make sure the health system is climate change-related disaster-resilient. There is a need to develop and implement the NHAP by mainstreaming to its various programs and by strengthening its partnership with relevant ministries, departments and stakeholders. The NHAP shall be implemented with the participation of communities from grassroot level through health awareness programs using healthcare professionals and workers. The implementation of a health plan should be supported and monitored at all levels so that it is successful in building a resilient health sector.

21.3 GLOBAL AND INDIAN EXPERIENCE

Climate change is a global issue as it affects agriculture, forestry, biodiversity, water resources, sanitation, transportation, communication, health, lifestyle, and so on. Currently, climate change receives a great deal of attention globally as its effect challenges both developed as well as developing nations. But still developing countries are more at risk of climate change impacts as they have less capacity to adapt to climate change (Azadi et al., 2019).

Although the impact of climate change is affected by ecological, human and social wellbeing and many other factors, recurring disasters lead to the emergence of new diseases and the re-emergence of diseases that had previously been eliminated. For example, the aggravation of existing vector-borne, food- and water-borne and respiratory infections is one of the common impacts of climate change.

Climate change alone is estimated to increase the number of people at risk by 2030 (60,000 additional deaths compared to a future without climate change). This is, however, likely to be outweighed by a reduction in the number of people at risk due to improved socioeconomic conditions and healthcare facilities (World Health Organization, 2014).

In one of the earliest studies for the Indian region in the context of contemporary global warming, it was reported that the mean annual temperature increased by about 0. 51°C/100 years in India from 1901 to 2007 (Kothawale & Singh, 2017). All-India mean annual temperature shows a significant warming trend of 0.05°C/10 years during the period 1901–2003 and 0.22°C/10 years during the recent period, 1971–2003. This represents a substantial acceleration of warming during the last three decades. The years 2015–2017 each had a global temperature departure from average that was more than 1.0°C above the 1880–1900 average, which is a period that is commonly used to represent pre-industrial conditions. However, the year 2018 also marks the 42nd consecutive year (since 1977) in which global land and ocean temperatures, at least nominally, were above the 20th-century average (National Centers for Environmental Information, National Oceanic & Atmospheric Administration (NOAA), 2018). India, being a developing country with high population density and varied temperature and climatic profile, might experience a myriad of human health effects because of climate change. These effects could include vector-borne and water-borne infectious diseases such as malaria, chikungunya, cholera and diarrhea. Increases in extreme weather events will also lead to several health consequences. Displacements due to the loss of housing, hunger and injuries are some of the adverse outcomes to the population.

21.4 HEALTH SECTOR VULNERABILITY

Across the world, the frequency of extreme events is increasing, by 46% between 2000 and 2013, along with continuing warming trends (IPCC, 2018; Watts et al., 2018). A variable changing climate is the highest global risk to populations, as it confers a direct and immediate danger to the health of society (World Economic Forum, 2018; World Meterological Organization, 2018). Human health is affected both directly and indirectly by climate change. Physiological effects due to exposure to high temperatures, increasing number of non-communicable diseases like cardiovascular and respiratory illnesses, and deaths and injuries due to extreme weather events of floods, droughts, storms and heat waves all constitute the direct health impacts of climate change. Various ecological changes like water and food insecurity, propagation of climate-sensitive infectious diseases and human response to climate change in the form of displacement and limited access to health services have many indirect impacts on human health (Figure 21.1) (Smith et al., 2014). The indirect impacts of climate change are usually hard to foresee as they are often the results of long complex pathways. The impact of climate change can be indirect or direct and long- or short-term in nature, often with chronic effects on individual wellbeing and health, for example, non-communicable diseases such as the mental effects of extreme weather events, human displacement due to climate change, culture loss and immigration. The shift in climate is even causing a hike in the disease-spreading capacity of various vectors; for example, the vectorial capacity of mosquitoes causing dengue fever has risen by about 10% since the 1950s (Watts et al., 2018). Climate change causes many ecological shifts by altering sanitation and water, giving rise to malnutrition and food insecurity which can further affect health (World Health Organization, 2015a). One of the major threats to human health from climate change is malnutrition, which most significantly affects the elderly and the young. Severe food crises are caused by weather extremes and climate variations. This amassed effect of climate change threatens all facets of food security – food access, availability, stability and use. Climate change-related disasters even affect food safety; for instance, a rise in temperature can raise the

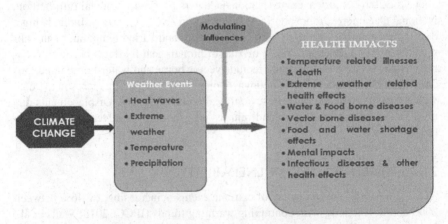

FIGURE 21.1   Health impact of climate change (adapted from Patz et al. 2000).

pathogen level in food and food sources, and the risk of pathogen spread from live-stock increases after floods.

The short-, medium- and long-term impacts of climate change and extreme events are mostly determined by broader dimensions, that can also affect health service delivery by health systems. It is well established that, although climate change will affect everyone, it will have the greatest health impact on the most vul-nerable and poorest population.

Health risks can further increase due to the effects of climate change and wea-ther variations on vulnerable infrastructure. For example, biological and chemical contamination of water supply and sanitation system can be caused by floods and storms and even result in energy distribution disruption (WHO, 2018). Extreme weather events and sea level rise, vector-borne and water-borne disease epidemics, population displacement, food insecurity and rise in demand all make health systems more vulnerable.

21.5   REGIONAL CONTEXT

The changing climate is heavily impacting the health sector and aggravating several communicable and non-communicable diseases such as malaria, dengue, yellow fever, diarrhea, meningitis, asthma, heat stroke, heart disease and lung cancer. The burden on health services will increase as climate change aggravates natural disasters causing social instability, physical damage, morbidity and mortality. There have been more flooding because of increased rain intensity, which will destroy health infrastructures unless preventive measures are taken prospectively.

21.6   DISASTER CONTEXT

Extreme weather events are expected to occur more often as an outcome of climate change. Human lives are devastated by these extreme weather events. For the most part these are precipitation fluctuation-related events like droughts, hurricanes and floods and temperature variation-related events like cold spells and heat waves (Hashim & Hashim, 2016). Droughts and floods have given rise to epidemics, famines and disasters in the past. Extreme weather events include unseasonal, unex-pected, severe and unusual weather. Climate variation also affects patterns of infec-tious diseases that are spread by means of food and water contamination. When fecal matter infects water after floods, many outbreaks of water-borne diseases like typhoid and cholera often occur (Zhong et al., 2018; Sood et al., 2020a).

It is difficult to estimate the health impacts of disasters due to poor reporting on long-term consequences and secondary effects. The organizations and units involved in direct disaster response and relief are the primary sources of infor-mation on natural disasters. Thus, often only information specifically required for operational purposes is collected and recorded. Documentation and data updation are very low priority in disasters because of competing demands (Jafar, 2020). This is particularly true for cyclones, hurricanes and floods, when direct injuries and deaths are very small in comparison to indirect impacts arising from infectious diseases and economic losses (Walker-Springett et al., 2017; Okaka & Odhiambo, 2018; Erickson et al., 2019).

A constant trend in natural disaster impacts has been seen globally. A threefold rise in the number of natural disaster events has been seen in the last ten years in comparison to the 1960s, based on analysis by Munich Re, a reinsurance company. This is not fundamentally due to a change in frequency of climatological events but rather due to rise in population vulnerabilities worldwide. Only a slight change in the number of people killed has been observed despite the recent rise in number of disasters. In 2000 alone, more than 400 disasters were seen affecting around 250 million people. This paradox may be the result of technological advances in early-warning systems, building construction and infrastructure strengthening. Despite fluctuations in the number of deaths each year due to disasters an increasing trend with more people affected and more deaths has been seen in recent decades (Munich Re Group, 2000).

21.7 HEALTH ADAPTATION PLAN

The major objectives of a Health Adaptation Plan (HAP) are to create an enabling environment; build a climate-resilient healthcare system; help institutions strengthen their preparedness, enhancing health system resilience under universal health coverage; and establish early-warning, surveillance and community mobilization in relation to health emergency risk management. The framework of the NHAP is shown in Figure 21.2. The methodology adopted for drafting the NHAP is given in Figure 21.3.

The primary intervention areas to implement in HAPs are strengthening and expanding health infrastructure, identifying and assessing health hazards and vulnerabilities associated with climate change-related disasters, building human resource capacity through policy planning, advocacy, research, training, education and knowledge management, promoting climate-resilient water and sanitation facilities, creating health insurance programs for the community, revising the building codes of health facilities, promoting climate change and health awareness programs as well as encouraging research and development programs on health and climate change.

The NHAP proposes a seven-pronged strategic approach to achieve its goal of developing a climate change-resilient health system (Figure 21.4).

21.8 IMPLEMENTATION STRATEGY

The public health activities required to address climate change challenges immediately should aim to strengthen the adaptive capacity to sustain change in the face of the increasing risks of climate change and also to build prevention for climate-related health vulnerabilities. Health systems are not properly adapted to deal with climate change consequences across the globe, specifically in low-medium-income

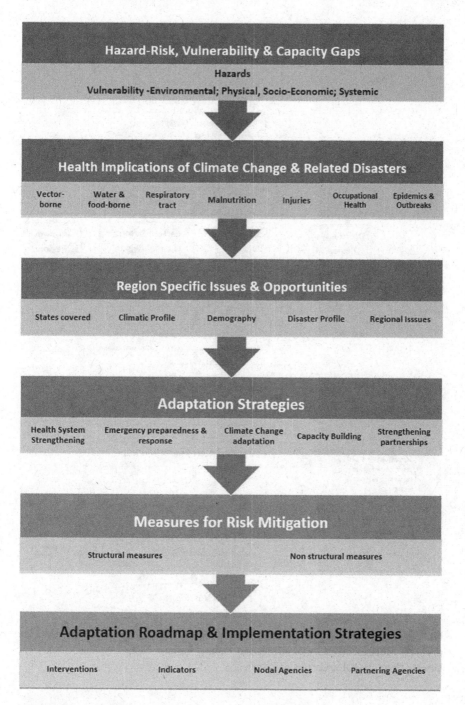

FIGURE 21.2 The framework of the National Health Adaptation Plan.

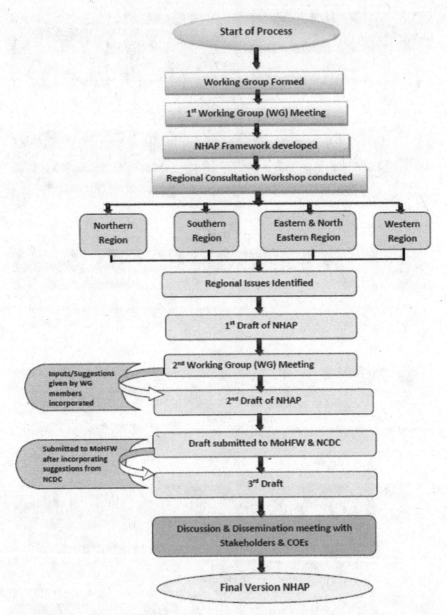

FIGURE 21.3 Methodology adopted for drafting the National Health Adaptation Plan (NHAP). MoHFW, Ministry of Health and Family Welfare; NCDC, National Centre for Disease Control; COEs, Centres of Excellence.

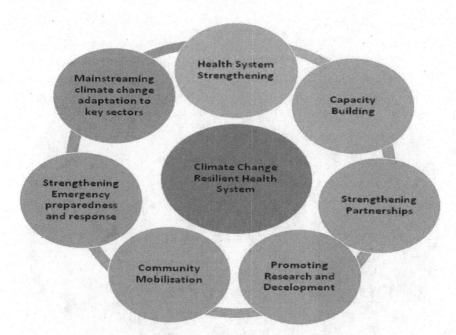

FIGURE 21.4 Seven-pronged strategic approach to developing a climate change- resilient health system.

countries. Although health is primarily affected by sectors like water, sanitation and food, climate change provides an added pressure. There is a need for a multisectoral response based on building upon the existing strengths of the system (Figure 21.5). Therefore, in various sectors like food systems, energy provision, water and sanitation, provisions from healthcare and public health should be integrated with added capacities and functions to build climate resilience (Chaturvedi & Siwan, 2020).

In the past few years, there has been increasing interest in strengthening the climate resilience of health systems. The most common features of adaptation strategies include a good understanding of the contribution of adaptation to development goals, more investment in capacity building and stakeholder engagement, multisectoral involvement, clear indicators for evaluation and monitoring and a cycle promoting continuous improvement.

21.9 RECENT LESSONS FROM COVID-19

Coronavirus disease 2019 (COVID-19) has changed the entire world forever. It has written new pages in world history. Worldwide countries are responding quite differently to the COVID-19 outbreak. While COVID-19 may be devastating in every aspect of life, we should not lose the opportunity to learn and grow. This is the time to evolve strategies to think in terms of overall population health, the healthcare system and infrastructure. Each country's healthcare system needs to be strong and

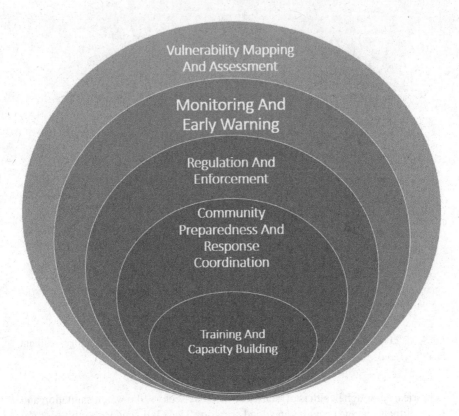

FIGURE 21.5 Implementation strategies.

effective. The general community should also be encouraged to provide information on infected people.

The need to plan for infectious disease outbreaks, whether naturally occurring or caused by bioterrorism, is now greater than ever. Any such outbreak constitutes a threat to national and international security, with the potential to cause a health disaster. Legal frameworks, protocols and HAPs need to be developed and adapted to handle such public health crises. This can delineate the scope of healthcare providers' and governments' responses to public health emergencies (Sood et al. 2020b).

21.10 FUTURISTIC AND FOLLOW-UP STRATEGIES

A healthcare facility comprises several subset facilities like Water Sanitation and Hygiene (WaSH), electricity, biomedical and hazardous waste management, transportation and kitchen services. These are critical to the functioning of the health system. Healthcare facilities need to develop resilience to climate-sensitive disasters by strengthening all these aspects.

All healthcare professionals and managers at all levels should receive training in capacity building on the health impacts of climate change and adaptation measures to be taken depending on the context and giving priority to regions or places frequently affected by disasters posed by climate change and climate-sensitive diseases. There is a need to strengthen the health management information system so that it can produce timely and quality information for decision making.

Capacity building and sensitization of medical and paramedical professionals are necessary at all levels – from policy makers and administrators at the top to doctors, nurses and even grassroot workers like Accredited Social Health Activists (ASHA) and aanganwadi workers – in facing up to the health implications of climate change and its related disorders. Medical professionals need to be trained in recognizing and managing climate-sensitive diseases, like heat stroke, and notifying them to the concerned authorities. Medical officers at district and state level also need to be trained regarding the optimal use of Integrated Disease Surveillance Programme (IDSP) data for the interpretation of climate-sensitive diseases to ensure timely action for their control and prevention.

Sensitization of two other sectors is critical to successfully building the capacity of the health system: the private health sector and Ayurveda, yoga and naturopathy, Unani, Siddha and homeopathy (AYUSH) practitioners. Integration with the private sector, including private clinics, nursing homes and hospitals, and practitioners of systems of indigenous medicine like AYUSH is important to develop and implement a holistic adaptation plan. In the current scenario, there is a need to integrate the systems to develop a common database that serves as an important policy and decision-making tool. Health facilities need to strengthen their surveillance systems to monitor food, air and water quality, vector breeding, malnutrition and other risk factors and behaviors which make the community more vulnerable to the effects of climate change-related disasters (Barwal et al., 2020).

REFERENCES

Austin, S. E., Biesbroek, R., Berrang-Ford, L., Ford, J. D., Parker, S., & Fleury, M. D. (2016). Public health adaptation to climate change in OECD countries. *International Journal of Environmental Research and Public Health*, 13(9), 889.

Azadi, Y., Yazdanpanah, M., & Mahmoudi, H. (2019). Understanding smallholder farmers' adaptation behaviors through climate change beliefs, risk perception, trust, and psychological distance: Evidence from wheat growers in Iran. *Journal of Environmental Management*, 250, 109456.

Barwal, A., Sood, A., Gupta, A. K., & Goyal, M. K. (2020). Lessons from trans-domain assessment of COVID 19 outbreak. In *Integrated Risk of Pandemic: Covid-19 Impacts, Resilience and Recommendations* (pp. 481–496). Springer, Singapore.

Chaturvedi, M., & Siwan, R. M. (2020). Resilience of healthcare system to outbreaks. In *Integrated Risk of Pandemic: Covid-19 Impacts, Resilience and Recommendations* (pp. 397–412). Springer, Singapore.

Erickson, T. B., Brooks, J., Nilles, E. J., Pham, P. N., & Vinck, P. (2019). Environmental health effects attributed to toxic and infectious agents following hurricanes, cyclones, flash floods and major hydrometeorological events. *Journal of Toxicology and Environmental Health, Part B, 22*(5–6), 157–171.

Hashim, J. H., & Hashim, Z. (2016). Climate change, extreme weather events, and human health implications in the Asia Pacific region. *Asia Pacific Journal of Public Health, 28*(2_suppl), 8S–14S. https://doi.org/10.1177/1010539515599030.

Intergovernmental Panel on Climate Change. (2018). Special report on global warming of 1.5°C. IPCC, Switzerland. *Population and Development Review, 45*(1), 251–252.

Jafar, A. J. (2020). Disaster documentation: Improving medical information-sharing in sudden-onset disaster scenarios. *Third World Quarterly, 41*(2), 321–339.

Kothawale, D. R., & Singh, H. N. (2017). Recent trends in tropospheric temperature over India during the period 1971–2015. *Earth and Space Science, 4*(5), 240–246.

Munich Re Group. (1999). *Topics 2000: Natural catastrophes – the current position.* Munich: Re Group.'

National Centers for Environmental Information, National Oceanic & Atmospheric Administration (NOAA). (2018). Annual NOAA Global Climate Report. www.ncdc. noaa.gov/sotc/global/201813.

National Health Adaptation Plan to Climate Change (2018). Federal Ministry of Health (2018–2020). www.who.int/globalchange/resources/wash-toolkit/national-health-adaptation-plan-to-climate-change.pdf.

Okaka, F. O., & Odhiambo, B. (2018). Relationship between flooding and out break of infectious diseases in Kenya: A review of the literature. *Journal of Environmental and Public Health, 17,* 5452938.

Patz, J. A., McGeehin, M. A., Bernard, S. M., et al. (2000). The potential health impacts of climate variability and climate change for the United States: Executive summary of the report of the health sector of the US National Assessment. *Environmental Health Perspectives, 108,* 367–376.

Smith, K. R., Woodward, A., Campbell-Lendrum, D., Chadee, D. D., Honda, Y., Liu, Q., et al. (2014). Human health: impacts, adaptation, and co-benefits. In: Field, C. B., Barros, V. R., Dokken, D. J., Mach, K. J., Mastrandrea, M. D., Bilir, T. E., et al., editors. *Climate Change 2014: Impacts, Adaptation, and Vulnerability. Part A: Global and Sectoral Aspects. Contribution of Working Group II to the Fifth Assessment Report of the Intergovernmental Panel of Climate Change.* Cambridge University Press, Cambridge; 709–754.

Sood, A., Barwal, A., Gupta, A. K., & Goyal, M. K. (2020a). Introduction to virus outbreaks. In *Integrated Risk of Pandemic: Covid-19 Impacts, Resilience and Recommendations* (pp. 3–20). Springer, Singapore.

Sood, A., Barwal, A., Gupta, A. K., & Kishore, J. (2020b). Novel coronavirus epidemic: New dimension for disaster management and health resilience. *Current Science, 118*(8), 1149–1150.

United Nations General Assembly. (1949). *Universal Declaration of Human Rights* (Vol. 3381). Department of State, United States of America.

Walker-Springett, K., Butler, C., & Adger, W. N. (2017). Wellbeing in the aftermath of floods. *Health & Place, 43,* 66–74.

Watts, N., Amann, M., Ayeb-Karlsson, S., Belesova, K., Bouley, T., Boykoff, M., Byass, P., et al. (2018). The Lancet countdown on health and climate change: From 25 years of inaction to a global transformation for public health. *Lancet, 391*(10120), 581–630.

World Economic Forum. (2018). The Global Risks Report 2018, 13th edition. World Economic Forum, Geneva. (www3.weforum.org/docs/WEF_GRR18_Report.pdf, accessed November 2018).

World Health Organization (WHO). (2014). Quantitative Risk Assessment of the Potential Effects of Climate Change on Health. World Health Organization, Geneva.

World Health Organization. (2015a). Connecting Global Priorities: Biodiversity and Human Health. A State of Knowledge Review. World Health Organization, Geneva; Secretariat of the Convention on Biological Diversity, Montreal.

World Health Organization (WHO). (2016). Second Global Conference: Health and Climate, Conference Conclusions and Action Agenda. World Health Organization, Geneva.World Health Organization. (2018). Chemical Releases Caused by Natural Hazard Events and Disasters. World Health Organization, Geneva.

World Meteorological Organization. (2018). WMO Statement on the State of the Global Climate in 2017 (WMO-No. 1212). World Meteorological Organization, Geneva.

Zhong, S., Yang, L., Toloo, S., Wang, Z., Tong, S., Sun, X., ... & Huang, C. (2018). The long-term physical and psychological health impacts of flooding: A systematic mapping. *Science of the Total Environment*, *626*, 165–194.

22 Monitoring an Environment and Human Health Perspective Using a Geospatial Approach

Shrey Rakholia, Abhinav Mehta* and Joystu Dutta

CONTENTS

22.1 INTRODUCTION

Multivariate healthcare datasets are not easy to represent using traditional methods (e.g. in the form of figures or statistics); however, using visualization tools like maps especially in the form of web applications can help visualize health performance combined with demographic data which can be directly used by health professionals and policy makers to present results. In particular, choropleth maps have been proven to be extremely useful for obtaining knowledge by representing geographical healthcare data (Sopan et al., 2012). Geospatial visualization techniques using open-source software tools can help health departments to build

* Corresponding author: Abhinav Mehta. mehta.abhinav01@gmail.com

DOI: 10.1201/9781003095422-22

healthcare information systems cost-effectively not only at state level but also at county or equivalent administrative division levels (Yi et al., 2008).

Our objective is to provide better maps that are easy to interpret and represent geographical healthcare multivariate data using open-source GIS (geographic information system) software like QGIS. In addition, we focus on discussing the effects of climate change and the changing environment of epidemic spread using the available literature. We aim to compare meteorological data with healthcare data taking the case study of the COVID-19 pandemic in the state of Gujarat in India in order to compare the natural variables and their effects on health-related variables.

The idea behind using geospatial techniques for public health is to understand how the spread of epidemics and pandemics depends on other factors using the form of combined maps to represent otherwise complex data. Moreover, the use of temporal analysis to understand changing conditions and the interactions between these variables is core to the objectives as it is highly necessary when studying if there is any rise in epidemics due to change in meteorological conditions or climate change over a longer temporal scale. Based on this information it will be easier to predict the spread of epidemics in future if these maps are compared over multiple times.

22.2 CONCEPTS ON CHANGING ENVIRONMENTAL CONDITIONS

As environment and public health are interconnected, any environmental degradation directly impacts human health negatively and thus it is a growing issue. Also, it is difficult to quantify the health impacts in terms of market values and therefore the health impacts from environmental degradation are likely to be neglected in the policy-making process (Remoundou & Koundouri, 2009).

The Intergovernmental Panel on Climate Change (IPCC) Fifth Assessment Report suggests changing weather patterns and climatic conditions such as heatwaves or floods can have a direct impact on public health (Field and Barros, 2014). Furthermore, the indirect impacts of changing climatic conditions can cause ecological imbalance which further results in crop destruction, endangering food security and leading to harmful increase in vector-borne diseases (Woodward et al., 2014).

Although currently the climate change factor poses less of a burden to human health compared to other factors, it is projected that there will be serious damage to public health because of the greater risk of malnutrition as a result of declining food production and reduced work productivity among vulnerable populations in underdeveloped regions (Smith et al., 2015). Furthermore, climate change and extreme weather events are often linked to major outbreaks of vector-borne diseases involving mosquitoes: one finding showed a strong and significant correlation between abundance of *Aedes aegypti* mosquitoes and higher night-time land surface temperatures (LSTs) based on field surveys and weather data (Moreno-Madriñán et al., 2014).

In order to achieve United Nations Sustainable Development Goal (SDG) 3, i.e. to ensure healthy lives and promote well-being, there is a necessity to address the disparities in socioeconomic classes in terms of universal health coverage and gaps in reporting and data collection mechanisms globally. This is because almost 23% of all deaths annually are related to environmental issues like degraded air quality or unavailability of clean water due to water pollution (Acharya et al., 2018).

There is an interdependence between SDGs including goals such as SDG 6, 7 and 13 as they are closely related to global environmental changes. SDGs also focus on addressing the environmental and social causes of human health. The urgency to mitigate climate change is a precondition to sustainable development as climate change is a serious health concern which requires community resilience, adaptation and an early-warning system to fulfill SDG 13 on climate action. World Health Organization (WHO) estimates suggest that more than half a million deaths could be prevented if there was universal access to potable water and better sanitation practices. Also, standard wastewater treatment and integrated water management are needed to achieve SDG 6 on clean water and sanitation (Prüss-Ustün et al., 2016).

22.3 IMPACT OF CHANGING ENVIRONMENT ON HUMAN HEALTH

Changing climatic conditions lead to extreme weather events such as floods, hurricanes and drought can have direct impacts like injuries and fatalities on public health. Also, climatic extremes can cause physical conditions like hypothermia (cold-induced condition) and hyperthermia (heat-induced condition) due to failure of thermoregulation mechanisms in the human body (Frumkin et al., 2008). Climate change plays an important role in the spread and distribution of vector-borne diseases like malaria, filariasis and dengue fever. Moreover, with the changing geographical distribution of vector-borne diseases, new populations are at higher risk of exposure to these diseases due to lack of immunity compared to populations in endemic regions which have developed immunity over time (Haines et al., 2006). Climate change is also found to enhance the exposure of allergens, e.g. elevated pollen distribution with temperature rise. Rising temperatures and humidity trigger fungal growth and can further lead to increased spread of fungal spores (carried by particulates) caused by climate-induced conditions like aridification and desertification, which can give rise to pulmonary infections and disease epidemics in humans (Bernard et al., 2001). It is evident from past studies that there is a positive correlation between the distribution and transmission of malaria vectors with changing environmental conditions based on environmental data derived from remote sensing satellites and transmission patterns (Kelly-Hope et al., 2009).

Furthermore, based on a potential dengue transmission study it is predicted that under a climate change scenario, e.g. the IPCC Fourth Assessment Report stating an increase of global temperatures up to 4°C, dengue transmission could increase to five times current transmission in India alone, especially with new introductions in many sub-Himalayan regions as well as southern parts of India.

This rate of temperature increase could put 3.5 billion people at risk of dengue globally (Dhiman et al., 2010).

In addition, other meteorological or climatological parameters such as the ultraviolet (UV) index have been found to affect the spread of influenza virus. A lower UV index along with lower temperatures has been associated with a surge in influenza activity, particularly in Europe. Low temperatures and low UV index can also contribute to increased mortality, affecting the over-65 age group (Ianevski et al., 2019).

22.4   PERSPECTIVES OF ENVIRONMENTAL HEALTH AND ITS MANAGEMENT

In recent times genetically modified crops have proved themselves handy if judged superficially. They provide us with a much wider selection of traits for improvement (not just pest, disease and herbicide resistance, which had already been achieved).

As part of a "no regrets" adaptive strategy the IPCC has recommended transforming the public health infrastructure. This is thought to be the most urgent and important solution that can be accomplished in an economically feasible manner, as the worsening of the public health infrastructure has led to a resurgence of infectious diseases despite medical advancements such as the introduction of antibiotics and vaccinations in recent times (Haines et al., 2006).

Although there has been research on climate change projections and findings related to the impacts of climate change on public health, the issue of enhancing public health capacity has been overlooked. Therefore, there is a need for new inventive management strategies which aim at the even distribution of resources, as well as institutional learning at all administrative levels for better understanding. Involved stakeholders need to be kept in mind for better decision making and coordination, especially where there is a need for a centralized body incorporating knowledge of models and tools for adaptive management to strengthen the resilience of public health at local levels (Hess et al., 2012).

Public health studies show that GIS techniques such as bivariate mapping have been underutilized even though they can be very simple and effective tools in public health decision making. GIS has been useful in cancer prevention and control planning as it incorporates other epidemiological parameters such as risk factors, incidence, screening and deaths for better resource allocation and target-based geo-specific solutions (Biesecker et al., 2020). These maps can represent larger and non-spatial regression findings and enable comparisons to be drawn between multiple administrative divisions and identification of geographical disparity patterns (Mobley et al., 2012).

In addition, choropleth maps have been used for epidemic studies including malaria incidence. In such cases these maps help identify highly affected areas and geographical locations demonstrating important relations between disease and risk factors. Thus, this benefits not only policy and decision makers but also health practitioners as they can decipher complex spatio-epidemiological data using simple maps for future predictions and assessing disparities (Nyadanu et al., 2019).

In order to reduce future predicted negative impacts on human health due to climate change, there is a need for evaluation, especially for expansion of present adaptive strategies and policy instruments. As present approaches to combat illnesses and deaths are insufficient due to unidentified options and delayed implementation of adaptive measures, the main focus should be on developing a win-win strategy which is cost-effective in terms of preventing diseases (Ebi et al., 2006). Improving air quality and reducing pollution in sources of water for human consumption can lead to better public health. It can massively reduce the number of respiratory and cardiovascular diseases caused by environmental degradation (Remoundou & Koundouri, 2009).

To achieve improved public health, actions that can provide significant benefits include the following:

- Replacing animal-based food products with plant-based products can yield both health and environmental benefits.
- Structuring better public transport systems can improve air quality and decrease usage of private vehicles, thereby reducing air pollution and increasing individual physical activities (Woodward et al., 2014).

As the challenges emerge of a growing population and greater environmental issues at local and global level, the demand to converge the public health and ecosystem services communities needs to be addressed. Therefore, a conceptual framework known as eDPSEEA (ecosystem-enriched Drivers, Pressure, State, Exposure, Effects, Actions) is proposed in order to integrate human and ecosystem health to mitigate these challenges. Based on the concept of ecological public health it is essential to consider human health as an integral part of the ecosystem as they are interrelated. The eDPSEAA model involves intensive stakeholder participation (e.g. workshops) which helps to identify the complex concerns related to ecosystem changes and public health (Reis et al., 2015).

22.5 CASE STUDY

We are evaluating a case study of COVID-19, the novel coronavirus (SARS-CoV-2), spread in Gujarat state in India to compare temporal differences in status between the months of June and October 2020 in order to understand the effects of climatic variables as well as the effects of COVID-19-related restrictions. Our model of geospatial analysis has three major classes of parameters: (1) epidemiological; (2) meteorological; and (3) demographic. The epidemiological class includes parameters such as COVID-19 cases categorized as active, deceased or recovered and the total number of cases. Parameters including temperature, precipitation and UV index constitute the meteorological class and demographic class includes population density data.

The timeframe for comparison is set between two months, as mentioned above, i.e. June to October, in order to understand the epidemics as there will be vast differences in terms of meteorological conditions.

22.5.1 METHODOLOGY

The mapping was carried out in the QGIS open-source environment. In order to compare data of cumulative COVID-19 cases with meteorological parameters bivariate choropleth maps were used. For instance, active cases were represented on one choropleth map layer and temperature on another choropleth map. Both layers were overlaid on each other using "Multiply" blend mode; the symbology was represented by the Jenks Natural breaks classification method and explained using a bivariate map legend.

In order to gain a general idea of the healthcare status of COVID-19 spread by district, pie-charts were generated by overlaying as shown in the figures below. These pie-charts contain three variables: active, recovered and deceased cases. In addition, to show the population density in the same map, the pie-charts were proportionately scaled in size according to population density; the symbols are showed in the key to each map, thereby all parameters are shown in a single map.

Since only two variables can be shown in a bivariate choropleth map, other maps were prepared based on the three meteorological variables, i.e. precipitation, temperature and UV index. Precipitation values were district monthly values (in mm) for June–July and cumulative for October, in order to obtain a general idea of rainfall distribution in those months. Also, temperature values were district average day-time LST based on the mean of MODIS (Moderate Resolution Imaging Spectroradiometer) Level-3 gridded cell values falling in each of the districts. As the cell values need to be converted to degrees Celsius (°C), values are multiplied by the scale factor (0.02) minus 273.15 (to convert from Kelvin to Celsius) after the land surface temperature (LST) raster is required to connect to the study area (i.e. Gujarat state). Similarly, average UV index was obtained for each district based on the mean of Aura-OMI (Ozone Monitoring Instrument) Level 3 gridded cell values.

22.5.2 DATASETS

Datasets were obtained to compare two months, i.e. June and October. Firstly, data were obtained on cumulative cases in three categories, as mentioned earlier from COVID19INDIA, a crowdsourced initiative for tracking COVID-19 cases. Secondly, temperature data were obtained from the MODIS Aqua eight-day Level 3 global gridded product which has 1 × 1-degree grid cells containing LST values.

Furthermore, precipitation data were obtained from the Indian Meteorological Department (IMD): this included cumulative district rainfall distribution (in mm) for June–July and October. Lastly, for UV index Level 3 daily gridded Aura-OMI Spectral Surface UVB irradiance and erythemal dose product were obtained, from

TABLE 22.1
Datasets and their respective source and data (ranges)

Datasets	Source	Date (or range)
Population density	2011 Census of India	2011
COVID-19 cases	COVID19INDIA crowdfunded initiative website	19 June 19 October
Land surface temperatures	MODIS (Moderate Resolution Imaging Spectroradiometer) Level 3 atmosphere gridded product	1–8 June 7–14 October
Precipitation	Indian Meteorological Department (IMD)	1 June–30 July 19 October
Ultraviolet index	Aura-Ozone Monitoring Instrument (OMI) Global gridded product	15 June 12 October

which the UV index was used. Also, population density data were based on the 2011 Census of India. Dates were chosen based on data availability and the optimal period close to the dates for comparison, i.e. 19 June and 19 October (Table 22.1).

22.5.3 DISCUSSION

In Figure 22.1, population density is represented roughly by the size of the pie-charts. Lighter to darker shades of cyan depict low-precipitation to high-precipitation categories respectively, whereas lighter to darker shades of yellow depict low to high number of active cases respectively, as shown in the bivariate key. As can be seen from Figure 22.1, districts in west and south Gujarat have high precipitation/low cases whereas most other districts in the state have low precipitation/low cases. The recovery rate is relatively higher in districts with higher numbers of cases (viz. Ahmedabad, Vadodara and Surat); precipitation in these districts is low to moderate but these districts also have higher population density. Districts with moderate precipitation (viz. Rajkot, Amreli, Junagadh, Jamnagar) have comparatively lower recovery rates in the state.

In October, precipitation was very low due to departure of the monsoon. However, in districts with a high-precipitation category there were low numbers of active cases in western and southern parts of the state, similar to data for June. Exceptions were Rajkot and Surat, where moderate precipitation and moderate numbers of active cases are observed (Figure 22.2). The key difference with June data is that active cases in high-case and high-density districts are relatively increased, whereas the proportion of active cases in districts with lower population density declined.

In Figure 22.3, from lighter to darker shades of green depict low-temperature to high-temperature categories respectively whereas lighter to darker shades of red depict low to high numbers of active cases respectively. High-temperature,

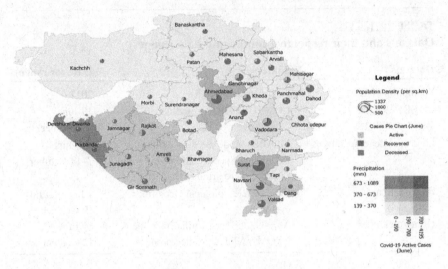

FIGURE 22.1 Bivariate choropleth map for June 2020 showing precipitation vs. active cases of COVID-19 in addition to pie-charts for each district.

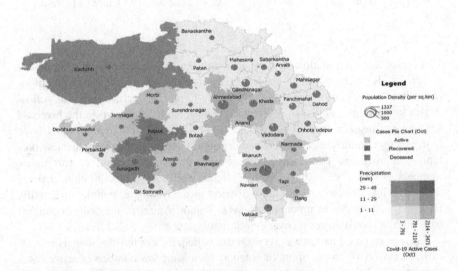

FIGURE 22.2 Bivariate choropleth map for October 2020 showing precipitation vs. active cases of COVID-19 in addition to pie-charts for each district.

low-case districts in the state are mostly found where the recovery rate is also higher. At this stage, districts with relatively lower population density have a lower number of active cases. As June is the end of the summer in this region, moderate to high temperatures prevail across the state. In addition, low-temperature districts

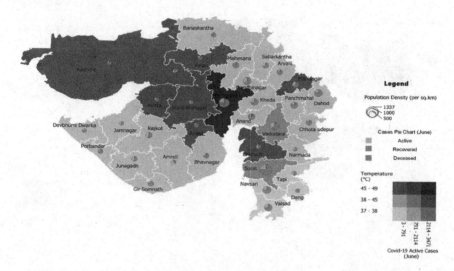

FIGURE 22.3 Bivariate choropleth map for June 2020 showing temperature vs. active cases of COVID-19 with pie-charts.

also have a small number of cases. The only exception is Ahmedabad in the high-temperature category which also has the highest number of cases.

Although the temperatures are lower June than in October, according to Natural Breaks there are more higher-temperature category districts in this category compared to June (Figure 22.4). Especially in these districts the recovery rate seems to be much higher and there are fewer active cases, with the exception of Rajkot district. In contrast, in districts in the low-temperature category with lower population density, the recovery rate is very high, with the exception of Surat, where there are higher cases than other districts in the same category.

In Figures 22.5 and 22.6, lighter to darker shades of blue depict low UV index to high UV index respectively whereas lighter to darker shades of purple depict low to high number of active cases respectively. Similar to temperature trends, UV index is also higher in those districts with higher temperature and lower cases relatively. The recovery rate is found to be lower in most districts with lower UV index. Even in districts with a high population density such as Gandhinagar and Mahisagar the number of active cases was lower.

22.6 CONCLUSION

Our model, including three major parameters – epidemiological, meteorological and demographic – presented in a single map can be used to present not only multi-variate healthcare data but also meteorological data such as precipitation, temperature and UV index. We found that population density is the most obvious and significant factor affecting COVID-19 spread. However, there are districts which,

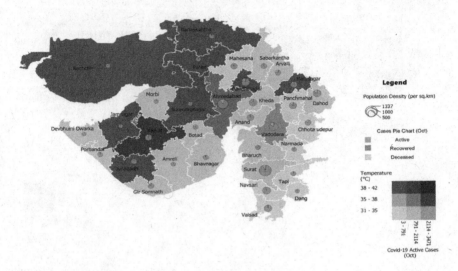

FIGURE 22.4 Bivariate choropleth map for October 2020 showing temperature vs. active cases of COVID-19 with pie-charts.

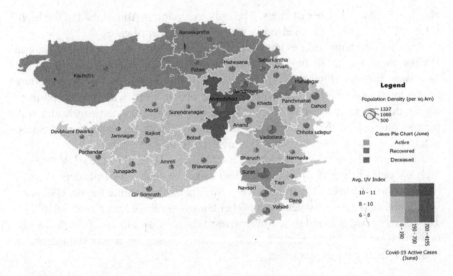

FIGURE 22.5 Bivariate choropleth map for June 2020 showing UV index vs. active cases of COVID-19 with pie-charts.

although densely populated, did not have spread to the same extent. Instead factors like temperature and UV index were responsible for fewer active cases and in some cases higher recovery rates compared to other districts. Although our district mapping is not statistically significant owing to small sample size and the direct

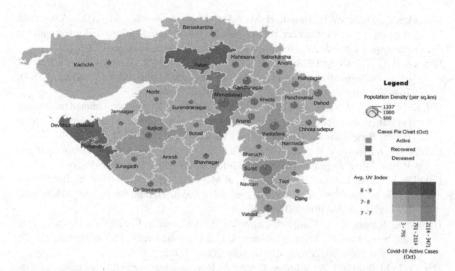

FIGURE 22.6 Bivariate choropleth map for October 2020 showing UV index vs active cases of COVID-19 with pie-charts.

effect of these meteorological parameters, it can provide general information to health professionals and policy makers regarding resource allocation and future spread based on multi-temporal – here, monthly – comparisons. Overall, our maps represent a complex mixture of health-related data and other environmental data in a simple and easy-to-use manner.

ACKNOWLEDGMENTS

We are grateful to NASA Earthdata portal for Aura-OMI and MODIS data and the Indian Meteorological Department for rainfall distribution data. We are also grateful for the COVID-19 data obtained from the crowdfunded initiative.[1]

NOTE

1 www.covid19india.org.

REFERENCES

Acharya, S., Lin, V., & Dhingra, N. (2018). The role of health in achieving the sustainable development goals. *Bulletin of the World Health Organization*, 96(9), 2018–2019. https://doi.org/10.2471/BLT.18.221432.

Bernard, S. M., Samet, J. M., Grambsch, A., Ebi, K. L., & Romieu, I. (2001). The potential impacts of climate variability and change on air pollution-related health effects in the United States. *Environmental Health Perspectives*, 109(Suppl. 2), 199–209. https://doi.org/10.2307/3435010.

Biesecker, C., Zahnd, W. E., Brandt, H. M., Adams, S. A., & Eberth, J. M. (2020). A bivariate mapping tutorial for cancer control resource allocation decisions and interventions. *Preventing Chronic Disease, 17*, 1–9. https://doi.org/10.5888/pcd17.190254.

Dhiman, R. C., Pahwa, S., Dhillon, G. P. S., & Dash, A. P. (2010). Climate change and threat of vector-borne diseases in India: Are we prepared? *Parasitology Research, 106*(4), 763–773. https://doi.org/10.1007/s00436-010-1767-4.

Ebi, K. L., Kovats, R. S., & Menne, B. (2006). An approach for assessing human health vulnerability and public health interventions to adapt to climate change. *Environmental Health Perspectives, 114*(12), 1930–1934. https://doi.org/10.1289/ehp.8430.

Field, C. B., & Barros, V. R. (eds.) (2014). *Climate Change 2014 – Impacts, Adaptation and Vulnerability: Regional Aspects.* Cambridge: Cambridge University Press.

Frumkin, H., Hess, J., Luber, G., Malilay, J., & McGeehin, M. (2008). Climate change: The public health response. *American Journal of Public Health, 98*(3), 435–445. https://doi.org/10.2105/AJPH.2007.119362.

Haines, A., Kovats, R. S., Campbell-Lendrum, D., & Corvalan, C. (2006). Climate change and human health: Impacts, vulnerability and public health. *Public Health, 120*(7), 585–596. https://doi.org/10.1016/j.puhe.2006.01.002.

Hess, J. J., Mcdowell, J. Z., & Luber, G. (2012). Review integrating climate change adaptation into public health practice. *Environmental Health Perspectives, 120*(2), 171–179.

Ianevski, A., Zusinaite, E., Shtaida, N., Kallio-Kokko, H., Valkonen, M., Kantele, A., Telling, K., Lutsar, I., Letjuka, P., Metelitsa, N., Oksenych, V., Dumpis, U., Vitkauskiene, A., Stašaitis, K., Öhrmalm, C., Bondeson, K., Bergqvist, A., Cox, R. J., Tenson, T., ... Kainov, D. E. (2019). Low temperature and low UV indexes correlated with peaks of influenza virus activity in northern Europe during 2010–2018. *Viruses, 11*(3). https://doi.org/10.3390/v11030207.

Kelly-Hope, L. A., Hemingway, J., & McKenzie, F. E. (2009). Environmental factors associated with the malaria vectors *Anopheles gambiae* and *Anopheles funestus* in Kenya. *Malaria Journal, 8*(1), 1–8. https://doi.org/10.1186/1475-2875-8-268.

Mobley, L. R., Kuo, T.-M., Urato, M., Subramanian, S., Watson, L., & Anselin, L. (2012). Spatial heterogeneity in cancer control planning and cancer screening behavior. *Annals of the Association of American Geographers, 102*(5), 1113–1124. https://doi.org/10.1080/00045608.2012.657494.

Moreno-Madriñán, M. J., Crosson, W. L., Eisen, L., Estes, S. M., Estes, M. G., Hayden, M., Hemmings, S. N., Irwin, D. E., Lozano-Fuentes, S., Monaghan, A. J., Quattrochi, D., Welsh-Rodriguez, C. M., & Zielinski-Gutierrez, E. (2014). Correlating remote sensing data with the abundance of pupae of the dengue virus mosquito vector, *Aedes aegypti*, in central Mexico. *ISPRS International Journal of Geo-Information, 3*(2), 732–749. https://doi.org/10.3390/ijgi3020732.

Nyadanu, S. D., Pereira, G., Nawumbeni, D. N., & Adampah, T. (2019). Geo-visual integration of health outcomes and risk factors using excess risk and conditioned choropleth maps: A case study of malaria incidence and sociodemographic determinants in Ghana. *BMC Public Health, 19*(1), 1–16. https://doi.org/10.1186/s12889-019-6816-z.

Prüss-Ustün, A., Wolf, J., Corvalán, C. F., Bos, R., Neira, M. P., & World Health Organization. (2016). Preventing disease through healthy environments: A global assessment of the environmental burden of disease. *Toxicology Letters* 259. https://doi.org/10.1016/j.toxlet.2016.07.028.

Reis, S., Morris, G., Fleming, L. E., Beck, S., Taylor, T., White, M., Depledge, M. H., Steinle, S., Sabel, C. E., Cowie, H., Hurley, F., Dick, J. M. P., Smith, R. I., & Austen,

M. (2015). Integrating health and environmental impact analysis. *Public Health*, *129*(10), 1383–1389. https://doi.org/10.1016/j.puhe.2013.07.006.

Remoundou, K., & Koundouri, P. (2009). Environmental effects on public health: An economic perspective. *International Journal of Environmental Research and Public Health*, *6*(8), 2160–2178. https://doi.org/10.3390/ijerph6082160.

Smith, K. R., Woodward, A., Campbell-Lendrum, D., Chadee, D. D., Honda, Y., Liu, Q., Olwoch, J. M., Revich, B., Sauerborn, R., Confalonieri, U., Haines, A., Chafe, Z., & Rocklov, J. (2015). Human health: Impacts, adaptation, and co-benefits. *Climate Change 2014 Impacts, Adaptation and Vulnerability: Part A: Global and Sectoral Aspects*, 709–754. https://doi.org/10.1017/CBO9781107415379.016.

Sopan, A., Noh, A. S. I., Karol, S., Rosenfeld, P., Lee, G., & Shneiderman, B. (2012). Community health map: A geospatial and multivariate data visualization tool for public health datasets. *Government Information Quarterly*, *29*(2), 223–234. https://doi.org/10.1016/j.giq.2011.10.002.

Woodward, A., Smith, K. R., Campbell-Lendrum, D., Chadee, D. D., Honda, Y., Liu, Q., Olwoch, J., Revich, B., Sauerborn, R., Chafe, Z., Confalonieri, U., & Haines, A. (2014). Climate change and health: On the latest IPCC report. *The Lancet*, *383*(9924), 1185–1189. https://doi.org/10.1016/S0140-6736(14)60576-6.

Yi, Q., Hoskins, R. E., Hillringhouse, E. A., Sorensen, S. S., Oberle, M. W., Fuller, S. S., & Wallace, J. C. (2008). Integrating open-source technologies to build low-cost information systems for improved access to public health data. *International Journal of Health Geographics*, *7*, 1–13. https://doi.org/10.1186/1476-072X-7-29.

23 Biosensors for Environmental Health

Exploring the Biological and Socioeconomic Impacts

Ashish Kumar*, Rameshwari A. Banjara,
Santosh Kumar Sethi, Alka Ekka and
Joystu Dutta

CONTENTS

* Corresponding author: Ashish Kumar. banjaraashish@gmail.com

DOI: 10.1201/9781003095422-23

23.1   INTRODUCTION TO BIOSENSORS

It is has been conclusively reported that various anthropogenic compounds are important for the release of various toxic pollutants into the environment. All over the world, environmental toxicants such as antibiotics, hazardous chemicals, insecticides and pesticides are released into the environment (Bilal et al., 2018). Although several procedures measure trace environmental pollutants through specialized techniques, undetected contaminants such as endocrine disruptors, pharmaceuticals, toxins and hormones need to be identified and quantified (Gaberlein et al., 2000). New prototypes urgently need to be developed to detect their existence in the environment. Low sample concentration, absence of sensitivity and lack of selectivity of traditional methods are among the major constraints of conventional methods. In addition, methods such as chromatography need long and specialized sample pre-treatment. From this perspective, biosensors are valuable tools to detect small sample sizes and minute concentrations of environmental pollutants (Arduini et al., 2017; El Harrad et al., 2018). The ability to design extremely accurate sites of recognition makes biosensors an appropriate alternative to conventional methods based on chromatography (Rodriguez et al., 2005). Biosensors has also been tested for detection and analysis of organic and inorganic environmental pollutants. Portability, on-site work, smaller size and ability to test pollutants in composite structures in minuscule sample preparations are the advantages provided by biosensors over traditional approaches for environmental implications. Many biosensors are specialized for a particular toxicant or may be used with a small range of pollutants (Roda et al., 2001; Rodriguez et al., 2006; Rogers, 2006).

Biosensors are typically categorized on the basis of bioreceptor factors such as whole cells (micro-organisms, plants, animals), DNA fragments and enzymes involved in the biological detection process, or on the basis of the physicochemical transducer used such as electrochemical, piezoelectric, optical or thermal. Microbes, antibodies, enzymes and DNA are the main types of bioreceptor component used in environmental pollutant analysis. It is also possible to develop these sensitive elements or biomaterials by applying genetic engineering techniques (Koedrith et al., 2014). In addition, the transducer and detector components work together according to different principles and convert the signal generated from communication of the analytes, i.e. biological sample materials, into a further signal which also can be quantified more easily. In general electrochemical transducer methods are applied in biosensors (Thevenot et al., 1999). The main component of the biosensor is the signal processor and it is mainly responsible for displaying results in a user-friendly manner.

The biosensor has three components: an organ of biological recognition material known as a bioreceptor, a transducer and a signal-processing mechanism (Sethi, 1994). Details of standard biosensors are shown in Figure 23.1. Further biosensors are grouped according to bioreceptor properties involved in the method of detection, such as whole cells (micro-organisms, plants, animals), DNA fragments and enzymes, or according to the physico-chemical character of transducers used

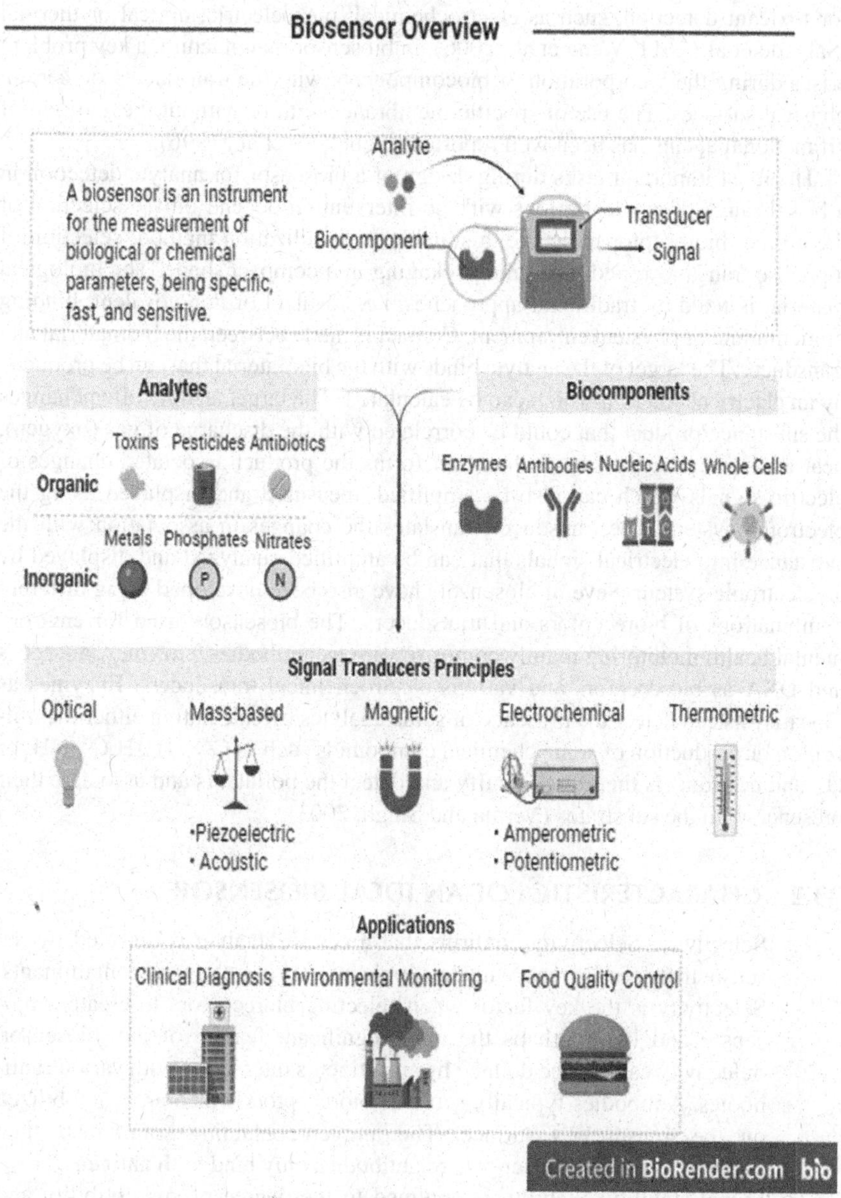

FIGURE 23.1 Potential biocomponents, signal transducers, principles and applications of biosensors.

for toxicant detection, such as electrochemical, piezoelectric, optical or thermal (Salgado et al., 2011; Wang et al., 2006). In biosensor manufacture, a key problem arises during the incorporation of biocomponents with the transducers on certain physical surfaces. The use of specific membranes with or without the addition of bifunctional agents has been well reported (Ikebukuro et al., 1996).

The most important tasks during design of a biosensor for analyte detection in a broad range of concentrations with no intervention depend on the selection of the correct bioreceptor molecule, a suitable immobilization method, selection of a precise transducer, and lastly the packaging in a compact shape. The biological material is fixed by traditional approaches, i.e. covalent or non-covalent, binding or membrane or physical entrapment. Contact is made between the biomaterial and transducer. The target of the analyte binds with the biomaterial that can be produced by an electrical reaction which can be calculated. The target analyte often changes the substance/product that could be correlated with the discharge of gas (oxygen), heat and ions. The transducer then transforms the product-associated changes of electric signals which can also be amplified, measured and displayed using the electronic system. The transducer translates the changes in association with the substance into electrical signals that can be amplified, analyzed and displayed by an electronic system. Several biosensors have also been developed using different combinations of bioreceptors and transducers. The biosensors used for environmental health monitoring mainly comprise various antibodies, enzymes, microbes and DNA as bioreceptors and various electrochemical transducers. Enzymes as biocatalysts can detect the presence of some analytes by calculating either the utilization or production of some chemical compounds such as CO_2, H^+, H_2O_2, NH_3 or O_2, and transducers therefore identify and detect the pollutants and associate their presence with the substrates (Verma and Singh, 2003).

23.2   CHARACTERISTICS OF AN IDEAL BIOSENSOR

1. Selectivity: Selectivity confirms that a certain analyte is detected by the sensor that does not react with the supplementary mixtures and contaminants. Selectivity is the key factor when selecting bioreceptors to create a biosensor and it is perhaps the most significant feature of any biosensor. Selectivity can best be defined by an antigen's interaction with various antibodies. Antibodies typically serve as bioreceptors which are immobilized on the transducer's surface. The antigen-containing solution is then exposed to the transducer, where antibodies only bind with antigens.

2. Signal stability: Stability is confined to the degree of susceptibility and the biosensing system to environmental disturbances. In the output signals of a biosensor under measurement, these disturbances can cause a drift. This can create an error in the calculated concentration and can also affect the detailed accuracy and precision of the biosensor. Stability is therefore the most important application for continuous monitoring and where long incubation details are necessary for a biosensor. The temperature-sensitive

response of electronics and transducers may affect the signal stability of a biosensor. Therefore, proper tuning of electronics is essential to ensure a constant sensor response. The affinity of the bioreceptor is another aspect that may affect stability; high-affinity bioreceptors enhance the strong electrostatic bonding application or the analyte's covalent linkage that strengthens the biosensor's stability.

3. Sensitivity (detection limit): This is the minimum analyte quantity (or concentration) that is detectable. The limit of detection or sensitivity is defined by the least number of analytes that can be quantified by a bio-sensor. In different environmental pollutant quality testing applications, to detect analyte concentration in the range of μg/ml or ng/ml, a biosensor is required to confirm the presence of different analyte traces in a sample. Sensitivity is therefore considered to be an important essential property of a biosensor.

4. Precision: This is the capacity of a biosensor to produce the same readings for repeated experimental set-ups under unchanged conditions. Changes of signals provide the detail inference which ensure the response of a bio-sensor has greater robustness and reliability.

5. Working range and regeneration time: This is the various ranges of concentrations of analytes at which the sensor can function, and the time needed to return the sensor to its working conditions after contact with the sample. The biosensor working range is characterized as the few changes in the analyte concentration that are needed to change the biosensor's response. Depending on the purpose, analyte concentration assessment over different working ranges is one of the main characteristics of a biosensor.

23.3 ENVIRONMENTAL APPLICATIONS OF BIOSENSORS

Various pollutants call for rapid and economic analytical tools and techniques to be used in comprehensive monitoring programs. Additionally, a few years ago, an increasing number of environmental pollution reduction policies and legislative measures were implemented in parallel with growing scientific and social interest (Rodriguez et al. 2004, 2005; Rogers, 2006; Rogers and Gerlach, 1996). The criteria for the application of most conventional analytical techniques studying environmental pollutants have been investigated; this often constitutes a major obstacle to their application on a daily basis. Recently the need for less time consuming and more ecofriendly techniques for environmental pollutant monitoring has been encouraged in implementing different formulations of technologies and more effective methodologies. From this perspective, biosensors appear to be a most suitable and effective alternative analytical tool.

Biosensors are a subgroup of chemical sensors that use a biological mechanism to detect analytes (Rodriguez et al., 2005; Rogers, 2006; Rogers and Gerlach, 1996). Biosensing process and techniques are being developed as effective tools for various applications, viz. agriculture, food quality analysis and in particular,

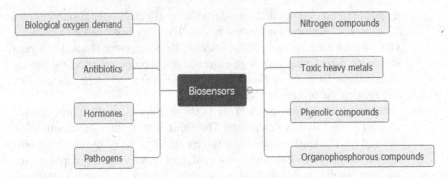

FIGURE 23.2 Different uses of biosensors for environmental pollutant monitoring and analysis.

environmental management and various sectors of medical applications. The key advantages provided by biosensors over traditional analytical techniques for environmental applications are miniaturization, portability, on-site work and the ability to evaluate pollutants in complex matrices with limited sample preparation.

The systems developed cannot yet compete, based on reproducibility and accuracy of analysis, with long-established analytical methods. However, regulatory authorities and industry can use them to provide adequate information for routine sample testing and screening (Rogers, 2006; Rogers and Gerlach, 1996; Sharpe, 2003). Biosensors also can be used as tools for environmental pollutant monitoring in the evaluation of environmental quality and for substance monitoring of organic and inorganic pollutants (Figure 23.2). In this chapter we present an overview of how the biosensor is useful for environmental monitoring, and describe various biosensors developed for various environmental applications, mainly air, water and soil quality monitoring and pathogen analysis.

23.4 GASEOUS POLLUTANT ANALYSIS AND AIR QUALITY MONITORING

There are various categories of air pollutants, including gases such as carbon monoxide, ammonia, chlorofluorocarbons, methane, sulfur dioxide and nitrous oxides, biological molecules and particulates like natural and inorganic products. Air pollutants can be produced by both natural processes and human interventions. Application of biosensors in air quality and gaseous pollutant monitoring has recently become an area of interest. Increased attention has been focused on in situ and real-time monitoring of pollutants, including the surveillance of agriculture, industrial waste and measurements of volcanic gases. For instance, in unmanned aerial vehicles and remotely piloted aircraft, a compact, sensitive and portable whole-cell biosensor has recently been incorporated (Phantom 2, Shenzhen, China) to monitor air and water quality and pollution in remote locations (Lu et al., 2015).

Air pollutants can be detected directly using biosensors, although the instruments developed for this purpose are very limited. Preliminary studies of environmental air pollutant monitoring were conducted for quantitative detection of volatile organic substances, such as methanol and formaldehyde using multiple-strain algal biosensors (Berno et al., 2004). In addition, the compound benzene has been analyzed and quantified in air samples by different biosensors (Lanyon et al., 2005).

23.5 SOIL AND WATER QUALITY MONITORING

Increasing numbers of potentially hazardous pollutants like chemical compounds, toxins and pathogens released to the soil and water bodies remain a critical global challenge (Salgado et al., 2011). In the soil and natural water bodies contamination of different toxic heavy metals and their subsequent ions poses significant hazards to human health, hence environmental safety is the most basic requirement for all living things on this earth. From this perspective, for the general protection and welfare of human beings, animals and plants, identification and control of environmental pollutants in the soil and water are essential.

23.6 TOXIC HEAVY-METAL ANALYSIS

Contamination by toxic heavy metals such as arsenic, lead, copper, zinc, cadmium and chromium is are one of the most hazardous soil and water pollutants even in trace amounts. It poses a severe risk to all living organisms, including to human health. Heavy metals are extensively present in polluted environments; for instance, many sites are substantially contaminated with chromium from tannery waste waters. In addition, fertilizers have become one of the contaminating sources of heavy metals. The heavy metals contained in chemical fertilizers can be harmful for human health as the crop will have heavy metals in its leaves and fruit (Atafar et al., 2010).

Existing approaches to detect various heavy metals include chromatographic spectroscopic, voltammetry methods that generally detect the species which could be at low concentrations or in single doses. These conventional techniques are typically costly and cannot easily be used for in situ analysis. Hence fast, compact and low-cost pollution analysis and monitoring tools are a global priority. Generally bacterial biosensors are applied for the recognition of toxic metals in soil and water samples, and their genes resistant to these target toxic metals are employed as bioreceptor molecules (Nigam and Shukla, 2015). Few bacterial species that have effective resistance against heavy metals have been assessed as potential biological receptors for the identification of zinc, copper, silver, tin, mercury, cobalt, etc. Some biosensors have also been evaluated by fusion of heavy genes that are resistant to different heavy metals with genes related to the expression of bioluminescent proteins, such as luciferin for the identification of elements present in soil and water samples. The detection of toxic heavy metal and its subsequent ion can also be recognized by enzyme-catalyzed reactions, as several ions directly suppress the activity of enzymes at low concentrations (Verma and Singh, 2003).

For the detection of highly toxic and pervasive environmental pollutants like heavy metal ions, mercury ions (Hg^{2+}) have been used as representative targets for testing in DNA optical biosensors. It is fast, economical and portable for on-site quantitative detection of mercury in various water samples within a fraction of minutes. Chromium ions may be accumulated by plants cultivated in such fields. Recently, using single-stranded DNA and magnetic substrates, the surface enhancement Raman spectrum (SERS) biosensor was reported for the rapid and effective recognition of Hg^{2+} (Madianos et al., 2018; Yang et al., 2017). The two fluorescence-dependent optical biosensors were mainly designed to use DNA aptamers (Chen et al., 2017) and DNAzymes/carboxylated magnetic beads (Ravikumar et al., 2017) to detect Pb^{2+} in lake and pond water samples. For the detection of Pb^{2+} and Cd^{2+} using mesoporous carbon nitride/self-doped polyaniline nanofibers a multi-analyte biosensor has been suggested where the limits of detection were 0.2 and 0.7 nM (Zhang et al., 2016). Similar detection limits of 0.33 and 0.24 nM were obtained respectively for Pb^{2+} and Cd^{2+}, using a wireless biosensor based on magnetoelastic theory, which enables real-time monitoring in remote places (Guo et al., 2018). A modern electrochemical biosensor has been proposed to detect Zn, using paper-based, graphene chitosan and oxide microfluidic channels (Li et al., 2017). In complex environmental samples, the biosensor was capable of detecting Zn^{2+} because it was found to be selective when the other seven cations (Cu^{2+}, Fe^{3+}, Cd^{2+}, Hg^{2+}, Mn^{2+}, Mg^{2+} and Ag^{2+}) were examined (Li et al., 2017). For the identification of Cu^{2+} by fusion of a Cu^{2+} inducible promoter with the *lacZ* gene, a microbial recombinant biosensor of amperometric kind has been developed (Law and Higson, 2005).

23.7   BIOCHEMICAL OXYGEN DEMAND

Biochemical oxygen demand (BOD) is a significant parameter used to assess the biodegradable organic pollutant's concentration in a water sample. In routine practice, BOD determination of any sample is a time-consuming process, i.e. it takes 5 days, and as a result it is not suitable for rapid and online monitoring of water samples. In order to shorten the time required to quantify BOD in water samples and to provide rapid input on the state of water quality, BOD biosensors have been developed using recombinant *Escherichia coli* and *Photobacterium phosphoreum* as potential signal indicators of BOD in domestic wastewaters (Cheng et al., 2010). Recombinant *E. coli* cells with *Vibrio fisheri* gene lux AE-dependent biosensors were developed for the measurement of BOD by Nakamura and Karube (Simona et al. 2011). Furthermore Kwok et al. (2005) developed simultaneously multi-sample assessment of BOD testing of wastewater samples using an optical biosensor. Biosensors used for BOD analysis using yeast with an oxygen probe have recently been developed to analyze the various organic contaminants more rapidly than traditional ones.

23.8 PATHOGENIC ORGANISMS

The presence of pathogenic organisms in the matrices of the environment, especially in water chambers, may pose a serious risk for human beings, and recently biosensors have been reported to monitor pathogenic organisms in the environment. Methods generally used to identify pathogenic species are dependent on traditional colony culture techniques and antibody-dependent assays, polymerase chain reaction (PCR) techniques. Such techniques are laborious, time consuming and expensive. An easy and sensitive aptamer-dependent biosensor for the detection of a particular *E. coli* outer membrane was designed using two different aptamers. The technique has also been used for magnetic bead enhancement, and another has been used as a signal reporter particularly for *E. coli*, which was amplified by isothermal strand displacement and further recognized through a flow biosensor. The pathogen recognition limit is as low as 10 units of colony formation per milliliter (CFU mL^{-1}). This technique may also be applied to detect other bacterial species using multiple bacterium-specific aptamers (Wu et al., 2015).

For complex environmental water sample analysis rapid and precise optical biosensors based on surface plasmon resonance have been reported to detect the metabolically active *Legionella pneumophila* (Enrico et al., 2013; Foudeh et al. 2015). In one report, the detection principle was dependent on the identification of bacterial RNA by the immobilized RNA-sensing element probe on the gold surface of a biochip (Foudeh et al., 2015). In another experiment, *E. coli* has been found in underground water supplies by a whole-cell imprinting biosensor dependent on piezoelectric and optical principles, providing capabilities of real-time identification (Yilmaz et al., 2015). As a detection factor, a polymerizable type of histidine (N-methacryloyl-L-histidine methyl ester) was used and immobilized on gold surfaces, achieving close recognition to that of natural antibodies. An entire cell-dependent micro-contact-imprinted capacitive biosensor dependent on gold electrodes for the identification of *E. coli* was obtained with an enhanced detection limit (70 CFU mL^{-1}) in river water samples (Idil et al., 2016). Also, in air-borne dust, specifically during Asian dust events, the detection of pathogenic bacteria (*Bacillus subtilis*) was reported through an electrochemical immunosensor which is based on single-walled carbon nanotube (SWCNT)-gold electrodes (Yoo et al., 2017).

23.9 ANTIBIOTICS

The existence of antibiotics in soil and water is troubling because they promote antibiotic resistance of bacterial species (Coille et al., 2002). The extensive applications of antibiotics pose significant environmental issues as antibiotic resistance may be passed to humans when infected milk and meat products are consumed (Setford et al., 1999). Most biosensors are therefore intended for the determination of antibiotics in biological and food samples, although their use for monitoring soil and water samples should be considered. For instance, the commercial biosensor BIACORE 3000 has been used to analyze the cross-reactivity of two sulfonamides: furosemide and sulfamethazine (Ahmad et al., 2002). The identified sulfamethazine has also been determined by Akkoyun et al. (2000) in animal urine with an optical immunobiosensor. In the development of three corresponding whole-cell biosensors, Hansen and Sorensen (2000) offered the choice of three distinct recombinant cells modified by a tetracycline-inducible promoter. Different biosensors are able to determine penicillin G (Setford et al., 1999) and tetracyclines (Hansen and Sorensen, 2000) in milk and food quality monitoring. In a review by Patel (2002), more reference to biosensors for the detection of antibiotic determination can also be found.

23.10 HORMONES

Owing to the rising population and more intensive farming, synthetic and natural hormone residues can be found in the soil and water as a result of human or animal excretion. Hormones like estradiol, ethinylestradiol and estrone have been detected at ng/L levels in water (Belfroid et al., 1999); some of these hormones may have endocrine-disrupting function in terrestrial and aquatic fauna even at these low concentrations. Estrone, progesterone and testosterone, along with the other organic pollutants, have also been determined with a fully automated optical immune biosensor in water samples, reaching limits of detection up to sub-ng/L (Hua et al., 2005; Rodriguez et al., 2004). In water samples, estrone, testosterone and progesterone, along with other organic contaminants, were determined by a fully automatic optical immune biosensor, exceeding detection limits up to sub-ng/L (Hua et al., 2005; Rodriguez et al., 2004).

23.11 PHENOLIC COMPOUNDS

Phenols and their derivatives are known to be poisonous substances and are present in various industrial effluents in which fibers, polymers, dyes, pharmaceuticals, pesticides, detergents and disinfectants are produced and synthesized (Rogers, 1995). These compounds have also been reported to exhibit significant toxic effects in plants and animals, causing mutagenicity and genotoxicity and reducing other biological processes and mechanisms, such as respiration, photosynthesis and enzyme-induced reactions at very low concentrations. Therefore, due to their high toxicity, phenols and their derivatives are defined as hazardous pollutants and are listed by the European Commission and the US Environmental Protection Agency as hazardous items and main pollutants.

Some significant enzymes such as laccase, peroxidase and tyrosinase, are exploited for the degradation of phenolic compounds and biosensor development. Toxic phenolic compounds in water usually interact with DNA. These interactions can be used in electrochemical DNA biosensors to generate a response signal. Based on this operation, a number of electrochemical DNA sensors for phenolic compound monitoring have been created. One of them is a disposable electrochemical

DNA biosensor made by immobilizing double-stranded DNA on to the surface of a disposable carbon screen-printed electrode. Amperometric biosensors with tyrosinase are immobilized in a hygrogel on a graphite electrode, which determines the phenol index in environmental samples. In addition, these organic pollutants can be oxidized by conventional carbonaceous electrodes generally at relatively high voltage (approximately 0.8 V).

Optical methods for determination of phenolic compounds have been developed in recent years. For example, chlorophenols can be detected with a chemiluminescence fiber-optic biosensor (Degiuli and Blum, 2000). Several phenol-detecting biosensors have been described using different micro-organisms either in immobilized form or in free state (Mehndiratta et al., 2013; Mulchandani et al., 1998; Theron and Cloete, 2002).

Cyanide is toxic to human health and inhibits the respiratory system by binding with cytochrome oxidase. *Saccharomyces cerevisiae* has been well reported as a potential microbe used as a sensor to analyze cyanide concentrations in water samples; the presence of cyanide inhibits the respiration process of yeast (Gavrilescu et al., 2015). Cyanide is very poisonous and by binding to cytochrome oxidase it suppresses respiration; *S. cerevisiae* has been developed as a microbial biosensor for tracking concentrations of cyanide in river water (Gavrilescu et al., 2015). An oxygen electrode that exploits immobilized bacteria has been developed to monitor the existence of cyanide (Attar et al., 2015; Lanyon et al., 2005).

23.12 NITROGEN COMPOUNDS

Nitrogen compounds, such as nitrite and nitrate, that are used to maintain the fertility of the soil, are the most ubiquitous chemical pollutants in soil and groundwater. They are not safe for living organisms, including in human health, since they irreversibly interfere with hemoglobin, inhibiting oxygen transport and causing methemoglobinemia, mutagenicity, carcinogenicity and blue-baby syndrome in infants. Thus, the intake of these ions in any form contributes to severe health complications. The high level of nitrate concentration in surface and groundwaters also damages aquatic environments. In accordance with this, measures have been enacted for municipal wastewater treatment to mitigate emissions, including nitrate pollution from domestic and commercial sewage of treatment plants (Rodriguez et al., 2005).

Over the past few decades, for determination of nitrate, spectrophotometric and ion exchange chromatography combined with spectrometric and conductometric approaches has been well reported (Cho et al., 2002). The majority of existing approaches used to detect nitrogen compounds include chromatographic spectroscopic, voltammetric methods that generally detect species at low concentrations. These conventional techniques are typically costly and not easy to use for in situ analysis. Hence fast, compact and low-cost pollution analysis and monitoring tools are a global priority.

A highly responsive, rapid and stable conductometric enzyme-dependent biosensor has been recorded for the detection of nitrate in water. An amperometric biosensor has been developed to evaluate nitrite by immobilizing cytochrome c nitrate reductase of *Desulfovibrio desulfuricans* and double-layered hydroxide containing anthraquinone-2-sulfonate (Chen et al., 2007). The reaction of the established sensor was rapid and the nitrite concentration was calculated in the 0.015–2.35 µmol range with a 4 nmol detection limit (Rogers, 1995). A disposable microbial sensor has been developed for the detection of urea in milk by combining an ammonium ion-selective electrode and urease enzyme-producing bacteria (Timur et al., 2004). For the detection of urea in milk, disposable microbial sensors have also been developed by combining an ammonium ion-selective electrode and urease enzyme-producing bacteria (Timur et al., 2004).

23.13 ORGANOPHOSPHORUS COMPOUNDS

Organophosphorus (OP) compounds are a kind of chemical substance commonly used in agriculture as insecticides to combat a variety of insect pests, carriers that spread diseases and weeds. For the evaluation of OPs in various samples enzyme-based biosensors have been evaluated on the basis of the inhibition of the particular enzyme by these OP compounds. Examples of biosensors for the recognition of carbamate pesticides and OPs, due to their inhibitory properties, include oncolin oxidase and acetyl cholinesterase (Andreou and Clonis, 2002; Andres and Narayanaswamy, 1997; Koedrith et al., 2014). Several biosensors were developed where pH electrode is connected with *E. coli* designed by recombinant DNA technology, and a wild-type OP-metabolizing bacterium of *Flavobacterium* sp. which induces the expression of the intracellular organophosphorus hydrolase on the cell surface (Espinosa-Urgel et al., 2015; Lehmann et al., 2000).

23.13.1 PESTICIDES

Of all the environmental toxins present in the atmosphere, plants, soil, water and food, pesticides are the most prevalent (Rodriguez et al., 2004). Owing to their broad scope of action pesticides (insecticides, herbicides and fungicides) are used all over the world. They are purposely introduced into the atmosphere and end up polluting it by different methods. The incidence of pesticide contaminants and metabolites in water, soil and fruit is among the largest problems and is a key concern (Mostafa, 2010). Pesticides are noticeable environmental pollutants because of their growing use in agriculture. The ongoing control of high pesticide levels in water, air and food has thus become a crucial practice for human health (Cesarino et al., 2012). Of all the pollutants in the environment pesticides are the most widespread and can be found in soil, water, air and plants. The European Community has imposed limits on concentration of pesticides in soil and water. The European Commission has also set residue thresholds for their use due to the toxicity of these pesticides and their existence in environmental samples. Conventional chromatographic approaches, such as high-performance liquid chromatography (HPLC), are efficient in environmental pesticide analysis, but some limitations are correlated with restrictions that prohibit their usage. Development of biosensors for the direct recognition of pesticide is of special importance because of the limitations of traditional approaches. The greatest use of biosensors for detection of pesticides found enzymatic biosensors which inhibit the choice of enzyme. The degradation of the pesticide parathion by the microbial enzyme parathion hydrolase was used by an amperometric sensor to detect the presence of pesticide. In the presence of acetylcholine esterase, the same approach was used to detect acetylcholine by biocatalytic degradation. Nanoparticles based on iridium oxide have been used in enzyme biosensors with tyrosinase based on low-cost printed carbon film electrodes for the detection of chlorpyrifos in river water samples (Mayorga et al., 2014).

23.13.2 HERBICIDES

Herbicides are mainly used to kill specific unwanted herbs and small plants, leaving the desired crop unharmed. There are reports on widely varying toxicity and possible carcinogenicity. Some herbicides have negative impacts on bird populations, although these can vary widely. Likewise, biosensors in which amperometric and optical transducers are used can detect herbicides (phenyl urea) and triazines which inhibit photosynthesis (Karube and Nakaniki, 1994). Biosensors have been developed for the recognition of herbicides, viz. triazines and phenyl ureas, which prevent photosynthesis through receptors of the membrane of chloroplasts, thylakoid or whole cell, such as single-cell algae, for which primarily optical transducers and amperometric biosensors are used (Cock et al., 2009); these inhibit photosynthesis. Photosynthesis process inhibition is an indicator that rapidly reflects the toxic effect of pollutants. Based on this feature, some biosensors have been developed to detect herbicides in the environment, such as phenylurea and triazines. The principle of operation of these sensors is based on water plastoquinone oxidoreductase (photosystem II). Amperometric biosensors have exhibited selective sensitivity to phenylurea and triazine herbicides (Jose et al., 2003).

23.13.3 INSECTICIDES

Dichlorvos (2,2-dichlorovinyl dimethyl phosphate, generally abbreviated as a DDVP) is an organophosphate broadly used as an insecticide to combat domestic pests and to protect stored goods from insects. For the recognition of dichlorvos in fruit samples, simple and fast fluorescence biosensors using a quantum dots method, bi-enzyme (acetylcholinesterase and choline oxidase) and acetylcholine as substrate have been suggested (Meng et al., 2013). Another enzymatic biosensor based on acetylcholinesterase–zinc oxide-modified platinum electrode was generated for the identification of dichlorvos with a 12 pM detection limit in orange samples (Sundarmurugasan et al., 2016). For the identification of carbamate insecticides (carbofuran), an electrochemical biosensor dependent on acetylcholinesterase immobilized on iron oxide-chitosan nanocomposite was used (Jeyapragasam and Saraswathi, 2014).

23.14 CHALLENGES IN BIOSENSOR RESEARCH FOR ENVIRONMENTAL MONITORING

Biosensors have been used for about 50 years, and the over the past 20 years research in this field has made tremendous contributions towards environmental health monitoring. However, in this field, despite numerous advances in bio-sensor development, relatively few biosensors have achieved global commercial growth at retail level for accurate, rapid and on-site monitoring of environmental pollutants. For the large-scale production of robust, sensitive and reliable biosensor devices with good specificity, it is a significant challenge to engage researchers from chemical, physical, biological and computer disciplines to work together. In addition, difficulties in transforming academic research into commercially feasible prototypes, complex regulatory systems in engineering of biological organisms and biomaterial are other challenges. Many elements of biosensors are composed of non-material; hence their exposure into the environment and accu-mulation in human beings through the agri-food chain are possible. The develop-ment of biosensors for on-site air pollutants and biological allergens or pathogen monitoring in air samples represents a challenge in environmental health analysis, where selectivity and specificity must be the main parameters to be controlled and optimized. Moreover, existing biosensors have a limited life expectancy, and due to the sensitive nature of biological material used in biosensor systems, they cannot tolerate adverse environmental conditions.

23.15 CONCLUSION

The environment is continuously burdened by the release of a number of toxic pollutants through anthropogenic activities that damage various ecological parameters; thus the integrity of various ecological system is under threat. The prevalence of these toxic pollutants is now a universal threat to protection of the environment and living beings. Presently, a large spectrum of biosensors such as aptasensors, electrochemical biosensors, enzymatic biosensors and immunosensors have been designed and utilized for various ecological quality as well as quantity monitoring devices in the evaluation of different harmful chemicals, or biological pollutants.

The use of novel and advanced biotechnological approaches such as recombinant-DNA technology and enzyme engineering has accelerated the efficacy of recognition factors and promoted biosensor research and development for future environmental applications. In addition, various computational biology approaches may be applied to program potential microbes for their enhancement of precision, accuracy and selectivity of biosensors, so that particular toxicity produced by various forms of pollutant may be sensed. Therefore, the use of biosensors has immense potential for the recognition and detection of toxic pollutants and ecological scrutiny in the environment.

REFERENCES

Ahmad, A., Ramakrishnan, A., McLean, M. A., Li, D., Rock, M. T., Karim, A., & Breau, A. P. (2002). Use of optical biosensor technology to study immunological cross-reactivity between different sulfonamide drugs. Anal. Biochem. 300, 177–184.

Akkoyun, A., Kohen, V. F., & Bilitewski, U. (2000). Detection of sulphamethazine with an optical biosensor and anti-idiotypic antibodies. Sens. Actuators B. 70, 12–18.

Andreou, V. G., & Clonis, Y. D. (2002). A portable fiber-optic pesticide biosensor based on immobilized cholinesterase and sol-gel entrapped bromocresol purple for in-field use. Biosens. Bioelectron. 17, 61–69.

Andres, R. T., & Narayanaswamy, R. (1997). Fibre-optic pesticide biosensor based on covalently immobilized acetylcholinesterase and thymol blue. Talanta 44, 1335–1352.

Arduini, F., Cinti, S., Scognamiglio, V., Moscone, D., & Palleschi, G. (2017). How cutting-edge technologies impact the design of electrochemical (bio) sensors for environmental analysis. A review. Anal. Chim. Acta. 959, 15–42.

Atafar, Z., Mesdaghinia, A., Nouri, J., Homaee, M., Yunesian, M., Ahmadimoghaddam, M., & Mahvi, A. H. (2010). Effect of fertilizer application on soil heavy metal concentration. Environ. Monit. Assess. 160, 83–89.

Attar, A., Cubillana-Aguilera, L., Naranjo-Rodríguez, I., Hidalgo de Cisneros, J. L., Palacios-Santander, J. M., & Aziz Amine, A. (2015). Amperometric inhibition biosensors based on horseradish peroxidase and gold sononanoparticles immobilized onto different electrodes for cyanide measurements. Bioelectrochem. 101: 84–91.

Belfroid, A. C., Van der Horst, A., Vethaak, A. D., Schafer, A. J., Rijs, G. B. J., Wegener, J., & Cofino, W. P. (1999). Analysis and occurrence of estrogenic hormones and their glucuronides in surface water and waste water in The Netherlands. Sci. Total Environ. 225:101–108.

Berno, E., Pereira Marcondes, D. F., Ricci Gamalero, S., & Eandi, M. (2004). Recombinant *Escherichia coli* for the biomonitoring of benzene and its derivatives in the air. Ecotoxicol. Environ. Saf. 57, 118–122.

Bilal, M., Rasheed, T., Sosa-Hernández, J. E., Raza, A., Nabeel, F., & Iqbal, H. M. N. (2018). Biosorption: An interplay between marine algae and potentially toxic elements – a review. Mar. Drugs. 16, 65.

Cesarino, I., Moraes, F. C., Lanza, M. R. V., & Machado, S. A. S. (2012). Electrochemical detection of carbamate pesticides in fruit and vegetables with a biosensor based on acetylcholinesterase immobilised on a composite of polyaniline-carbon nanotubes. Food Chem. 135, 873–879.

Chen, H., Mousty, C., Cosnier, S., Silveira, C., Moura, J. J. G., & Almeida, M. G. (2007). Highly sensitive nitrite biosensor based on the electrical wiring of nitrite reductase by [ZnCr-AQS] LDH. Electrochem. Commun. 9, 2240–2245.

Chen, Y., Li, H., Gao, T., Zhang, T., Xu, L., Wang, B., Wang, J., & Pei, R. (2017). Selection of DNA aptamers for the development of light-up biosensor to detect Pb(II). Sens. Actuators B Chem. 254, 214–221.

Cheng, C. Y., Jong, T. K., Yu, C. L., & Yi, R. L. (2010). Comparisons of *Vibrio fischeri*, *Photobacterium phosphoreum*, and recombinant luminescent using *Escherichia coli* as BOD measurement. J. Environ. Sci. Health Part A 45(2), 233–238.

Cho, S. J., Sasaki, S., Ikebukuro, K., & Karube, I. (2002). A simple nitrate sensor system using titanium trichloride and an ammonium electrode. Sens. Actuators B 85, 120–125.

Cock, L. S., Arenas, A. M. Z., & Aponte, A. A. (2009). Use of enzymatic biosensor as quality indices: A synopsis of present and future trends in the food industry, Chilean J. Agri. Res. 69, 2–270.

Coille, I., Reder, S., Bucher, S., & Gauglitz, G. (2002). Comparison of two fluorescence immunoassay methods for the detection of endocrine disrupting chemicals in water. Biomol. Engin. 18 (6), 273–280.

Degiuli, A., & Blum, L. J. (2000). Fiberoptic biosensors based on chemiluminescent reactions. Appl. Biochem. Biotechnol. 89 (2–3), 107–115.

El Harrad, L., Bourais, I., Mohammadi, H., & Amine, A. (2018). Recent advances in electrochemical biosensors based on enzyme inhibition for clinical and pharmaceutical applications. Sensors 18, 164.

Enrico, D. L., Manera, M. G., Montagna, G., Cimaglia, F., Chiesa, M., Poltronieri, P., Santino, A., & Rella, R. (2013). SPR based immunosensor for detection of *Legionella pneumophila* in water samples. *Optics Commun.* 294, 420–426.

Espinosa-Urgel, M. E., Seranno, L., Ramos, J. L., & Fernandez Escamilla, A. M. (2015). Engineering biological approaches for detection of toxic compounds: A new microbial biosensor based on the *Pseudomonas putida* TtgR repressor. Mol. Biotechnol. 57, 558–564.

Foudeh, A., Daniel, B., Maryam, T., & Teodor, V. (2015). Rapid and multiplex detection of Legionella's RNA using digital microfluidics. Lab on a Chip 15, 1609–1618.

Gaberlein, S., Spencer, F., & Zaborosch, C. (2000). Microbial and cytoplasmic membrane-based potentiometric biosensors for direct determination of organophosphorus insecticides. Appl. Microbiol. Biotechnol. 54, 652–658.

Gavrilescu, M., Demnerova, K., Aamand, J., Agathos, S., & Fava, F. (2015). Emerging pollutants in the environment: Present and future challenges in biomonitoring, ecological risks and bioremediation. New Biotechnol. 32, 147–156.

Guo, X., Sang, S., Jian, A., Gao, S., Duan, Q., Ji, J., Zhang, Q., & Zhang, W. (2018). A bovine serum albumin-coated magnetoelastic biosensor for the wireless detection of heavy metal ions. Sens. Actuators B Chem. 256, 318–324.

Hansen, L. H., & Sorensen, S. J. (2000). Detection and quantification of tetracyclines by whole cell biosensors. FEMS Microbiol. Lett. 190 (2), 273–278.

Hua, P., Hole, J. P., Wilkinson, J. S., Proll, G., Tschmelak, J., Gauglitz, G., Jackson, M., Nudd, R., Griffith, H., Abuknesha, R., Kaiser, J., & Kraemmer, P. (2005). Integrated optical fluorescence multisensory for water pollution. Optics Express 13, 1124–1130.

Idil, N., Martin, H., Denizli, A., & Mattiasson, B. (2016). Whole cell based microcontact imprinted capacitive biosensor for the detection of *Escherichia coli*. Biosens Bioelectron 15(87), 807–815.

Ikebukuro, K., Miyata, A., Cho, S. J., Nomura, Y., Chang, S. M., & Yamauchi, Y. (1996). Microbial cyanide sensor for monitoring river water. J. Biotechnol. 48, 73–80.

Jeyapragasam, T., & Saraswathi, R. (2014). Electrochemical biosensing of carbofuran based on acetylcholinesterase immobilized onto iron oxide-chitosan nanocomposite. Sens. Actuators B Chem. 191, 681–687.

Jose, I., Reyes, D. C., & Ralph, P. C. (2003). Biosensors. In Encyclopedia of Agricultural, Food, and Biological Engineering. Pullman, WA: Marcel Dekker. DOI: 10.1081/E-EAFE 120007212

Karube, I., & Nakaniki, K. (1994). Immobilized cells used for detection and analysis. Curr. Opin. Biotechnol. 5, 54–59.

Koedrith, P., Thasiphu, T., Weon, J. I. I., Boonprasert, R., Tuitemwong, K., & Tuitemwong, P. (2014). Recent trends in rapid environmental monitoring of pathogens and toxicants: Potential for nanoparticle based biosensor and applications. Sci. World J. 1–12.

Kwok, N. Y., Dongb, S., & Loa, W. (2005). An optical biosensor for multi-sample determination of biochemical oxygen demand (BOD). Sens. Actuators B Chem. 110, 289–298.

Lanyon, Y. H., Marrazza, G., Tothill, I. E., & Mascini, M. (2005). Benzene analysis in workplace air using an FIA based bacterial biosensor. Biosens. Bioelectron. 20, 2089–2096.

Law, K., & Higson, S. P. J. (2005). Sonochemically fabricated acetylcholinesterase microelectrode arrays within a flow injection analyser for the determination of organophosphate pesticides. Biosens. Bioelectron. 20, 1914–1924.

Lehmann, M., Riedel, K., Alder, K., & Kunze, G. (2000). Amperometric measurement of copper ion with a deputy substrate using a novel *Saccharomyces cerevisiae* sensor. Biosens. Bioelectron. 15, 211–219.

Li, L., Zhang, Y., Zhang, L., Ge, S., Yan, M., & Yu, J. (2017). Steric paper based ratio-type electrochemical biosensor with hollow-channel for sensitive detection of Zn^{2+}. Sci. Bull. 62, 1114–1121.

Lu, Y., Macias, D., Dean, Z.S., Kreger, N. R., & Wong, P. K. (2015). A UAV-mounted whole cell biosensor system for environmental monitoring applications. IEEE Trans. Nanobiosci. 14, 811–817.

Madianos, L., Tsekenis, G., Skotadis, E., Patsiouras, L., & Tsoukalas, D. (2018). A highly sensitive impedimetric aptasensor for the selective detection of acetamiprid and atrazine based on microwires formed by platinum nanoparticles. Biosens. Bioelectron. 101, 268–274.

Mayorga, M. C., Pino, F., Kurbanoglua, S., Rivas, L., Ozkan, S. A., & Merkoci, A. (2014). Iridium oxide nanoparticles induced dual catalytic/inhibition based detection of phenol and pesticide compounds. J. Mater. Chem. B. 2, 2233–2239.

Mehndiratta, P., Jain, A., Srivastava, S., & Gupta, N. (2013). Environmental pollution and nanotechnology. Environ. Pollut. 2, 49–58.

Meng, X., Wei, J., Ren, X., Ren, J., & Tang F. (2013). A simple and sensitive fluorescence biosensor for detection of organophosphorus pesticides using H_2O_2-sensitive quantum dots/bi-enzyme. Biosens. Bioelectron. 47, 402–407.

Mostafa, G. A. (2010). Electrochemical biosensors for the detection of pesticides. Open Electrochem. J. 2, 22–42.

Mulchandani, A., Mulchandani, P., Keneva, I., & Chen, W. (1998). Biosensors for direct determination of organophosphate nerve agents using recombinant *E. coli* with surface expressed organophosphorus hydrolase. Anal. Chem. 70: 4140–4145.

Nigam, V. K., & Shukla, P. (2015). Enzyme based biosensors for detection of environmental pollutants: a review. J. Microbiol. Biotechnol. 25(11), 1773–1781.

Patel, P. D. (2002). (Bio)sensors for measurement of analytes implicated in food safety: A review. Trends Anal. Chem. 21, 96–115.

Ravikumar, A., Panneerselvam, P., Radhakrishnan, K., Morad, N., Anuradha, C. D., & Sivanesan, S. (2017). DNAzyme based amplified biosensor on ultrasensitive fluorescence detection of Pb(II) ions from aqueous system. J. Fluoresc. 27, 2101–2109.

Roda, A., Pasini, P., Mirasoli, M., Guardigli, M., Russo, C., & Musiani, M. (2001). A sensitive determination of urinary mercury (II) by a bioluminescent transgenic bacteria-based biosensor. Anal. Lett. 34, 29–41.

Rodriguez, M. S., Marco, M. P., Alda, M. J. L., & Barcelo D. (2004). Biosensors for environmental applications: Future development trends. Pure Appl. Chem. 76, 723–752.

Rodriguez, S., de Alda, M. J. L., Marco, M. P., & Barcelo D. (2005). Biosensors for environmental monitoring: A global perspective. Talanta 65, 291–297.

Rodriguez, S., Maria, J., De, A. L., & Barcelo, D. (2006). Biosensors as useful tools for environmental analysis and monitoring. Anal. Bioanal. Chem. 386, 1025–1041.

Rogers, K. R. (1995). Biosensors for Environmental Applications. Las Vegas: US EPA, Environmental Monitoring Systems Laboratory.

Rogers, K. R. (2006). Recent advances in biosensor techniques for environmental monitoring. Anal. Chim. Acta 568, 222–231.

Rogers, K. R., & Gerlach, C. L. (1996). Environmental biosensors – A status report. Environ. Sci. Technol. 30, 486–491.

Salgado, A. M., Silva, L. M., & Melo, A. F. (2011). Biosensor for environmental applications. In Somerset V. (ed.). Environmental Biosensors. InTech.

Setford, S. J., Van Es, R. M., Blankwater, Y. J., & Kroger, S. (1999). Receptor binding protein amperometric affinity sensor for rapid β-lactam quantification in milk. Anal Chim Acta 398:13–22

Sethi, R. S. (1994). Transducer aspects of biosensors. Biosens. Bioelectron. 9, 243–264.

Sharpe, M. (2003). It's a bug's life: Biosensors for environmental monitoring. J. Environ. Monit. 5, 109–113.

Simona, C. L., Sandra, A. V., Eremia, M. D., Andreia, T., & Gabriel-Lucian R. (2011). Biosensors applications on assessment of reactive oxygen species and antioxidants. In Somerset V. (ed.). Environmental Biosensors. InTech.

Sundarmurugasan, R., Gumpu, M. B., Ramachandra, B. L., Nesakumar, N., Sethuraman, S., Krishnan, U. M., & Rayappan, J. B. B. (2016). Simultaneous detection of monocrotophos and dichlorvos in orange samples using acetylcholinesterase-zinc oxide modified platinum electrode with linear regression calibration. Sens. Actuators B Chem. 2230, 306–313.

Theron, J., & Cloete, T. E. (2002). Emerging waterborne infections: contributing factors, agents and detection tools. Crit. Rev. Microbiol. 28, 1–26.

Thevenot, D. R. K., Toth, K., Durst, R. A., & Wilson, G. S. (1999). Electrochemical biosensors: Recommended definitions and classification. Pure Appl. Chem. 71, 2333–2348.

Timur, S., Seta, L. D., Pazarlioglu, N., Pilloton, R., & Telefoncu, A. (2004). Screen printed graphite biosensors based on bacterial cells. Process Biochem. 39, 1325–1329.

Verma, N., & Singh, M. (2003). A disposable microbial based biosensor for quality control in milk. Biosens. Bioelectron. 18, 1219–1228.

Wang, X., Dzyadevych, S. V., Chovelon, J. M., Jaffrezic-Renault, N., Chen, L., Xia, S., & Zhao, J. (2006). Conductometric nitrate biosensor based on methyl viologen/nafion®/nitrate reductase interdigitated electrodes. Talanta 69, 450–455.

Wu, C., Sun, H., Li, Y., Liu, X., Du, X., Wang, X., & Xu, P. (2015). Biosensor based on glucose oxidase-nanoporous gold cocatalysis for glucose detection. Biosens. Bioelectron. 66, 350–355.

Yang, X., He, Y., Wang, X., & Yuan, R. A. (2017). SERS biosensor with magnetic substrate $CoFe_2O_4$@Ag for sensitive detection of Hg^{2+} Appl. Surf. Sci. 16, 581–586.

Yilmaz, E., Majidi D., Ozgur E., & Denizli, A. (2015). Whole cell imprinting based *Escherichia coli sensors*: a study for SPR and QCM. Sens. Actuators B Chem. 209, 714–721.

Yoo, M. S., Minguk, S., Younghun, K., Min, J., Choi, Y. E., Park, S., Jonghoon, C., Jinyoung, L., & Chulhwan, P. (2017). Development of electrochemical biosensor for detection of pathogenic microorganism in Asian dust events. Chemosphere 175, 269–274.

Zhang, C., Zhou, Y., Tang, L., Zeng, G., Zhang, J., Peng, B., Xie, X., Lai, C., Long, B., & Zhu, J. (2016). Determination of Cd^{2+} and Pb^{2+} based on mesoporous carbon nitride/ self-doped polyaniline nanofibers and square wave anodic stripping voltammetry. Nanomaterials 6, 7.

Printed in the United States
by Baker & Taylor Publisher Services